# INSIGHT
# AND
# PSYCHOSIS

# INSIGHT
# AND
# PSYCHOSIS

*Edited by*

XAVIER F. AMADOR

ANTHONY S. DAVID

New York   Oxford   •   Oxford University Press   1998

## Oxford University Press

Oxford    New York    Athens    Auckland    Bangkok    Bogota    Bombay    Buenos Aires
Calcutta    Cape Town    Dar es Salaam    Delhi    Florence    Hong Kong
Istanbul    Karachi    Kuala Lumpur    Madras    Madrid    Melbourne
Mexico City    Nairobi    Paris    Singapore    Taipei    Tokyo    Toronto    Warsaw

and associated companies in
Berlin    Ibadan

## Copyright © 1998 by Oxford University Press, Inc.

Published by Oxford University Press, Inc.,
198 Madison Avenue, New York, New York 10016

Oxford is a registered trademark of Oxford University Press

Library of Congress Cataloging-in-Publication Data
Insight and psychosis / edited by Xavier F. Amador and Anthony S. David.
p.    cm.
Includes bibliographical references and index.
ISBN 0-19-508497-7
1. Psychoses—Diagnosis.    2. Insight.    3. Mental status examination.    I. Amador, Xavier Francisco.
II. David, Anthony S. [DNLM: 1. Psychotic Disorders—psychology.    2. Awareness.
WM 200 I59 1996] RC512.I49    1998
616.89—dc20        96-18781

1 3 5 7 9 8 6 4 2
Printed in the United States of America
on acid-free paper

*To my brother Henry Amador*
*for being my friend*
*and teacher*

XFA

*To Patsy, Michael,*
*and Rebecca for*
*tolerating my own*
*lack of insight*

ASD

# Foreword

When I was growing up, during the era when Freudian influence reigned supreme in psychiatry, I would frequently hear remarks suggesting that a major difference between neurotic and psychotic illnesses was in their internal experience: the neurotic person suffered intensely, while "the insane" were so ill that they didn't understand how sick they really were. In this atmosphere, interest in the topic of insight in psychosis was lost along with interest in the study of psychosis itself. This book is a wonderful first step toward redressing that loss. It clearly demonstrates that thinking about the subjective experience of illness and a patient's understanding and awareness of his or her illness should be addressed from both the perspective of research investigation and from that of clinical care.

This book, *Insight and Psychosis*, has been carefully and imaginatively constructed. The first section, covering phenomenology, introduces readers to the issues and problems that arise when one attempts to measure subjective experience; it also proposes some solutions, such as the application of rating scales to the assessment of insight. The possible origins of symptoms such as delusions from a context of poor insight are discussed. Empirical data about negative symptoms are presented, illustrating that objective measurement is feasible. The second section of the book, exploring the origins of poor insight, is especially intriguing, helping readers think about insight within the context of contemporary neuroscience and philosophy of mind. The third section provides an interesting exploration of cross-cultural differences in awareness of illness and attitudes toward it. The final two sections of the book examine the implications of the topic. Insight impinges on a variety of practical aspects of clinical care, including compliance, violence, and education.

It is sometimes said that "mental suffering is even worse than physical suffering." When the topic of insight in psychotic patients was ignored, few entertained the possibility that patients might be aware of their suffering, let alone studied regarding the extent to which they suffered or the effects of that suffering on the manifestations of their illness. *Insight and Psychosis* will restore the study of the subjective experience of suffering in the seriously mentally ill to the central position that it deserves.

*Iowa City, Iowa*                                                Nancy C. Andreasen, M.D., Ph.D.
*September 1997*

# Preface

As clinicians and scientists, the problem of poor insight into illness was one that was impossible for either of us to ignore. When faced with a psychotic patient who believes that he is not ill, we have had to grapple with difficult ethical, clinical, and legal conundrums. Do we collude with the patient's idiosyncratic view of himself and circumstances in order to persuade him to accept treatment? Or should we attempt to coerce him into accepting our perspective on his situation? Do we decide that our view of his needs should supersede his own? And if this is the conclusion we come to, do we then enlist the help of the courts to impose the treatment he believes he does not need? These are only a handful of questions faced by every clinician who treats individuals "suffering" from psychotic disorders. As scientists, the questions we had were even more numerous and complex.

Empirical research that focuses on the problem of poor insight in psychotic disorders is a relatively new endeavor. Less than a decade ago, independent of one another and on opposite sides of the Atlantic, we reviewed the extant research literature and found only a handful of studies. There are several reasons why so few studies have been done. First among them, perhaps, were the behavioral and biological movements in psychiatry and psychology, which made the study of consciousness unpopular.

The history of the topic is addressed by Berrios and Marková in this volume. However, our immediate conceptual forebears were those who were deeply interested in the study of such things as consciousness and awareness. At the turn of the century, Wundt in Europe and Titchner in the United States had their laboratories staffed with trained "introspectionists" who laboriously chronicled their perceptions and thoughts in response to various controlled stimuli. Perceptual thresholds were documented and laws of sensation promulgated. At the same time, practice of psychoanalysis had taken root and flourished on both continents, resulting in countless published papers detailing the nature of consciousness. Theories were developed to explain the mechanisms involved in relegating one's feelings and thoughts into the unconscious and the process by which they could be retrieved into consciousness. Indeed, the process of developing insight was (and still is) believed to be a central component to the mutative effects of psychoanalysis. Psychoanalytic theories were validated in clinical practice, and the data relied upon was, like that from the introspectionists, usually based on the experiences of one individual. However, with the advent of behaviorism in the middle part of this century, the focus shifted to phenomena that could be objectively and reliably measured. Because the data relied upon by the introspectionists and psychoanalysts were inherently subjective and not readily, much less reliably, accessible to outside observers, the study of consciousness was not destined to become a popular topic among the newer researchers. The biological movement inadvertently added to our neglect of the study of consciousness and insight for the same reasons.

The problem wasn't that no one was interested in the topic of insight in psychotic disorders, because papers on the topic continued to appear in the published literature. However, the majority of these papers, with the exception of people like Aubrey Lewis at the Maudsley Hospital, came from the psychoanalytic perspective. They did not address one of the main obstacles to conducting reliable empirical research in this area—the problem of measurement.

In the last seven years there has been a tremendous resurgence of interest in the topic among clinical researchers because of advances in measurement and terminology. It is now well accepted that insight into illness is a multidimensional phenomenon, involving many discrete and measurable acts of cognition. Several assessment tools have been developed and have begun to gain widespread acceptance. It was because of this latter development that we felt the time was ripe for a volume such as *Insight and Psychosis*. In this volume, we have brought together experts in psychology, psychiatry, sociology, philosophy, anthropology, and neuropsychology to address the problem of poor insight in psychotic disorders. It is this multidisciplinary effort that has been so enlightening for us. It serves as a perfect reminder of the breadth and scope of scholarship demanded in the study of psychosis that first attracted us to the field. The chapters range from reviews of recent studies to theoretical treatises on important topics such as the neurological underpinnings of insight.

There are many people we would like to thank for their contributions to this volume. First and foremost, we want to thank the individuals with psychotic disorders and neurological illnesses that participated in the research studies and case reports described in this book. The fact that many of them suffer tremendously from the added burden of conflict with their loved ones and society, because they do not believe that they are ill, is not lost on us. We want to thank the National Institute of Mental Health, the National Alliance for Research in Schizophrenia and Affective Disorders, the Medical Research Council of Great Britain, the Scottish Rite Foundation, and the Stanley Foundation, which had the foresight to support new research in the area of insight and psychosis. We also want to express our gratitude to the following people who made direct and indirect contributions to this volume: Scott Yale, David Strauss, Jack Gorman, Thomas McGlashan, Nancy C. Andreasen, William T. Carpenter, Robin Murray, and Roisin Kemp. Special thanks to our editor, Joan Bossert, who shares our enthusiasm for the topic of insight and psychosis.

X.F.A.
A.S.D.

# Contents

# Contributors

**Xavier F. Amador**
Department of Clinical Psychobiology, New York State Psychiatric Institute and Department of Psychiatry, Columbia University

**William B. Barr**
Departments of Neurology and Psychiatry, Hillside Hospital, Long Island Jewish Medical Center

**Morris D. Bell**
West Haven V.A. Medical Center and Department of Psychiatry, Yale University School of Medicine

**German E. Berrios**
Department of Psychiatry, University of Cambridge

**Robert J. van den Bosch**
University of Groningen, Groningen, The Netherlands

**Alec Buchanan**
Department of Forensic Psychiatry, Institute of Psychiatry, Denmark Hill, London

**Ellen Corin**
Division of Social and Transcultural Psychiatry, McGill University and Psychosocial Research Unit, Douglas Hospital, Verdun, Quebec

**Anthony S. David**
Department of Psychological Medicine, King's College School of Medicine and Dentistry and the Institute of Psychiatry, London.

**K. William M. Fulford**
Department of Philosophy, University of Warwick

**Phillipa A. Garety**
ISIS Education Center, Warneford Hospital, Oxford

**Richard S.E. Keefe**
Department of Psychiatry, Duke University, North Carolina

**Judith E. Kiersky**
Department of Social Work, Memorial Sloan-Kettering Cancer Center and

Department of Biological Psychiatry, New York State Psychiatric Institute

**Yoshiharu Kim**
Division of Adult Mental Health, National Institute of Mental Health of Japan

**Marcel Kinsbourne**
Department of Psychology, New School for Social Research, New York

**Laurence J. Kirmayer**
Division of Social and Transcultural Psychiatry, McGill University and Institute of Community and Family Psychiatry, Sir Mortimer B. Davis—Jewish General Hospital, Montreal, Quebec

**Henry Kronengold**
Department of Psychology, New York University and New York State Psychiatric Institute

**Ellen P. Lukens**
Columbia University School of Social Work, Department of Clinical Psychobiology, New York State Psychiatric Institute

**Paul H. Lysaker**
Outpatient Rural Outreach, Hamilton Center, and Department of Psychology, Indiana University and Purdue University at Indianapolis

**Ivana S. Marková**
Department of Psychiatry, University of Cambridge

**Joseph P. McEvoy**
Adult Admission Unit, John Umstead Hospital, Butner, North Carolina

**William R. McFarlane**
Department of Psychiatry, Maine Medical Center

**Harold A. Sackeim**
Department of Biological Psychiatry, New York State Psychiatric Institute

**Jean-Paul C.J. Selten**
Rosenburg Psychiatric Hospital, The Hague, The Netherlands

**A.E.S. Sijben**
Consultant for Mental Health Organizations, Velp, The Netherlands

**John S. Strauss**
Department of Psychiatry, Yale University

**E. Fuller Torrey**
NIMH Neuroscience Center, St. Elizabeth's Hospital

**Simon Wessely**
Department of Psychological Medicine, King's College Hospital, Denmark Hill, London

# INSIGHT
# AND
# PSYCHOSIS

HAROLD A. SACKEIM

# Introduction

## The Meaning of Insight

CASE A is a talented linguist. He has translated books into scores of languages, earning an international reputation. Casual conversation reveals that A is an elderly, engaging man and indicates little else that is peculiar. It is a mystery that he has been continuously hospitalized since receiving his undergraduate degree at Oxford. However, during this time A has had the fixed delusion that he is the Duke of Windsor. Nothing seems to shake this belief.

CASE B claims that he has been followed by a "devil" for 20 years. This devil persecutes him, calling him demeaning names and otherwise ridiculing him. In the course of an interview, B walks past a mirror. He becomes agitated and states, "There is that devil looking right at me."

CASE C has a gross movement disorder, with spastic movements of the face and upper limbs. These movements are continuous and commented on by others. When asked about this abnormality, C firmly denies there is anything wrong. C has no difficulty in discerning such abnormalities in other patients.

CASE D is socially active and a pillar of her church and community. She gradually stops her social activities. Concomitantly, she develops insomnia, loss of appetite, and weight loss, and she has marked difficulty carrying out everyday activities. Interspersed between long periods of good functioning, this is her third episode of this characteristic phenomenology. When asked what is troubling her, D indicates that she does not understand why she is in the hospital, as there is nothing wrong with her.

CASE E had a long career as a law-enforcement official, with no previous psychiatric history. He is well aware that he is suffering from profound depression, as he describes his

3

symptoms in exquisite detail. E believes that his state is a punishment brought on by his caressing a woman's breast 20 years previously. Because of this act, he is beyond redemption, is worthless, and will suffer interminably. His guilt and associated suffering seem dramatically out of proportion to the "heinousness" of the act.

It is one thing for people to have strange or impossible beliefs or bizarre perceptions, or to act inappropriately. It is another thing for people to fail to appreciate that these mental contents or behaviors are atypical or, even more, to deny their very existence. As illustrated in the vignettes, day-to-day clinical interactions with psychiatric patients are rife with examples of gross disturbances of insight.

It makes sense that, historically, disturbed insight has been at the core of many conceptions about the nature of psychopathology and insanity. When we state that the "insane" are "out of touch with reality," the focus is often not simply on the unusual nature of perception, thought, or action but on the failure to appreciate the bizarreness of the symptom or to acknowledge its existence. Indeed, fundamental to the distinction between the "neurotic" and "psychotic" thought processes is the differentiation between ego syntonic and ego dystonic disturbance. Patients with obsessive-compulsive disorder are afflicted by recurring, bizarre thoughts that appear alien to them and are unwanted. In essence, they view the strange thoughts as symptoms. In contrast, patients with schizophrenia may steadfastly affirm the veracity of impossible ideas (e.g., thought insertion, paranoid delusions) and deny the existence of abnormality.

Notions of insight have also permeated conceptions of therapeutics. In the realm of psychological treatment, the argument can be made that virtually all forms of psychotherapy hinge on the assumptions that failures of insight are causative in generating psychological illness and that restoration of insight is curative. Clearly, this view is expounded in the dynamic, insight-oriented psychotherapies. Here the traditional conception has been that a motivated lack of awareness of drives and wishes generates symptoms, and that uncovering the unconscious conflicts is restorative (Sackeim, 1983). When stripped to bare bones, such approaches argue that the accuracy of knowledge about the self (truth) and psychological well-being (happiness) are highly positively correlated. It may not be so evident that similar premises underlie other psychotherapeutic approaches. However, when we broaden the concept of insight to embrace accurate representation (self-awareness) of our contributions in the world, it can be argued that virtually all the psychotherapies assume a positive correlation between truth and happiness. The cognitive-behavioral therapist helps patients think "accurately" about their contributions to events and to not overgeneralize from failure. The interpersonal therapist helps patients recognize how their "dysfunctional" patterns of social interaction generate conflict and symptoms. In essence, one can argue that the psychotherapies and their associated theories of psychopathology undercut a qualitative distinction between neurosis and psychosis and, with a broad definition of insight, view all psychopathology as failures of accurate awareness of the self or of one's involvement with the external world.

Against this background, it is surprising, then, that until recently the empirical study of insight in psychosis has been neglected. This neglect is seen in several areas. Our understanding of the phenomenology of impaired insight has been impoverished. For instance, at this point we are uncertain whether impaired insight in schizophrenia is an expression or consequence of the positive symptoms of the disorder—that is, is it itself a type of delusion—an outcome of core cognitive deficits and perhaps covarying with the magnitude of negative symptoms—or does impaired insight reflect an independent dimension of symptomatology? Indeed, our standard approaches for rating the severity of psychotic disturbance have rarely included consideration of patients' appreciation of and attributions for their symptoms. Consequently, it can be argued that our standard approaches to quantifying symptomatic improvement and response often ignore a seemingly fundamental feature of the illness. Further, it is uncertain whether deficits in insight are themselves unidimensional, with patients varying only in the severity of a core, prototypic abnormality, or heterogeneous, with patients varying in the nature of deficits in self-awareness. In her psychotic depression, patient D seemed to be unaware of symptoms and had a global denial of illness. In his psychotic depression, patient E was acutely aware of symptoms, but his explanations for their genesis seemed grossly inappropriate. Did both patients have impaired insight, and were these impairments on a continuum or wholly distinct?

Progress in our knowledge of the phenomenology of insight disturbance will constrain and sharpen the models used to explain the neurobiological and psychological bases of this disturbance. Similarly, as we refine our attempts to conceptualize and assess insight disturbance, the significance of impairments in this domain for prognosis should become clearer. Intuitively, it makes sense that patients who fail to recognize symptoms are less likely to seek and comply with treatment, and much of the evidence discussed in this volume indicates that this is the case. However, beyond this correlation, one wants to know whether impaired insight conveys special prognostic information, independent of implications for access to and use of treatment. For example, there have been longstanding suggestions that depressed patients who minimize or deny symptoms are particularly responsive to electroconvulsive therapy (ECT; see Fink, 1979; Sayer et al., 1993). Why might this be?

In recent years there has been a renaissance in the empirical study of impaired insight and in theoretical attempts to model the disturbance. This volume reflects these efforts and conveys our current state of knowledge. To help frame these presentations, I will briefly raise theoretical concerns about what is meant by insight, how impaired insight might be modeled, and the implications of impaired insight for theories of psychopathology and theories of mind.

## The Meaning of Impaired Insight in Psychopathology

Often the term *insight* is used differently in ordinary language than in characterizations of psychopathology. In ordinary usage, insight is usually defined as the capacity to apprehend or intuit the inner nature of things. We can describe an analysis of world political affairs or a treatise on physics as "insightful." In contrast, in psychopathology the term is often restricted to aspects of self-awareness. When patients have fundamental difficulties in discerning the feelings experienced by others or in interpreting the significance of events in the outside world, we do not necessarily characterize the deficits as reflecting impaired insight. Rather, we typically view these problems as reflecting deficits in the processing of affective information or in reasoning. In essence, usage of the term *insight* in the psychopathology literature often implies a bifurcation between knowledge of the self and knowledge of the outside world.

This fact suggests a critical theoretical distinction. The presumption is that impairments of self-knowledge in psychopathology are distinct from impairments of knowledge of the outside world. In turn, models of the genesis of impaired insight commonly posit that the core deficits that give rise to impaired insight pertain to the processing of information about the "self." For example, historically, psychodynamic formulations offered the first putative explanations of impaired insight, and they presumed that the unawareness of symptoms was motivationally based, owing to the special affective significance of information about the self. As we will see, other theories presume that the core problem resides in limited access to information about inner experience, in disturbance in the quality of this information, or in some aspect of a discrete self-monitoring function.

At the outset, one should question whether this self-other distinction is justified. Put simply, is it true that in psychosis knowledge about the self is dissociated from knowledge of the outside world? At face value, this would seem to be so. For instance, we have evidence that many patients with tardive dyskinesia will deny that they have abnormal involuntary movements, but will recognize such movements in others (Caracci, Mukherjee, Roth, & Decina, 1990). More generally, it is common for psychotic patients to deny they exhibit a broad range of symptomatology, yet discern such symptoms in others. Even more striking are isolated delusions (patient A), where knowledge about the self and the world appears to be intact, with specific lacunae about special self-related topics.

Nonetheless, as evidenced in this volume, much of current theorizing includes in the domain of impaired insight not just the prototypic case where patients are unaware of their symptoms but also instances in which patients make inappropriate attributions for the source of their symptoms (patient E). The patient who acknowledges psychotic symptoms but views them as a result of poison in the water, alien forces, vitamin deficiency, tiredness, or marital difficulties might be said to have impaired insight. In this case, the evidence of impairment of insight lies in the patient's explanation of why he or she is symptomatic or ill. However, whether the self-other distinction applies as readily to these "faulty" models of madness is uncertain. It is not known whether psychotic patients use these "faulty" theories only when accounting for their own symptoms or whether these theories typically embrace the behaviors of others.

An alternative approach to defining the phenomena of impaired insight rejects the requirement of impairment and concerns only knowledge of the self. Instead, what is emphasized is the implausibility of patients' perceptual experiences or their statements about themselves or the world—that is, being "out of touch with reality." The patient who believes he is the Duke of Windsor (patient A) and the patient who believes that the other patients on the ward are spies from an alien intelligence service might both be said to lack insight. In this case, one could argue that either because their beliefs are highly implausible or, additionally, because they fail to appreciate the implausibility of the beliefs, such patients lack insight. If we equate the lack of insight simply with the holding of implausible beliefs, all instances of delusions or grossly false beliefs become examples of impaired insight. This approach is unsatisfying because it is insufficiently restrictive. It equates faulty knowledge about the self or the world (or faulty perceptual experiences) with lack of insight, and it fails to capture the value of the ego syntonic-dystonic distinction. For example, when individuals report that they have an implausible perceptual experience, but are aware that such an experience is an hallucination, we do not ascribe an insight disturbance. However, when individuals state that the people around them all have the heads of rats, and additionally believe that this perceptual experience is veridical, we are more likely to question the quality of their insights.

This suggests that the basis for ascribing impaired insight often hinges on the individual's appreciation of the implausibility or bizarreness of perceptual experiences and beliefs. In turn, this approach suggests that the core deficit in insight resides in the capacity to entertain self-doubt. In information-processing terms, there is dysregulation in error checking, whereby the contents of perceptual experience or beliefs are compared to the available evidence or to consensual knowledge. As opposed to the models specifically emphasizing faulty knowledge of the self, this approach centers on deficits in the psychological processes involved in testing and establishing the certainty of our knowledge (about self or others).

This approach to defining insight is also not without its limitations. Among those limitations is the failure to capture instances in which patients acknowledge symptoms and provide consensually appropriate attributions, but appear to be unaware or unconcerned about their implications. Babinski (1914) first introduced the terms anosognosia and anosodiaphoria. Originally, *anosognosia* referred to the phenomenon, commonly seen acutely following right-hemisphere lesions, in which brain-damaged patients deny that they are paralyzed on the left side of the body. At least superficially, the phenomenology of anosognosia shares features with the gross denial of symptoms commonly observed in functional psychoses. By *anosodiaphoria*, Babinski was referring to an inappropriate lack of dysphoria. Specifically, he noted that some patients with left hemiplegia acknowledged sensorimotor and other deficits, but appeared inappropriately placid and unconcerned. The patient with anosodiaphoria does not present with implausible perceptual experiences or beliefs. Consequently, there is no failure to "appreciate implausibility." Rather, these patients appear to have an inappropriate emotional response in the context of an accurate representation of their neurological status.

Similarly, some have suggested impaired insight in psychosis may involve disturbance not only in the recognition and appropriate attribution of deficits but also in the appreciation of the implications of deficits (David, 1990). Failure to appreciate the implications of deficits may itself have various manifestations. Some individuals may acknowledge specific symptoms, yet fail to recognize the implication that they have an illness needing intervention. This lack of insight may be akin to the everyday example of the physician who suffers from repeated chest pain but fails to entertain the possibility of an impending heart attack. Alternatively, some individuals may be cognizant of symptoms and disease, but have an inappropriate affective response. Indeed, in the case of psychopathology, it is common to question insight not simply when patients are seemingly lackadaisical in the face of their own debilitating conditions, as in anosodiaphoria, but more generally when affective responses are inappropriate to the circumstances. Surely there is a problem with insight when the psychotic patient giggles and appears gleeful on being informed that a loved one has died. Finally, failure to appreciate implications may be manifested in behavior. Some patients may acknowledge illness, appear intellectually and affectively cognizant of the implications, yet fail to act appropriately. In the case of psychopathology this is often observed as lack of compliance with treatment.

This approach broadens the concept of insight to include appreciation of the cognitive, affective, and behavioral implications of knowledge. In turn, a host of new models can be generated to account for impaired insight. Likely at issue are the psychological processes involved in inductive reasoning (i.e., given these signs and symptoms, *x* must be the case), the processes involved in linking thought to affect, and/or the processes involved in generating and monitoring plans and action, or all of these things. In sum, this discussion suggests that a variety of phenomena might be considered as reflecting impaired insight in psychosis. With respect to patients' insights into their illness, these phenomena include:

1. Failure to recognize signs, symptoms, or disease (lack of awareness)
2. Misattribution of the source or cause of signs, symptoms, or disease
3. Failure to appreciate the implausibility of perceptual experiences or beliefs
4. Failure to derive appropriate cognitive representations despite recognition of pathological signs, symptoms, or disease
5. Inappropriate affective reactions despite recognition of pathological signs, symptoms, or disease
6. Inappropriate behavioral responses (actions) despite recognition of pathological signs, symptoms, or disease

## Models of Impaired Insight

The neurobiological and psychological models generated to account for impaired insight will likely differ depending on the phenomena included as instantiating this disturbance. For example, some of the earliest accounts of anosognosia in the neurological literature were restricted to the denial of hemiplegia and emphasized decreased sensory input to higher corical centers (Battersby, Bender, & Pollack, 1956), a disturbance in capacity to alter body schema (Brain, 1941), or deficits in the capacity to integrate multiple sensory stimuli (Denny-Brown & Banker, 1954). In essence, the view was that the brain damage left patients unable to alter their representations of their physical state and consequently resulted in denial of the paralysis on one side of the body. However, a central challenge to such formulations has been the contention that some anosognosic patients deny more than disabilities that pertain to one side of the body. Some anosognosic patients may also deny memory deficits, incontinence, the fact of a recent stroke, or that an operation has been performed (Weinstein & Kahn, 1955). These forms of denial are not readily explained as failures to integrate sensorimotor feedback or to alter body schema. Similarly, models that seemingly account for the failure to be aware of the symptoms of psychosis may not be sufficiently broad to cover failures to appreciate or act on the implications of symptoms that are acknowledged. Clearly, achieving consensus on what is meant by impaired insight will impact on the attempts to understand its genesis and correlates.

It might be worthwhile to outline the general thrust of some theoretical approaches taken to explain impaired insight. These theories might be organized as follows:

1. *Inferential processes are intact, but perceptual input is disturbed.* The classic form of this type of theorizing is the view that hearing loss can result in paranoid ideation—that is, the belief that people are whispering behind your back. Similarly, dysregulation of auditory or visual pathways can result in abnormal perceptual experiences (halluci-

nations). Since virtually all waking perceptual experiences are veridical, a long personal history of validated perception would dictate accepting hallucinations as veridical.

2. *There is a breakdown in inferential processes.* This leads to absurd ideas, misattributions, and a failure to recognize implications. The view emphasizes the failure of patients with delusions to alter beliefs in the face of countervailing evidence or to appreciate the import of evidence.

3. *There is a breakdown in the process of self-monitoring.* This view may assert that the experience of consciousness is altered, and for instance, the distinction between internally and externally generated phenomena may be impaired. For example, the patient with auditory hallucinations may be engaged in subvocal speech, but be unaware that the speech is self-generated.

4. *There is a breakdown in the processes involved in error checking.* The "capacity to doubt" is impaired owing to deficits in matching the product of information processing against consensual information as to what is definite, likely, possible, and improbable.

5. *The linkage between thought and affect is impaired.* In this view, affective responses are inappropriate relative to the content of mentation.

6. *There are deficits in the capacity to.* This view involves the ability to maintain a representation in memory over time (maintain a mental set), organize behavior sequentially, and sustain effort to establish and achieve a goal or plan. Deficits in these domains lead to a mismatch between intellectual appreciation of the implications of beliefs and subsequent behavior.

At this gross theoretical level, it is evident that disturbance in multiple classes of psychological processes could result in apparent disturbances of insight. Further, depending on the nature of heterogeneity in manifestations of impaired insight, there may be heterogeneity in the nature of underlying neuropsychological deficits. Thus it may not be useful to ask whether disturbed insight reflects impaired "executive" or self-monitoring functions, impairments in the allocation of attention, or the adequacy of working memory. Rather, linkage with neuropsychological profiles may be heavily dependent on how the dimensionality of insight impairments is resolved.

These approaches to modeling the nature of impaired insight are limited in their capacity to address the issue of the selectivity in the mental contents subject to impaired insight. It is difficult to accommodate these theories that link impaired insight to disturbance in specific aspects of information processing with the observation that only some discrete domains of self-representation may be subject to insight impairment. For example, it is common for psychotic patients to have enduring persecutory delusions or specific and repeated hallucinatory experiences that they deny are bizarre or unexpected. Our difficulty here may be analogous to the problem of individual differences in lying to others. Some people may engage in deceptions more than others do, and indeed a number of "lie scales" have been developed to assess variation in this proclivity. But it is also true that individuals differ with some consistency in the content of what they lie to others about (e.g., accomplishments, wealth, sexual prowess, eating habits).

Note that we often characterize patients as having grossly impaired insight as if this were a generalized deficit, like subnormal intelligence. The concern here is not only with possibility that there may be heterogeneous manifestations of impaired insight but that within a particular domain of impaired insight (e.g., denial of signs, symptoms, disease) there may be selectivity in the content. This presents additional empirical and conceptual challenge for the field. At the data level, we need to know the extent to which impairments of insight do, in fact, reflect dimensions of individual difference and generalize across different content areas. Is it the case that patients who deny that they are characterized by movement disorders also deny hallucinations, bizarre behavior, and illness (Caracci et al., 1990)? Do such patients also fail to acknowledge broader classes of disability and shortcoming? What is the consistency over time of such insight impairments?

Conceptually, the challenge is to devise methods that allow us to identify the factors that modulate the selectivity in mental content subject to lack of insight. Traditional psychodynamic formulations assumed that lack of insight pertained especially to conflictual ideation. In essence, some have thought that lack of insight serves a mood-regulatory purpose in preserving self-esteem or warding off unacceptable ideas or urges (Sackeim, 1983, 1986). This type of formulation is drastically different from models that view lack of insight as a breakdown in a motivationally neutral aspect of information processing. A fundamental problem with this dynamic theorizing has concerned not the breadth of its explanatory power but the limitations in testing its validity. As a start, we would like to know whether patients with impaired insight register and respond to personally threatening information in a different manner than do patients with preserved insight. At the practical level, we need to know the consequences for mood and self-esteem when patients recover insight into the nature of their devastating illnesses.

## Theories of Psychopathology and Mind

No one champions the view that gross distortions of insight reflect psychological health. Indeed, as noted, notions of insanity have often been grounded in formulations of what it means to lack insight. Neuropsychological models of impaired insight typically attribute the disturbance to any of a variety of core deficits in the processing of information. In this respect, lack of insight is on a conceptual par with alogia, apraxia, or aphasia in reflecting disturbed cognitive processing. Psychodynamic and other theories of the psychological causation of symptoms typically go a step further and view inaccurate knowledge of the self as itself pathogenic. In many respects, such theorizing shares the core premise that accurate representation of the self (and of our contributions in the world) is paradigmatic of psychological health (or of a properly working neurobiological machinery).

In entertaining models of insight, it is important to note a contrary view. It is an indisputable fact about humanity that what we think can determine what we feel. Our abstract representations of ourselves and of the world impact on our emotions. In turn, a cognitive apparatus that invariably results in accurate representations would leave us vulnerable to undesirable and, at times, dangerous mood alteration. Undoubtedly, one of the functions of the brain is mood regulation. This may be accomplished, in part, by biasing and distorting the products of information processing, particularly what we believe to be true about ourselves (Sackeim, 1986). In essence, inaccuracy in self-knowledge and acts of self-deception may reflect the operation of adaptive mechanisms in mood regulation.

A number of studies have observed that individual differences in the tendency to engage in self-deception covary with reports of depressive mood. Less of a tendency to lie to oneself is associated with greater dysphoria (Kiersky, this volume). A large body of literature has documented self-serving biases among normal individuals and a seemingly more accurate and even-handed realism among depressed patients (Sackeim & Wegner, 1986). The argument has been made that some degree of "impaired insight" characterizes normal function, and that some forms of psychopathology may be associated with excessive insight.

This perspective complicates matters. It presumes that the relations between the accuracy of self-knowledge and mental health are complex and that the correlation between "truth" and "happiness" is not invariably positive. At the mechanistic level, gross failures of insight, as reflected in anosognosia or in denial of illness in psychosis, may not be negative symptoms in the Hughlings Jackson sense, reflecting a deficit in normal psychological processes. Rather, such phenomena may reflect the release, overutilization, or rigidification of basic mood-regulatory operations. If we are built so as to be able to lie to ourselves, some gross manifestations of impaired insight may reflect an adaptive process gone awry.

It is exciting that the problem of insight has returned to the forefront in research on psychotic illness. Impaired insight confronts the clinician regularly and bedevils attempts to treat and rehabilitate. Nonetheless, determining what we mean by impaired insight remains a challenge, and we are far from consensus on the genesis of this disturbance. Undoubtedly, progress in this area will not only address this peculiar clinical problem but will more broadly contribute to our theories of psychopathology and our theories of mind.

*References*

Babinski, J. (1914). Contribution à l'étude des troubles mentaux dans l'hémiplégie organique cérébrale (Anosognosie). *Revue Neurologique, 27*, 845–848.

Battersby, W. S., Bender, M. B., & Pollack, M. (1956). Unilateral spaqtial agnosia (inattention) in patients with cerebral lesions. *Brain, 79*, 68–93.

Brain, W. R. (1941). Visual disorientation with special reference to lesions of the right cerebral hemisphere. *Brain, 64*, 224–272.

Carraci, G., Mukherjee, S., Roth, S. D., & Decina, P. (1990). Subjective awareness of abnormal involuntary movements in chronic schizophrenia patients. *American Journal of Psychiatry, 147*, 295–298.

David, A. S. (1990). Insight and psychosis. *British Journal of Psychiatry, 156*, 798–808.

Denny-Brown, D., & Banker, B. Q. (1954). Amorphosynthesis from left parietal lesion. *Archives of Neurology and Psychiatry, 71*, 302–313.

Fink, M. (1979). *Convulsive therapy: Theory and practice.* New York: Raven Press.

Sackeim, H. A. (1983). Self-deception, self-esteem and depression: The adaptive value of lying to oneself. In J. Masling (Ed.), *Empirical studies of psychoanalytic theory* (pp. 101–157). Hillsdale, NJ: Erlbaum.

Sackeim, H. A. (1986). A neuropsychodynamic perspective on the self: Brain, thought, emotion. In L. M. Hartman and K. R. Blankstein (Eds.), *Perception of self in emotional disorder and psychotherapy* (pp. 51–83). New York: Plenum.

Sackeim, H. A., & Wegner, A. (1986). Attributional patterns in depression and euthymia. *Archives of General Psychiatry, 43*, 553–560.

Sayer, N. A., Sackeim, H. A., Moeller, J. R., Prudic, J., Devanand, D. P., Coleman, E. A., & Kiersky, J. E. (1993). The relations between observer-rating and self-report of depressive symptomatology. *Psychological Assessment, 5,* 350–360.

Weinstein, E. A., & Kahn, R. L. (1955). *Denial of illness: Symbolic and physiological aspects.* Springfield, IL: Charles C. Thomas.

# PART I

*Phenomenology
of
Insight*

# 1

XAVIER F. AMADOR

HENRY KRONENGOLD

# The Description and Meaning of Insight in Psychosis

Clinicians treating individuals with schizophrenia and other psychoses have long been struck by the seeming indifference or unawareness many of these patients display in regard to their own illness. People diagnosed with psychotic disorders have similarly been frustrated with their friends, family members, and doctors who insist they have a serious mental illness when they know that they do not. Owing to its prevalence and to disruption of the therapist-patient relationship, this type of discrepancy in perspective—or what we in the mental health field have labeled "poor insight"—has become integral to our conception of particular psychoses. Poor insight often frustrates attempts by clinicians and concerned family members to render assistance and treatment. Such patients, feeling coerced into accepting medications for an illness they don't believe they have, understandably resist cooperating with prescribed treatments.

For years, the published literature related to poor insight in psychotic disorders reflected a largely theoretical and psychoanalytic perspective. Though valuable, this literature offered few guidelines regarding the phenomenology or measurement of the psychological processes conceptualized to constitute insight (Amador, Strauss, Yale, & Gorman, 1991). Furthermore, the analytic literature's almost exclusive reliance on the subjective interpretation of case material resulted in a premature consensus that poor insight was the result of psychological defense. The lack of empirical methods and data, coupled with preconceptions as to the causes of poor insight, has hampered progress in this area. However, over the past several years the topic of insight has become increasingly popular among researchers studying psychotic disorders. Investigators have begun to develop more sophisticated methods to assess the psychological and social

15

processes underlying insight, providing a clearer understanding of the causes of poor insight and its role in the expression of psychosis.

In this chapter, we will discuss the theoretical and empirical data related to insight, with particular emphasis on schizophrenia. We will begin by discussing the meaning of insight and the history of the use of this term in psychiatry, followed by a review of current methods and challenges related to its assessment. We will then consider the relationship between insight and symptoms of psychosis before moving on to suggest the unique role of poor insight in schizophrenia. Finally, we will conclude this chapter by discussing the etiological factors underlying the development of idiosyncratic and isolating perspectives on the self (i.e., poor insight) that are all too common in schizophrenia.

## What Is Insight?

Undertaking a survey of the literature on insight requires the skill to navigate through an often bewildering sea of terms that have been applied to the observed unawareness of illness (or lack of a consensual perspective) in psychotic disorders. Terms such as *poor insight, sealing over, defensive denial, attitudes about illness, indifference reaction, evasion,* and *external attributions* (e.g., David, 1990; Greenfeld, Strauss, Bowers, & Mandelkern, 1989; Wciórka, 1988; McGlashan, Levy, & Carpenter, 1975) reflect important underlying conceptual differences in addition to semantic preferences. On one end of the spectrum poor insight is understood as a psychological defense mechanism, while at the other extreme it denotes a theoretical position implicating cognitive deficit. In between lies a quagmire of related constructs that vary with the orientations of their authors. For example, researchers grounded in cognitive psychology have examined the "external attributions about illness" (Wciórka, 1988), while psychodynamically oriented authors have distinguished emotional versus intellectual forms of insight (Richfield, 1954). A more detailed discussion of the conceptual history of insight in psychotic disorders can be found in the chapter by Berrios and Marková in this volume.

Furthermore, as suggested by the various terms, insight is a complex and multidimensional phenomenon. For example, Wciórka et al. (1988) and others (Greenfeld et al., 1989; David, 1990, Amador et al., 1991) have argued that insight comprises a variety of phenomena, including retrospective and current insight. As we shall discuss in greater detail, Amador et al. (1991) have stressed the distinction between awareness and attribution of psychotic symptoms, as some patients may recognize signs of illness but attribute their presence to reasons other than mental dysfunction. Furthermore, some patients may recognize certain symptoms while remaining unaware of others. In a recent article, Marková & Berrios (1993) proposed further complexity by conceptualizing awareness of illness as a subcategory of self-knowledge rather than an independent feature of psychotic disorders. Finally, any discussion of insight raises epistemological presumptions about the nature of reality (David, 1990). Philosophical considerations aside, the phenomenon of insight relevant to mental health professionals is one in which *an individual's perception of him- or herself is grossly at odds with that of his or her community and culture.* Indeed, as we shall discuss with particular reference to individuals with schizophrenia, this perception may even differ from the views of similarly affected psychiatric patients (Wing, Monck, Brown, & Carstairs, 1964).

At the most fundamental level, then, poor insight in psychosis has been described as a seeming lack of awareness of the deficits, consequences of the disorder, and need for treatment. We will use the term *unawareness of illness* in this broadest sense. However, since we are in agreement with those authors who propose that insight is best conceptualized as a multidimensional construct, we will comment on the specific methods and definitions used to assess insight in the studies we review below. With that said, we nonetheless recognize that what we are speaking of are essentially radical differences between psychotic individuals and others in their subjective experience, self concept, and perception.

## The Measurement of Insight

Much of the early literature on insight in schizophrenia relied heavily on case material describing patients' beliefs regarding their illness. While this method offered a rich context in which to view each patient's self-assessment, it offered little in the way of replicable research. As a result, investigators began to devise standardized interviews or systematized scoring methods to assess insight. Unfortunately, few researchers combined a standardized interview with a systematic scoring system, and many early studies struggled with either a continued reliance on subjective clinical observations or a preconceived scoring system that did not always do justice to patients' free responses. In addition, early attempts to rate insight typically relied on crude global ratings that classified patients as having "good" or "poor" insight based on whether the patient "vigorously denied he was disturbed." Approximately four years ago, two semistructured interviews with systematized scoring systems and proven psychometric strengths were devised to measure insight.

The Insight and Treatment Attitudes Questionnaire (ITAQ) developed by McEvoy, et al. (1981) has been used in large samples of patients with schizophrenia and has been shown to be reliable and valid. An 11-item questionnaire, the ITAQ assesses patients' attitudes (or beliefs) about whether they have a mental illness and whether they need treatment. Though predictive of several measures of clinical outcome and compliance (McEvoy, et al., 1981; McEvoy, Apperson, et al., 1989; McEvoy, Freter, et al. 1989), the ITAQ fails to assess many of the psychological domains that investigators believe constitute "insight." Indeed, although this scale represents progress in the assessment of insight, it continues in the tradition of viewing insight as a simple, or unitary, phenomenon.

Adopting a multidimensional view, Amador et al. (1991; Amador, Strauss, Yale, Gorman, & Endicott, 1993; Amador & Strauss, 1993) have proposed a more complex terminology that distinguishes two main component dimensions of insight: awareness of illness and attribution regarding illness. *Unawareness of illness* reflects an individual's failure to acknowledge the presence of a specific deficit or sign of illness even when confronted with it by an examiner. *Incorrect attribution* reflects the individual's expressed belief that the specific deficit, sign, or consequence of illness does not stem from mental dysfunction. For example, a patient with severe flat affect who does not recognize the presence of this negative symptom illustrates unawareness of flat affect. A patient who is aware that her or his expressions of emotion were flattened, but is certain that this was due to a recent course of antibiotics, would be said to be aware but would display incorrect attribution regarding this sign of illness.

Consistent with this conception of insight, Amador & Strauss (1990) have developed the Scale to assess Unawareness of Mental Disorder (SUMD). In addition to the independent assessment of awareness and attribution, the SUMD distinguishes current and retrospective awareness of (1) having a mental disorder, (2) the effects of medication, (3) the consequences of mental disorder, and (4) the specific signs and symptoms. The SUMD, therefore, represents a departure from other published measures that assess whether the patient accepts a diagnostic label or whether the patient believes in the need for treatment. The assessment of insight regarding specific symptoms offers at least two important benefits: First, it can provide data on moderating variables useful for studies of psychoeducational strategies (e.g., are patients more likely to be unaware of particular symptoms?); second, these assessments are of importance theoretically, as they can provide data on the nature and pervasiveness of poor insight. In two independent studies, the SUMD has proved both reliable and valid (Amador et al., 1993).

Despite the SUMD's comprehensiveness, patients may still express subtle variations of insight that defy easy categorization. Furthermore, some patients may object to answering what they perceive as intrusive questions about their past and present experiences, especially if these experiences leave the patient feeling stigmatized. Perhaps to allow for a simpler and gentler method of measuring awareness, Selten and colleagues and Marková and Berrios have each developed self-rating scales to assess insight. Interested in negative symptoms, Selten, Sijben, van den Bosch, Omloo-Visser, & Warmerdam (1993) developed a self-rating scale that measures the patient's Subjective Experience of Negative Symptoms (SENS). An interviewer describes each symptom to the patient and then asks the patient to rate him or herself compared to other people who have not been admitted to the hospital. Designed to complement the Scale for the Assessment of Negative Symptoms (SANS) (Andreasen, 1989), the SENS allows for a fairly simple measure of insight that can be readily compared to an interviewer's clinical ratings. In a recent study, the SENS was found to have good internal consistency and test-retest reliability.

Marková and her colleagues also developed a self-rated Insight Scale (Marková & Berrios, 1993). Consisting of 32 items that are answered yes, no, or don't know, the Insight Scale attempts to broaden the measurement of insight by assessing deficits in self-knowledge not only related to illness but also to how the illness affects a patient's interaction with the world. While most measures of insight focus on having a "mental disorder" or assess symptoms such as hallucinations, Marková et al. present the patient with statements such as "I feel different from my normal self" or "I want to know why I am feeling like this" to address the process of insight along a continuum of self-knowledge. Patients may realize that a change has occurred within them without being able to label this change as a mental disorder. Marková and Berrios's emphasis on insight as a dynamic process offers an important contribution to the understanding of poor insight. Recent research has attempted to establish insight as an identifiable symptom of psychotic disorders, and later in this chapter we will present evidence to support this contention. At the same time, poor insight may reflect a broader disturbance of a patient's self-representation or self-schema, as Marková and Berrios imply. Though preliminary, the Insight Scale will encourage further research into insight as it relates to the complexity of self-experience in individuals with psychotic disorders.

Any method of assessing awareness of illness must take the individual's culture and subculture into account. While early studies by the World Health Organization (WHO), which we will discuss shortly, suggested that insight can be consistently measured cross-culturally, a recent study by Johnson and Orrell argues for greater sensitivity to sociocultural bias in the assessment of insight. Johnson and Orrell examined casenote summaries of 357 inpatients and compared demographic variables including gender, age, previous psychiatric history, and ethnic origin with comments describing the patients' levels of insight. Classifying these comments as indicating either little or no insight, partial insight, or full insight, Johnson and Orrell found that Caucasian British patients were rated as displaying significantly greater insight than patients from ethnic minority groups. Only 47% of the Caucasian British patients compared to 70% of the patients from other ethnic groups were viewed as having little or no insight. Furthermore, when entered into a regression analysis with the other variables, ethnicity emerged as the most significant independent factor influencing perceived insight.

Discussing various explanations to account for these results, Johnson and Orrell consider the possibility that patients from social groups where mental illness is especially stigmatized may be more likely to deny their illness or that different sociocultural groups may entertain different models of mental illness from that of Western psychiatry. They also suggest that patients from ethnic minorities may not be admitted to the hospital unless they are more severely ill than Caucasian British patients, and that more severely ill patients display poorer insight—a debatable position that we will discuss in the next section of this chapter.

The most important possibility from a methodological perspective concerns the possible sociocultural bias related to ratings of insight. Perhaps, as Johnson and Orrell point out, patients from ethnic minorities are more likely to be viewed by clinicians as lacking insight. If so, we need to understand the causes of such distortions as well as the means with which to correct them. Clearly, further research into the cross-cultural aspects of insight is needed. Sociocultural factors may influence patients' views of themselves, and in the process affect the levels of insight that are perceived by Western-trained clinicians and raters. These factors may also influence our understanding of what we consider psychotic symptoms. Though sociocultural factors should be examined as they relate to all aspects of psychiatric assessment, they seem especially pertinent to the measurement of an individual's potentially cultural-bound experiences of self that constitute our understanding of insight in psychotic disorders.

## The Relationship Between Insight and Symptoms of Psychosis

As alluded to earlier, a fair degree of controversy surrounds the relationship between level of insight and severity of symptoms. The earliest studies to examine this relationship yielded inconsistent results (Whittman & Duffey, 1961; Small, Small, & Gonzalez, 1965). Subsequent reports, using standardized assessments of symptoms, [e.g., Brief Psychiatric Rating Scale (BPRS), (Overall & Gorham 1962); Scale to Assess Positive Symptoms (SAPS), (Andreasen, 1984); and Scale to Assess Negative Symptoms (SANS), (Andreasen, 1984)] suggest that insight and severity of symptoms are independent factors (Bartko, Herczeg, & Zádor, 1988; McEvoy, Apperson, et al., 1989; Amador et al., 1993). These studies found no significant correlations between insight and positive or negative symptoms, general measures of symptoms, depressive symptoms, or manic symptoms. However, the issue has become clouded once again by recent findings of a relationship between poor insight and more severe scores of general psychopathology (Marková et al., 1992; Takei, Uematsu, Ueki & Sone, 1992; Young, Davila, & Scher, 1993).

A large-scale study by Amador et al. (1994) failed to completely clarify the nature of the relationship between poor insight and symptoms of psychosis. Amador et al. concluded that level of awareness was generally unrelated to symptom severity. Nonetheless, increased delusionality, thought disorder, and disorganized behavior were all modestly correlated with decreased awareness of mental disorder, the social consequences of mental disorder, and several positive symptoms. While these correlations achieved significance, they remained rather modest, with $r$'s ranging from +.18 to +.24. That said, the significance of the findings likely reflected the large sample size rather than the strength of the associations.

The relationship between insight and symptom severity has important ramifications for our understanding of insight. One may view poor insight as a reflection of symptom severity or delusional beliefs — in other words, more symptomatic or delusional patients should display less awareness of having a mental disorder or of having a specific sign of a mental disorder. If so, poor insight would qualify as an important consequence of psychopathology rather than as a sign of illness in its own right. If as many studies suggest, however, poor insight is not related to severity of symptoms, then we can consider insight as an independent phenomenological feature. While we should continue to examine this possible relationship, the studies cited above that support poor insight as independent of symptom severity, coupled with some of the evidence we will present regarding the prevalence of poor insight in the psychoses, suggest that poor insight is not merely a consequence of increased symptomatology.

Though not necessarily related to general symptomatology, diminished insight appears characteristic of schizophrenia patients with the deficit syndrome. Recently, we assessed a group of patients at the Maryland Psychiatric Center in collaboration with Drs. William T. Carpenter and Brian Kirkpatrick. These patients had been previously assessed with respect to the deficit syndrome. Utilizing the SUMD to assess insight, we found that schizophrenia patients with the deficit syndrome displayed significantly poorer insight compared to nondeficit schizophrenia patients. The associations between poor insight and primary negative symptoms were much stronger than the associations found previously between poor insight and both positive and negative symptoms. Such findings suggest that while poor insight may not simply reflect global severity of symptoms, it may nonetheless relate to individual or specific groups of symptoms. From a theoretical vantage point, the relationship between insight and primary negative symptoms may suggest that poor insight is reflective of an individual's inability to experience emotion, a potentially vital and challenging breakthrough for research that has thus far emphasized the cognitive aspects of insight. As shall be discussed later, lack of emotional response to illness, the "la belle indifference" reaction, has potentially identifiable neuropsychological underpinnings. We have hypothesized that the neuropsychological deficits associated with the deficit syndrome, resulting in part in an inability to experience emotion, may also account for the indifference reaction seen in schizophrenia (Amador et al., 1994). We are currently conducting a study of this question in a sample of schizophrenia patients with and without the deficit syndrome.

### Are Particular Aspects of Poor Insight Unique to Schizophrenia?

We agree with those investigators who view schizophrenia as a disorder involving multiple domains of psychopathology (e.g., Carpenter & Kirkpatrick, 1988; Andreasen, 1990). In this section, we will examine the question of whether poor insight can be conceptualized as a sign of schizophrenia. As reviewed previously by Amador et al. (1991; Amador & Strauss, 1993), and as discussed in this volume by Dr. Anthony David, research suggests the prognostic value of insight with regard to treatment compliance and course of illness. However, in order to establish insight as a sign of schizophrenia, we still need to answer two more questions: What is the prevalence of poor insight in schizophrenia? And, is poor insight unique to schizophrenia?

In an attempt to better identify more distinct subtypes of schizophrenia, Carpenter and his associates (1976) employed cluster analytic techniques on quantified sign and symptom data. This study, based on data collected from the International Pilot Study of Schizophrenia (IPSS) (WHO, 1973), provided a unique opportunity to determine whether subtype diagnoses effectively categorize groups of patients across culture. Examining the data from 811 subjects, 680 of whom were diagnosed as schizophrenic, Carpenter et al. (1976) found poor insight to be a prevalent feature of schizophrenia as well as an important discriminating factor in making subtype diagnoses.

Along these lines, Carpenter et al. (1976) identified four mathematically defined subtypes culled from the 27 dimensions of the Present State Examination (PSE). They labeled these four subtypes, consisting of 573 patients, as typical, flagrant, insightful, and hypochondriacal schizophrenia. *Typical schizophrenia* was characterized by poor insight, persecutory and passivity delusions, auditory hallucinations, restricted affect, and social withdrawal. *Flagrant schizophrenia* included aberrant, agitated, or bizarre behavior, incomprehensibility, unkempt appearance, incongruent or restricted affect, and the absence of anxiety or depression. *Insightful schizophrenia* shared many of the features of typical schizophrenia, but had good rather than poor insight and did not include behavioral aberrance other than social withdrawal. The fourth subtype, *hypochondriacal schizophrenia*, was characterized by intermediate insight and was distinguished by increased somatic concerns and visual hallucinations. The authors raised several methodological difficulties regarding the use of cluster analytic techniques to define diagnostic groups and cautioned that their results should be considered preliminary, pending replication and validity studies. Despite these limitations, Carpenter's findings strongly support the importance of insight as a common feature of schizophrenia.

In a more recent multinational study, entitled Classification of Chronic Hospitalized Schizophrenics (CCHS), the 12 signs and symptoms of the Flexible System Criteria (Carpenter, Strauss, & Bartko, 1973) were assessed in a relatively chronic sample of 768 patients (Wilson, Ban, & Guy, 1986). The results of this study replicated the IPSS finding of high rates of poor insight in schizophrenia. Across both the CCHS and IPSS samples, poor insight occurred more often than did any other dimension and ranked among the least variable dimensions of schizophrenia across subtypes. While the study by Johnson and Orrell discussed earlier raises the question of sociocultural bias in the assessment of insight, both of these multicultural studies found comparable rates of insight and, as such, support the notion of insight as a cross-culturally stable and identifiable characteristic of mental illness.

In both the CCHS and the IPSS studies, insight was defined as present "if there was some awareness of emotional illness" and absent if the patient "vigorously denied he was disturbed" (WHO, 1973). Such a conservative definition of insight requires only that the patient express some awareness of emotional illness. In the IPSS, awareness did not need be accompanied by correct attribution for specific signs and symptoms (e.g., aware that they have specific symptoms and accurately identify these as a consequence of mental illness) in order to be called insight. Similarly, their definition of insight did not include recognition of the need for treatment. One can argue that a patient who vigorously denies the existence of a mental illness may display a defensive response to escape the depressing reality of his or her situation (Van Putten, Crumpton, & Yale, 1976). Consequently, the definition of insight used in these studies may have identified something other than lack of awareness. Furthermore, as a result of the global and unitary definition of insight used in the above studies, we cannot determine if any of the patients displayed at least partial awareness of various aspects of the disorder. We also cannot determine whether any of the patients were aware of the particular signs or symptoms of schizophrenia, the consequences of the disorder, or the effects of medication.

Such limitations aside, these studies offered clear support for a consideration of poor insight as a common feature of psychotic disorders. Moreover, Carpenter et al. (1973) reported that poor insight was one of 12 signs and symptoms that were "especially discriminating between schizophrenia and other psychiatric disorders (p. 1275)." Though not clear-cut, this finding at least suggests that poor insight is a unique feature of schizophrenia.

Recently, we reported on a large-scale study using the SUMD to examine the prevalence and specificity of poor insight in schizophrenia. We completed a collaboration with the Schizophrenia and Psychotic Disorders Work Group empaneled by the American Psychiatric Association to revise the diagnostic criteria for schizophrenia in the *Diagnostic and Statistical Manual for Mental Disorders* (*DSM-III-R*) (APA, 1987). An abbreviated version of the SUMD was used in the assessment procedure for the DSM-IV field trials. In this study, more than 400 patients from geographically diverse regions of the United States were evaluated for a wide range of symptoms. The main objective of the insight study was to determine the prevalence of poor insight in psychotic disorders and to examine its specificity to schizophrenia (Amador et al., 1994).

The results indicated that nearly 60% of the patients with schizophrenia displayed moderate to severe unawareness of having a mental disorder. This finding replicates the IPSS report and the CCHS study results, which both indicated that a majority of patients with schizophrenia believe they do not have a mental disorder. In addition, in the *DSM-IV* field trial sample, between 27 and 87% of the patients with schizophrenia were also unaware of specific symptoms, for example, delusions, thought disorder, blunt affect, anhedonia, asociality, and other dimensions of illness. The prevalence of unawareness of symptoms has not previously been reported in the literature. Importantly, patients with schizophrenia were significantly less aware of: having a mental disorder, the efficacy of medication, various aspects of delusion, and anhedonia than were psychotic mood-disorder patients. Similarly, patients with schizophrenia also had poor awareness of various symptoms (i.e., hallucinations, delusions, anhedonia, and asociality) relative to schizoaffective patients. Furthermore, patients with schizophrenia had poor insight into many aspects of their illness compared to patients with a psychotic or nonpsychotic major depressive disorder. Items where these two groups did not differ tended to have small sample sizes that drastically reduced the statistical power necessary to adequately compare the two groups. These results suggest that at least some aspects of poor insight (i.e., severe and pervasive deficits in self-awareness) are uniquely characteristic of schizophrenia when compared to other psychotic disorders—the one exception to this rule being patients with bipolar disorder.

Qualifications in hand then, the literature on insight reviewed earlier and the *DSM-IV* field trial data support the commonly held belief that patients with schizophrenia, as well as other psychotic disorders, display poor insight and that level of insight is an important dimension on which patients can be subtyped. The field trial data also provide the first direct evidence suggesting that poor insight, or self-awareness deficits, is more severe and pervasive among individuals with schizophrenia. These results, taken together with the data reviewed above regarding the relations between level of insight and severity of psychopathology, suggest that poor insight is not simply a consequence of increased symptom severity. If poor insight appeared solely on the basis of psychotic symptoms, we would not expect to find any difference between patients with schizophrenia and other patients with psychotic disorders. Instead, poor insight appears to be an independent feature of the schizophrenia syndrome that may help distinguish schizophrenia from other psychotic disorders. Further rationale for this conceptualization will be presented in the next section, where we will consider the possible causes of poor insight.

## The Etiology of Poor Insight in Schizophrenia

While a variety of hypotheses exist to explain poor insight in schizophrenia, two approaches tend to predominate. One of these approaches considers poor insight in schizophrenia as a psychological defense or adaptive coping mechanism. The other, more contemporary view suggests the role of neurological abnormalities and neuropsychological deficit in the etiology of poor insight in schizophrenia.

### Psychological Defense

Historically, self-awareness deficits in schizophrenia have typically been understood as stemming from psychological defenses or adaptive coping strategies (e.g., Lally, 1989; Levy et al., 1975; Mayer-Gross, 1920; McGlashan & Carpenter, 1976; Semrad, 1966; Searles, 1965; Van Putten et al., 1976). In 1920, Mayer-Gross classified the defensive strategies of patients with schizophrenia and offered two categories highly relevant to the present discussion: denial of the future and denial of the psychotic experience. In the *denial of the future category*, patients were observed to deny the possibility of positive future events (i.e., they expressed "despair"), even when such events were of high likelihood. Meanwhile, in the *denial of the psychotic experience category*, patients were typically unaware of the signs and symptoms of the illness. This latter stage is of direct relevance to the present discussion, while the former combines unawareness phenomena (e.g., denial of relevant data for making predictions about the future) with attributional processes. Essentially, Mayer-Gross identified various domains for which patients with schizophrenia displayed awareness deficits and interpreted this finding as evidence for distinct categories of psychological defense.

Similarly, McGlashan and Carpenter (1976) identified the relationship between postpsychotic depression (PPD) and denial in schizophrenia. In their review of the literature, they cite several authors who consider PPD as a stage of recovery from psychosis that either follows a more "primitive" defensive state characterized by denial or precedes the reinstatement of psychotic denial. Despite their differences, these authors share the view that PDD stems from a lessening of defensive denial, resulting in the patient's awareness of the tragic circumstances of his or her illness. In short, this view states that patients who accept rather than deny the reality of their psychotic experiences are prone to depression. In the process, this view of PPD implies a defensive function for denial in schizophrenia.

In other work, McGlashan, Levy, & Carpenter (1975) have suggested a continuum of recovery styles: on one end lies *integration*, and on the other *sealing over*. Fourteen neuroleptic withdrawn, "generally nonpsychotic" *DSM-II* diagnosed patients with schizophrenia were interviewed 12 months following an acute psychotic episode. Patient responses during a taped structured interview were reliably categorized into either the integration or sealing over categories. The raters employed the following criteria for making this distinction:

> (1) Some patients prefer not to think about their psychotic experience during recovery and adopt an attitude of "the less said the better." Such individuals were referred to as sealing over patients. (2) Some patients manifest an interest in their psychotic experiences during recovery and are willing to discuss their experiences in an effort to learn more about themselves. These patients would be considered integrators. (McGlashan et al., 1975, p. 1270)

Responses from each group were evaluated and led the authors to conclude that integrators displayed an awareness of the continuity of their personality before, during, and after their psychotic episode. These patients "took responsibility" for their psychotic symptoms and were flexible in their thoughts about them. Meanwhile, patients that sealed over were either unaware of their psychotic experience or viewed their psychotic experiences as alien, caused by some force outside themselves.

While psychoanalytic approaches emphasize the role of unconscious defense in poor insight, more cognitively oriented research emphasizes the importance of attribution in understanding poor insight. Evidence suggests that depressed college students and psychiatric outpatients may be more accurate than normal controls in some aspects of self-evaluation, such as in judging social competency and evaluating contingencies between their own behaviors and certain outcomes (Alloy & Abramson, 1979; Lewinsohn, Mischel, Chaplain, & Barton, 1980). Similarly, in a study contrasting depressed with nondepressed college students (i.e., mean Beck Depression Inventory Scores for depressed = 16.12, and nondepressed = 1.19), Sackeim and Wegner (1986) found that depressed subjects were more accurate in their self-evaluations (i.e., did not utilize the same self-serving biases) than nondepressed subjects. In a second study, they contrasted depressed inpatients and outpatients with inpatients with schizophrenia and a group of normal controls. Sackeim and Wegner found that the latter two groups utilized "self-serving biases" in their appraisals of their behaviors and their outcomes, while the depressed patients did not. The self-serving biases were characterized as follows: "If an outcome is positive, I controlled it, I should be praised, and the outcome was very good. If an outcome is negative, I did not control it (as much), I should not be blamed, and it was not so bad anyway." The authors go on to say that the cognitive distortions displayed by normal controls and patients with schizophrenia represent a "normal" pattern of functioning. In fact, there is an abundance of work with nonpsychiatric samples that supports this position (see Taylor & Brown, 1988, for a review).

Interestingly, Sackeim and Wegner found no differences between normals and patients with schizophrenia. This finding suggests that in at least some areas of self-awareness, patients with schizophrenia, like most people, utilize a generally adaptive self-serving bias to evaluate their behaviors and their outcomes. Taken a step further, these findings may influence our theories about the etiology of poor insight in schizophrenia. The gross unawareness of illness observed in schizophrenia could be explained as a result of the disinhibition of normally adaptive cognitive biases rather than as a cognitive or psychodynamic deficit state. Meanwhile, the more accurate self-appraisals identified in depressives can be understood as a failure of these cognitive biases to influence their normal inhibitory effect on dysphoric mood. In other words, the self-awareness deficits evident in schizophrenia may result from overuse of normally adaptive cognitive biases. Indeed, Sackeim (1983) has proposed that self-deception (or denial) is adaptive and essential to the regulation of euthymic mood states. Interestingly, a report on insight and medication compliance from Van Putten et al. (1976) seems to support this view. They found a significant inverse relation between grandiosity and insight, leading the authors to hypothesize that medication refusers may prefer a grandiose psychotic state (i.e., extreme self-serving cognitive bias) to the more normal state induced by psychotropic medicine.

The above studies support the notion of poor insight as a form of psychological defense or as a cognitive coping mechanism. However, empirical research has yet to directly measure the relationship between poor insight and defense. Currently, we are involved in two studies that measure self-deception and social desirability among patients with schizophrenia. If patients with lower levels of insight display increased levels of self-deception, then evidence suggesting the role of defense or coping mechanisms in the etiology of poor insight will have been obtained. Furthermore, in the self-deception study, we will be able to correlate self-rated self-deception scores, insight ratings, and depression scores, providing a direct test of the relationships among poor insight, a self-deceptive cognitive style, and depressive symptoms. If, indeed, poor insight reflects psychological defense or cognitive distortion, we would expect a high correlation between poor insight and increased self-deception, as well as a three-way relationship among greater insight, decreased self-deception, and increased levels of depression.

## Neuropsychological Deficit

Amador et al. have suggested that at least some forms of poor insight stem from neuropsychological deficit (Amador et al., 1991, 1993). Babinski's description of anosognosia, the unawareness of illness in neurological disorders, bears a striking resemblance to poor insight in schizophrenia. He characterizes the anosognostic patient as displaying a lack of knowledge, awareness, or recognition of disease. This has most frequently been observed in patients suffering from hemiplegia and hemianopia following stroke. Gerstmann (1942) offers the following description:

> The hemiplegia is usually on the left side of the body. The patient behaves as though he knew nothing about his hemiplegia, as though it had not existed, as though his paralysed limbs were normal, and insists that he can move them and walk as well as he did before. (pp. 891–892)

As in schizophrenia, unawareness of illness in neurological disorders is largely intractable to direct confrontation. For example, when an anosognostic patient with hemiparesis is confronted with the affected limb, the patient may express indifference (Gerstmann, 1942) or even reveal delusional ideas (e.g., insist that the limb is not his) to account for his or her condition.

As with unawareness of illness in schizophrenia, anosognosia has been understood in varying ways. Terms used besides anosognosia include lack of insight, imperception of disease, denial of illness, and organic depression. McGlynn and Schacter (1989) have provided an extensive review of this literature and the theoretical implications of the various terms. Regardless of the etiology, one thing is certain: anosognosia in neurological disorders arises directly following injury to the brain. Consequently, anosognosia is generally thought to stem from a neuropsychological deficit leaving one unaware of the signs of illness (McGlynn & Schacter, 1989).

In neurological disorders, neuroanatomically based theories of anosognosia can be broadly divided into those that attribute this deficit to focal brain lesions and those that emphasize diffuse brain damage (McGlynn & Schacter, 1989). Researchers subscribing to the focal lesion viewpoint generally attribute anosognosia to right-hemisphere lesions of the parietal area and its connections (Gerstmann, 1942; Geschwind, 1965; Von Hagen & Ives, 1939; Warrington, 1962; Critchley, 1953; Stuss & Benson, 1986). Although some reports of anosognosia implicate left-hemisphere insult, the bulk of evidence suggests right-hemisphere lesions (McGlynn & Schactner, 1988; Stuss & Benson, 1986). The findings implicating right-hemisphere involvement in self-awareness deficits have led to several theories suggesting that anosognosia may stem from the isolation of cortical speech areas (Geschwind, 1965), a disconnection from awareness of body scheme or image representation (e.g., Gerstmann, 1942; Schilder, 1935), or a neurologically based affective disturbance (e.g., Bear, 1982).

The frontal lobes have also been implicated in anosognosia. Stuss and Benson (1986) suggest that awareness deficits share an inability to self-monitor or self-correct, and that self-awareness demands intact prefrontal function. They note the similarities among different forms of anosognosia, Capgras syndrome, reduplicative paramnesia, and confabulations frequently seen in Korsakoff syndrome. Specifically, they suggest that these deficits in reality testing stem from a disorder of self-awareness and the ability to self-correct. Although structural damage to the frontal lobe has not been demonstrated in reported disorders of awareness, Stuss and Benson cite a large body of literature implicating prefrontal function as necessary for self-awareness.

Anosognosia has also been observed in patients who have had diffuse brain damage, usually following a stroke (Cole, Saexinger, & Hard, 1968; Sandifer, 1946; Ullman, 1962). In these patients, self-awareness deficits are most often understood as stemming from an overall decline in cognitive function. This seems unlikely, however, since anosognosia has been observed in patients without general intellectual impairment (Gerstman, 1942; Cutting, 1978; Babinski, 1914) and in patients with unawareness of specific dysfunctions coinciding with intact awareness of other deficits (Von Hagen & Ives, 1939). If anosognosia stemmed from general intellectual impairments, then we would expect awareness deficits for multiple rather than for specific defects.

Of particular interest is the finding of domain specificity for anosognosia (e.g., Bisiach, Valler, Periani, Papogano, & Berti, 1986). For example, Von Hagen and Ives (1939) described a 76-year-old patient who denied paralysis of the left leg and yet was aware of the paralysis of the left upper limb and of severe memory impairment. Such observations have led some investigators to postulate that these deficits involve modality-specific disorders of thought that arise from a dysfunction of a modular central processing system rather than a single higher order system responsible for self-awareness. Schacter (1989) disagrees with this view and offers a descriptive model for unawareness phenomena referred to as Dissociable Interactions and Conscious Experience (DICE). This model involves a centralized conscious awareness system (CAS) that interacts with modular systems concerned with language, memory, perception, and so forth. In order for unawareness to occur in a particular domain, the input to the CAS from the relevant module would need to drop to a sufficiently low level of activation to become functionally disconnected from awareness.

The literature on unawareness of tardive dyskinesia in schizophrenia (Rosen, Mukherjee, Olarte, Varia, & Cardenas, 1982; Caracci, Mukherjee, Roth, & Decina, 1990) suggests that self-awareness deficits in schizophrenia may also be domain specific. Rosen and his associates (1982) found that of 70 patients with schizophrenia who displayed tardive dyskinesia, 47 (67%) were unaware of the deficits produced by the movement disorder. Similarly, Caracci et al. (1990) found that 15 of 20 (75%) patients with schizophrenia with tardive dyskinesia were unaware of their movement disorder. Interestingly, verbal and visual feedback resulted in a short-term increase in awareness, though this was not sustained for longer than two weeks. Moreover, when the relation between awareness of tardive dyskinesia and awareness of psychiatric disorder was examined, they observed that 13 patients were unaware of having a psychiatric disorder, indicating that although the two measures strongly correlated, there was no complete overlap.

The literature suggesting neuropsychological underpinnings of self-awareness deficits may offer profound implications for understanding poor insight in schizophrenia. From the literature reviewed, we can draw certain parallels between the unawareness phenomena described in neurological disorders and schizophrenia. For example, in a letter addressed to his friend Lucilius (Liber V, Epistula IX), L. A. Seneca, writing on the moral implications of self-beliefs 2,000 years ago, described what appears to be a case of anosognosia following hemianopia: "Incredible as it might appear . . . she does not know that she is blind. Therefore, again and again she asks her guardian to take her elsewhere. She claims that my home is dark." Similarly, individuals with schizophrenia are frequently observed to attribute their hospitalizations solely to fights with parents, misunderstandings, and so on. In addition, patients with both disorders are frequently rigid in their unawareness, unable to integrate new information contrary to their erroneous beliefs, and they display affective indifference. Affective unawareness has also been described in neurological patients—for example, "Other cases exist in which deficient knowledge of illness is inferred from the apparent lack of adequate emotional reactions, the condition Babinski named "anosodiaphoria" (Bisiach et al., 1986, p. 19)—and in schizophrenia—for example, "What always surprises the observer anew is the quiet complacency with which the most nonsensical ideas can be uttered by them and the most incomprehensible actions carried out" (Kraepelin, 1919/1971, p. 25), and "the patients have, at first at least, no real understanding of the gravity of the disorder. . . . To all representations of the incomprehensibility and morbidity of their conduct the patients give as answers explanations which say nothing" (Kraepelin, 1919/1971, p. 151). Finally, the unawareness phenomena observed are frequently heterogeneous in their presentation in both anosognosia and schizophrenia. For example, the anosognostic patient may be aware of a memory deficit but unaware of paralysis. Similarly, we have found that patients with schizophrenia can be aware of having hallucinations and delusions, but not of having a thought disorder or negative symptoms.

Until recently, studies had yet to directly measure the relationship between poor insight and neurological deficit. However, in a recent study of 31 chronic patients, Young et al. (1993) found a significant correlation between unawareness of illness as measured by the SUMD and two variables on the Wisconsin Card Sorting Task (WCST), a neuropsychological test sensitive to frontal lobe dysfunction. The percentage of perseverative responses and number of categories completed on the WCST were found to significantly correlate with the total symptom awareness and total symptom attribution scores as measured by the SUMD. Young et al. also classified the sample into high and low awareness groups and performed a discriminant function analysis to determine which of a set of variables most significantly distinguished the high and low groups. From a group of variables including inpatient vs. outpatient status, IQ, WCST categories completed, WCST percentage perseverative responses, and average symptom severity, Young et al. found that a combination of perseverative errors and average symptom severity correctly categorized 83.9% of the high and low awareness groups. This study offered the first empirical support of Amador et al.'s (1991) hypothesized relationship between poor insight and frontal lobe dysfunction. Further support comes from Lysaker and Bell, who in their chapter in this volume report that poor-insight schizophrenia patients with neuropsychological dysfunction of the frontal lobes did not show improved insight following psychosocial treatment compared to a poor-insight schizophrenia group that did not display frontal lobe dysfunction. Finally, further support for the neurological basis of at least some aspects of poor insight comes from Takai et al.'s (1992) finding of a relationship between poor insight and structural brain abnormalities such as ventricular enlargement. MRI examination of 57 male patients with chronic schizophrenia revealed a significant relationship between ventricular enlargement and lack of insight. Nonetheless, these studies have their limitations. In the Young et al. study, poor insight was not related to other measures of frontal lobe performance administered in the study. Furthermore, a relatively low percentage of patients in the sample displayed poor insight. Consequently, we need to consider the possibility that the Young et al. study used a nonrepresentative sample. Similarly, Takai et al.'s sample of males with a chronic course of illness may not accurately represent the range of patients with schizophrenia. Despite these limitations, the above studies should encourage research to more fully explore the relationship between poor insight and both neuropsychological disturbance and structural brain abnormalities. In light of such promising preliminary findings, further research may indeed shed light on a potentially vital relationship.

## Conclusions

Generally speaking, the literature concerning the etiology of poor insight in schizophrenia reveals a rift between proponents of psychological defense and those of neuropsychological dysfunction as the basis of poor insight. Exacerbating their conceptual differences, the two schools of thought rely on often mutually exclusive forms of evidence to support their hypotheses. While neuropsychological approaches use objective methods amenable to replicable research, supporters of the psychological defense approach rely on the subjective interpretation of case material. The above review of the literature suggests that both approaches may offer important contributions to our understanding of poor insight in schizophrenia. In our own interviews with patients with schizophrenia, we have seen different patients manifesting distinct expressions of poor insight into their illness. While some patients may show consistently little awareness of their illness, other patients may display levels of insight that vary with the content of an interview. For example, a patient may articulate an especially vehement denial when confronted directly by a question such as "Have you ever heard voices that other people could not hear?" When asked directly about a symptom, some patients may instead discuss their past achievements in an apparent effort to avoid, consciously or not, discussing their experiences. With this in mind, we need to consider the possibility that poor insight may stem from more than one etiological process. Perhaps both psychological defense and neuropsychological deficit account for the phenomenon of poor insight. Furthermore, the above example highlights the importance of utilizing clinical material in our examination of poor insight. Often, it is from listening carefully to what our patients have to say that we can learn new directions for investigating and understanding psychological phenomena. It is hoped that future research will continue to combine rigorous standardization with an appreciation of the richness of clinical material to better understand the phenomenon of poor insight.

As we mentioned earlier, insight is a complex and multidimensional phenomenon. In the past several years, investigators have increasingly turned their attention to poor insight as an important feature in schizophrenia. In the process, research has demonstrated that poor insight is a prevalent feature of psychotic disorders in general and of schizophrenia in particular. While the etiology of poor insight in schizophrenia remains unclear, recent studies have strengthened the hypothesis that neuropsychological deficits, particularly in the frontal lobe, may account for at least some cases of poor insight. Studies of poor insight have seemingly blossomed over the past several years. As investigators continue to report their findings, we should be able to paint a clearer picture of poor insight. As we bolster our own awareness of this phenomenon, we hope to begin to consider ways in which we can illuminate patients' awareness of their illness and its consequences. As we continue to explore this area of research, we hope to improve not only our understanding of insight but also our capacity to improve the lives of our patients with schizophrenia and other psychoses.

*References*

Alloy, L. B., & Abramson, L. Y. (1979). Judgment of contingency in depressed and nondepressed students: Sadder but wiser? *Journal of Experimental Psychology, 108,* 441–485.

Amador, X. F., & Strauss, D. H. (1990). The Scale to assess Unawareness of Mental Disorder (SUMD). Columbia University and New York State Psychiatric Institute.

Amador, X. F., Strauss, D. H., Yale, S. A., & Gorman, J. M. (1991). Awareness of illness in schizophrenia. *Schizophrenia Bulletin, 17,* 113–132.

Amador, X. F., & Strauss, D. H. (1993). Poor insight in schizophrenia. *Psychiatric Quarterly, 64,* 305–318.

Amador, X. F., Strauss, D. H., Yale, S., Gorman, J. M., & Endicott, J. (1993). The assessment of insight in psychosis. *American Journal of Psychiatry, 150,* 873–879.

Amador, X. F., Andreasen, N. C., Flaum, M., Strauss, D. H., Yale, S. A., Clark, S. & Gorman, J. M. (1994). Awareness of illness in schizophrenia, schizoaffective and mood disorders. *Archives of General Psychiatry, 51,* 826–836.

American Psychiatric Association. (1987). *Diagnostic and statistical manual of mental disorders* (3rd ed. rev.) Washington, DC: Author.

Andreasen, N. C. (1984). The Scale for the Assessment of Negative Symptoms (SANS). Iowa City, IA: University of Iowa.

Andreasen, N. C. (1984). The Scale for the Assessment of Positive Symptoms (SAPS). Iowa City, IA: University of Iowa.

Andreasen, N. C. (1989). Scale for the assessment of negative symptoms (SANS). *British Journal of Psychiatry, 155,* 53–58.

Andreasen, N. C. Schizophrenia. (1990, August/September). *DSM-IV Update.* Washington, DC: American Psychiatric Association.

Babinski, J. (1914). Contribution à l'étude des troubles mentaux dans l'hemiplégie organique cérébale (Anosognosie). *Revue Neurologique, 27,* 845–888.

Bartko, G., Herczeg, I., & Zádor, G. (1988). Clinical symptomatology and drug compliance in schizophrenic patients. *Acta Psychiatrica Scandinavica, 77,* 74–76.

Bear, D. M. (1982). Hemispheric specialization and neurology of emotion. *Archives of Neurology, 40,* 195–202.

Bisiach, C., Valler, G., Periani, D., Papogano, C., & Berti, J. (1986). Unawareness of disease following lesions of the right hemisphere: Anosognosia for hemiplegia and anosognosia for hemianopia. *Neuropsychologia, 24,* 471–482.

Caracci, G., Mukherjee, S., Roth, S., & Decina, P. (1990). Subjective awareness of abnormal involuntary movements in chronic schizophrenic patients. *American Journal of Psychiatry, 147,* 295–298.

Carpenter, W. T., Jr., Bartko, J. J., Carpenter, C. L., & Strauss, J. S. (1976). Another view of schizophrenia subtypes. *Archives of General Psychiatry, 33,* 508–516.

Carpenter, W. T., Jr., & Kirkpatrick, B. (1988). The heterogeneity of the long term course of schizophrenia. *Schizophrenia Bulletin, 14,* 645–651.

Carpenter, W. T., Jr., Strauss, J. S., & Bartko, J. J. (1973). Flexible system for the diagnosis of schizophrenia: Report from the WHO International Pilot Study of Schizophrenia. *Science, 182,* 1275–1277.

Cole, M., Saexinger, H. G., and Hard, A. (1968). Anosognosia: Studies using regional intravenous anasthesia. *Neuropsychologia, 6,* 365–371.

Critchley, M. (1953). *The parietal lobes.* New York: Hafner Publishing.

Cutting, J. (1978). Study of anosognosia. *Journal of Neurology, Neurosurgery, and Psychiatry, 41,* 548–555.

David, A. S. (1990). Insight and psychosis. *British Journal of Psychiatry, 161,* 599–602.

Gerstmann, J. (1942). Problem of imperception of disease and of impaired body territories with organic lesions. Relation to body scheme and its disorders. *Archives of Neurology and Psychiatry, 48*, 890–913.

Geschwind, N. (1965). Disconnexion syndromes in animals and man. *Brain, 88*, 237–294, 585–644.

Greenfeld, D., Strauss, J. S., Bowers, M. B., & Mandelkern, M. (1989). Insight and interpretation of illness in recovery from psychosis. *Schizophrenia Bulletin, 15*, 245–252.

Johnson, S., & Orrell, M. (1995). Insight and psychosis: A social perspective. *Psychological Medicine, 25*, 515–520.

Kraepelin, E. (1919/1971) *Dementia praecox and paraphrenia.* Huntington, NY: Robert E. Krieger.

Lally, S. J. (1989). "Does being in here mean there is something wrong with me?" *Schizophrenia Bulletin, 15*, 253–265.

Lewinsohn, P. M., Mischel, W., Chaplain, W., & Barton, R. (1980). Social competence and depression: The role of illusory self-perceptions? *Journal of Abnormal Psychology, 89*, 203–212.

Marková, I. S., & Berrios, G. E. (1992). The assessment of insight in clinical psychology. *Acta Psychiatrica Scandinavica, 86*, 159–164.

Mayer-Gross, W. (1920). Ueber die Stellungnahme zur abgelaufenen akuten Psychose. *Zeitschrifte fur die Gesmate Neurologie und Psychiatrie, 60*, 160–212.

McEvoy, J. P., Aland, J. Jr., Wilson, W. H., Guy, W., & Hawkins, L. (1981). Measuring chronic schizophrenic patients' attitudes toward their illness and treatment. *Hospital and Community Psychiatry, 32*, 856–858.

McEvoy, J. P., Apperson, L. J., Appelbaum, P. S., Ortlip, P., Brecosky, J., & Hammill, K. (1989). Insight in schizophrenia. Its relationship to acute psychopathology. *Journal of Nervous and Mental Disorders, 177*, 43–47.

McEvoy, J. P., Freter, S., Everett, G., Geller, J. L., Appelbaum, P., Apperson, L. J., & Roth, L. (1989). Insight and the clinical outcome of schizophrenics. *Journal of Nervous and Mental Disorders, 177*, 48–51.

McGlashan, T. H., & Carpenter, W. T., Jr. (1976). Postpsychotic depression in schizophrenia. *Archives of General Psychiatry, 33*, 231–239.

McGlashan, T. H., Levy, S. T., & Carpenter, W. T., Jr. (1975). Integration and sealing over. Clinically distinct recovery styles from schizophrenia. *Archives of General Psychiatry, 32*, 1269–1272.

McGlynn, S. M., & Schacter, D. L. (1989). Unawareness of deficits in neuropsychological syndromes. *Journal of Clinical and Experimental Neuropsychology, 11*, 143–205.

Overall, J. E., and Gorham, D. R. (1962). The brief psychiatric rating scale. *Psychological Reports, 10*, 799–812.

Richfield, J. (1954). An analysis of the concept of insight. *Psychoanalytic Quarterly, 23*, 390–408.

Rosen, A. M., Mukherjee, S., Olarte, S., Varia, V., & Cardenas, C. (1982). Perception of tardive dyskinesia in outpatients receiving maintenance neuroleptics. *American Journal of Psychiatry 139*, 372–373.

Sackeim, H. A. (1983). Self-deception, depression, and self-esteem: The adaptive value of lying to oneself. In J. Masling (Ed.), *Empirical studies of psychoanalytic theory* (pp. 101–157). Hillsdale, NJ: Erlbaum.

Sackeim, H. A., & Wegner, A. Z. (1986). Attributional patterns in depression and euthymia. *Archives of General Psychiatry, 43*, 553–560.

Sandifer, P. H. (1946). Anosognosia and disorders of body scheme. *Brain, 69*, 122–137.

Schacter, D. L. (1989). On the relation between memory and consciousness. In H. Roediger & F. Craik (Eds.), *Varieties of memory and consciousness.* Hillsdale, NJ: Erlbaum.

Searles, H. F. (1965). *Collected papers on schizophrenia and related subjects*. New York: New York International University Press.

Selten, J. P. C. J., Sijben, N.E.S., van den Bosch, R. J., Omloo-Visser, J., & Warmerdam, H. (1993). The subjective experience of negative symptoms: A self-rating scale. *Comprehensive Psychiatry*, 34, 192–197.

Semrad, E. V. (1966). Longterm therapy of schizophrenia. In G. Usdin, (Ed.), *Psychoneuroses and schizophrenia* (pp. 155–173). Philadelphia: Lippincott.

Schilder, P. (1935). *The Image and Appearance of the Human Body*. London: Kegan, Paul, Trench & Trubner.

Small, I. F., Small, J. G., & Gonzalez, R. (1965). The clinical correlates of attitudinal change during psychiatric treatment. *American Journal of Psychotherapy*, 19, 66–74.

Stuss, D. T., & Benson, D. F. (1986). *The frontal lobes*. New York: Raven Press.

Takai, A., Uematsu, M., Ueki, H., & Sone, K. (1992). Insight and its related factors in chronic schizophrenic patients: A preliminary study. *European Journal of Psychiatry*, 6, 159–170.

Taylor, E. T., & Brown J. D. (1988). Illusion and well-being. A social psychological perspective on mental health. *Psychological Bulletin*, 103, 193–210.

Ullman, M. (1962). *Behavioral changes in patients following strokes*. Springfield, IL: Charles C. Thomas.

Van Putten, T., Crumpton, E., & Yale, C. (1976). Drug refusal in schizophrenia and the wish to be crazy. *Archives of General Psychiatry*, 33, 1443–1446.

Von Hagen, K. O., & Ives, E. R. (1939). Two autopsied cases of anosognosia. *Bulletin of the Los Angeles Neurological Society*, 4, 41–44.

Warrington, E. K. (1962). The completion of visual forms across hemianopic defects. *Journal of Neurology, Neurosurgery, and Psychiatry*, 25, 208–217.

Wciórka, J. (1988). A clinical typology of schizophrenic patients' attitudes towards their illness. *Psychopathology*, 21, 259–266.

Whittman, J. R., & Duffey, R. F. (1961). The relationship between type of therapy received and a patient's perception of his illness. *Journal of Nervous and Mental Disease*, 133, 288–292.

Wilson, W. H., Ban, T. A., & Guy, W. (1986). Flexible system criteria in chronic schizophrenia. *Comprehensive Psychiatry*, 27, 259–265.

Wing, J. K., Monck, E., Brown, G. W., & Carstairs, G. M. (1964). Morbidity in the community of schizophrenic patients discharged from London mental hospitals in 1959. *British Journal of Psychiatry*, 110, 10–21.

World Health Organization (WHO). (1973). *Report of the international pilot study of schizophrenia*. Geneva: WHO Press.

Young, D. A., Davila, R., & Scher, H. (1993). Unawareness of illness and neuropsychological performance in chronic schizophrenia. *Schizophrenia Research*, 10, 117–124.

# 2

GERMAN E. BERRIOS
IVANA S. MARKOVÁ

# Insight in the Psychoses

## A Conceptual History

Attempting a history of insight (and its clinical derivative, lack of insight) illustrates the problem of chronicling the evolution of an ambiguous notion. Should the historian use as a guiding object, or *invariant*, a narrow definition such as the correct attitude to being ill (Lewis, 1934), or the equally narrow view implicit in most current empirical studies (Marková & Berrios, 1995) or in configurational learning (Hartmann, 1931; Sternberg & Davidson, 1994)? Or perhaps the historian should embrace the wider idea of insight as self-knowledge (Marková & Berrios, 1992; Gillett, 1995), mystical intellection (Lonergan, 1970, pp. 406–408), creative moment (Hutchinson, 1939; 1941), or psychoanalytic comprehension (Richfield, 1954). And how about the cognitive view that insight is a function of a putative mind-reading system (Baron-Cohen, 1995)? The difficulty concerns not the history of these views in particular but the composition of a general history of insight. In other words, the problem is to determine whether such views are *conceptually cognate* (i.e., have a common ancestor) or whether their only link is the usage of the word *insight*.

## The Object of Inquiry

It is important to specify what the main object of the inquiry is. Failure to distinguish between the history of the *term* insight (and its equivalents in other languages) and the pertinent *behaviors* (however termed) and *concepts* (however theoretically underpinned) can only lead to confusion. As in empirical work, the choice in historical research is never totally an objective one. Behavior is not an atheoretical object but the result of overt or (often enough) covert conceptualization. Furthermore, the behaviors

33

corresponding to insight are likely to have less ontological mass than do other medical objects, such as moles, murmurs, or hallucinations. This is not to say that insight has no neurobiological basis, but only that the capture of its behavioral core (ontology) depends on concepts, or epistemological devices. Hence, a history of insight must study the contextualized interaction of etymology, concepts, and behaviors. In accordance with this rule and the theme of this book, we shall concentrate on the history of insight (and lack of insight) in relation to the psychoses. It should not be forgotten, however, that the history of insight in dementia, obsessional disorder, hysteria, and the like is still to be written.

## Historical Contexts

### Insanity and Awareness of Illness

Until the early 19th century, the official view of insanity—as had been first offered by Hobbes and Locke during the 17th century (Berrios, 1994)—was based on the presence of delusions, and in this conceptual lattice, the crucial substructure was lack of insight. In other words, between the late 17th century and the early 19th century, the statement "he is aware of being deluded" would have been a logical contradiction and considered nonsensical. Insight was thus not a variable but a parameter in the definition of insanity. This very fact makes it difficult to find a writer from this period who actually discusses the importance of varying insightlessness in insanity. But there is also a second reason subjective or introspective facts such as insight were not yet a central part of the definition of madness: such additions took place only during the middle of the 19th century.

Only occasionally during the 18th century was the issue of awareness of illness raised by lawyers, in their relentless attack on the notion—and defense—of total insanity. The eventual success of such challenges led to the concept of partial insanity. At the beginning of the 19th century, partial insanity had two meanings: *intermittent* (i.e., periods of madness interspersed with lucid intervals),[1] and *incomplete* (i.e., madness affecting one region of the psyche, or monomania) (Kageyama, 1984).

In addition to partial insanity, there was at the beginning of the 19th century another development, also important to the history of insight. This was the challenge to Locke's intellectual (i.e., delusional) definition of madness.[2] Pinel, Prichard, and Esquirol, among others, proposed a definition of insanity in terms of faculty psychology, which in due course made possible the creation of new clinical categories such as the *emotional* and *volitional* insanities (Berrios & Gili, 1995). It was soon realized that the latter were not necessarily linked to insightlessness, even if in practice patients with severe depression, or mania, or abulia might refuse to accept that they were ill. In other words, the concept of partial madness and of monomania allowed for the existence of an insanity that, to paraphrase Baillarger, was aware of itself. This is the historical moment in which insightlessness ceased to be a substructure (or parameter or constant) in the conceptual lattice of insanity, and for the first time it became meaningful to treat it as a variable.

Changes in views on the causes of insanity opened up yet more space for the possibility of insight into mental illness. As an anonymous historian put it in 1840: "all explanations of mental illness boil down to three options: they are localized in the brain . . . or in the soul . . . or in both" (Fabre, 1840, p. 118). The former two options had interesting implications. In general, notions of monomania and partial insanity (and hence insight) were more readily accepted by supporters of the anatomoclinical view of madness (Ackerknecht, 1967; López Piñero, 1983) than by those who believed that insanity was exclusively sited in the mind or soul (*l'âme*). It was difficult, in terms of the philosophical psychology of the period, to accept that the soul was divided up, and hence could become partially diseased. Such was the very argument that Jules Falret used before the Société Médico-Psychologique in 1866.[3]

These categorical changes were made possible by a deeper shift in the notion of disease. Until the 18th century, total insanity was but a reflection of what has been called the ontological definition of disease—that is, being mad and losing one's reason was a sort of permanent state that affected the entire person. In a way, the problem at the time was to explain recovery. On the other hand, the notion of partial insanity, which took hold after the momentous changes brought about by the ideas of Bichat,[4] assumed a modular model for the mind and more or less specific cerebral localization.[5] This allowed for the coexistence of sanity and insanity in the human mind (Kageyama, 1984). Alienists during the 1830s were fully aware of the implications of this change, and an important debate ensued on the legitimacy of such a mosaiclike model of the mind (SMP, 1866). Others, like Maudsley, accepted this view, but felt that in the insane all regions of the mind were affected: "when an insane delusion exists in the mind, however circumscribed the range of its action may seem to be, the *rest of the mind is certainly not sound*" (our italics) (Maudsley, 1885, p. 220).

## Consciousness and Insight

Yet more conceptual space was provided with the incorporation in the late 19th century of noble concepts such as *consciousness* (awareness) and *introspection* (Boring, 1953; Danziger, 1980), and of *self* (Berrios, 1993)—without which the notion of insight would be difficult to understand.[6] Acceptance of these concepts was facilitated by determined efforts to incorporate *subjectivity* (i.e., descriptions of inner experiences) into the definition of insanity. Moreau de Tours (Bollotte, 1973) was important in articulating this need (Moreau de Tours, 1845). Encouraged by his work, alienists accepted the view that the way patients actually experienced their illness was essential for diagnosis and classification. This belief paved the way for development of a language of description, of interviewing techniques, and of scientific questions as to the value and legitimacy of introspection (Lyons, 1986). During the 19th century, the psychological concept of consciousness was couched in terms of *perception* (an inner eye). Not surprisingly, the old English term *insight* was preferred to *inwit*, which could have been as useful but carried less visual connotations.

## Insight and Verstehen

The final facilitator for a development of a science of insight was the arrival of the concept of *comprehension* (*Verstehen*), and later of *self-consciousness* (Marková, 1988). Important to the former were the ideas of Brentano (1874/1973), Fancher (1977), Dilthey (1976), Martin-Santos (1955), and eventually Freud, Husserl, and Jaspers

(Berrios, 1992). These grander concepts were more ambitious than the mere "looking into one's mind," as suggested by introspection: they attempted to grasp the totality of one's mental and existential state (which includes regions of information that are not conscious or volitional). Within this new conceptual frame, *full insight* needs more than a mere definition as the intellectual knowledge of being ill; it demands attitudinal processes involving emotions and volitions. The mechanisms that make such holistic insight possible vary according to school of thought, however. In Brentano, it concerned intentionality and his mechanism of a third consciousness.[7] In Dilthey, it pertained to grasping the totality, or *Verstehen* (Apel, 1987; McCarthy, 1972; Makkreel, 1975; López Moreno, 1990).[8] In the psychoanalytical movement, it varied according to model of the mind (Richfield, 1954).

## Insight: A Convergence Manqué?

We have now described three (no doubt there are more) conceptual spaces within which the history of insight could be explored. The question is, have they converged into a unitary phenomenon? Or have they remained parallel developments? Current empirical studies seem to assume the former—namely, that there is such a thing as insightless behavior, as an ontological given. What has been said so far suggests that the latter is the case, and that the so-called insightlessness of schizophrenia (even if the latter is the expression of organic disorganization) is in fact *concept driven*—that is, it reflects the way in which it is portrayed in contemporary culture. This generates a mild form of relativism, and that will be the perspective used in this chapter.[9]

The reason for this relativism is that the process of symptom construction, when historically studied, results from the convergence at a point in time of a term (insight, *Einsicht, conciencia de enfermedad*, etc.), a concept ("looking into," *Verstehen*, etc.), and a behavior (which is partly dependent on the existence of deeper conceptual frames). Strictly speaking, insightlessness should not be viewed as a symptom in the traditional sense of hallucination or anxiety. Its construction as an entity can be considered as analogous to symptom construction (in addition, current practice tends to treat it as a symptom), and hence it parallels the convergence model. This convergence may last only a short period or may became stable—a veritable word-concept-behavior complex. Some symptoms, such as depression, hallucination, and so on, have proved to be longer-lasting complexes. The model also suggests that convergence can be unstable. We propose that this is the case with insightlessness, which can be said to belong to the category of convergence *manqué*.

## History of Words

A history of the word *insight* and its equivalents is informative. The term exists only in the North and West Germanic families of languages. The Italic family (French, Spanish, Italian, Portuguese, etc.) does not have a corresponding unitary term, and so translation of *insight* into any of these languages is according to verbal function; for example, a well-known 19th-century German-French dictionary translates *Einsicht* as: *inspection, examen, connaissance de cause, bon sens, jugement* (Rose, 1878). This linguistic fact would be of little import were it not that it corresponds with a more marked interest in insight in the countries of the Germanic families. More research is needed to determine to what extent having a unitary term (*insight* or *Einsicht*) causes a referential or ontological mirage—that is, the belief that the term refers to one rather than to a family of objects.

For the German term *Einsicht*, Grimm and Grimm propose as equivalents the Latin terms *intelligentia* and *judicium*, and suggest that the term gained wider usage in the work of Goethe and Kant (Grimm & Grimm, 1862; Pauleikhoff & Mester, 1973). Adelung, at the very beginning of the 19th century, defines it as *Das sinneinsehen in eine Sache* ("understanding the sense of something") (Adelung, 1811, Vol. 1). Ritter adds that the Middle German term *însehen* is present in medieval mystical writings meaning *hineinsehen* ("looking into"). J. C. Günther, at the beginning of the 18th century, discarded the religious denotation to use *Einsicht* as equivalent to personal evidence (Ritter, 1972, Vol. 2). This writer also suggests that the psychological meaning introduced by Köhler (see below) was a departure, in that it simply meant "intelligence" and hence approached the old Aristotelian meaning of φρονηζιζ ("thought or understanding").[10]

As far as English is concerned, the *New Oxford English Dictionary* provides a set of definitions governed by the same metaphor: internal sight, with the eyes of the mind, mental vision, perception discernment or the fact of penetrating with the eyes or the understanding into the inner character or hidden nature of things; a glimpse or view beneath the surface; the faculty or power of thus seeing.

On the other hand, the earliest clinical usage of the term insightlessness we have been able to identify dates back to Krafft-Ebing: "in the later stages of insanity, where delusions have become organized or mental disintegration has ensued, the patient is completely insightless about his disease state (Krafft-Ebing, 1893, p. 103).[11]

## History of Concepts

The history of the concept of insight is also illuminating, particularly in relation to the evolution of notions of reason, consciousness, and self-knowledge. In this section we shall deal only with its psychiatric aspects. Because of the special nature of the behaviors corresponding to insight (i.e., they can be only accessed via concepts), their history will be dealt with together with the history of concepts.

### French Views

*Despine and Dagonet*     Prosper Despine distinguished two meanings for the term *lucidity*: one concerned the state of recovery, the other the sparing of the intellectual faculty. The first, in turn, Despine divided up into two: improvement after the illness had lifted and *lucidité pendant la folie même*. The latter included an inchoate form of the current concept of insight as awareness of illness. This state, according to Despine, arose when delusions were limited to specific topics and there was absence of a *passion pathologique* affecting the mind (Despine, 1875, pp. 312–314); others disagreed. Perhaps the best known work defending the old-fashioned view of delusion as an insightless phenomenon was *Les Folies Raisonnantes*, in which Sérieux and Capgras, already during the early 20th century, described approximately 19 cases with circumscribed delusional disorder, none of whom had any insight into their condition. Indeed, when exploring the natural history of their delusions, the authors do not consider the question of insight (Sérieux & Capgras, 1909).

In a classic paper, "Conscience et Aliénation mentale," Dagonet (1881) recommended that alienists accepted a new definition of consciousness: "to comprehend mental illness further it is indispensable to examine the mental symptoms *in themselves* . . . the first to study amongst the latter should be the disorders of consciousness" (our italics) (Dagonet, 1881, p. 369). Defined by Littré as "the intimate, immediate, and constant monitoring of the activities of the self," consciousness had as one of its functions the detection of change: "consciousness captures all the phenomena of our internal life, and commits them to memory: this includes the feeling of totality of the person. Consciousness should be subject to any transformation in the latter caused by mental illness" (Dagonet, 1881, p. 370); "in the different forms of mental illness, the disorders of consciousness will depend upon what other faculties are involved . . . only in exceptional cases can cerebral automatism occur in clear consciousness" (Dagonet, 1881, p. 389). For example, in the case of hallucinated patients, some have no awareness of illness while others "preserve the sense of the strangeness of the hallucination and search for explanations" (Dagonet, 1881, p. 393). Dagonet explained such awareness of illness on the basis of Luys's hypothesis that "one cerebral hemisphere remained normal whilst the other was pathological" (Dagonet, 1881, p. 20). The notion of consciousness proposed by Littré (1877) and Parant (1888) was less popular in England. Maudsley, in his usual acerbic tone, wrote:

> It has been very difficult to persuade speculative psychologists who elaborate webs of philosophy out of their own consciousnesses that consciousness has nothing to do with the actual work of mental function; that it is the adjunct not the energy at work; not the agent in the process, but the light which lightens a small part of it. . . . We may then put consciousness aside when we are considering the nature of the mechanism and the manner of its work. . . . (Maudsley, 1895, p. 8).

*Parant*    Seven years after Dagonet, Parant offered a full analysis of the problem.[12] *La Raison dans La Folie* is an important book, for it directly tackles the issue of legal responsibility in insanity. Parant called one approach to this problem *la conscience de soi dans la folie*. Awareness of illness in the context of insanity, he wrote, "concerns the state in which the patient is aware of his experiences, acts, of all internal changes and of their consequences. . . . Thus understood, this awareness implies not only knowledge of illness but capacity by degrees to judge it" (Parant, 1888, p. 174).

Parant discussed awareness of illness early in, during, and after the mental illness. In the second group, and using combinations of awareness relating to quality of acts, to illness, and to the emotional response to such knowledge, he recognized patients who may have awareness: (1) of the goodness or badness of their acts but not of disease; (2) of being ill but that the illness was not insanity; (3) of being insane but not fully accepting it; (4) of being insane but unable to do something about it; and (5) like item 4 but involved in serious acts (Parant, 1888, pp. 177–179).[13] In regard to group 3, Parant made the important point that "the awareness of these patients is complex in that it probably results from conscious and unconscious factors" (Parant, 1888, p. 196).

The question of the role and state of consciousness in insanity continued to trouble writers well into the 20th century. For example, Claye Shaw inquired whether there was a disturbance of consciousness during the acute episode, and whether it could explain the lack of memory shown by psychotic patients of symptoms experienced during the attack. Indeed, he came close to explaining why there was no awareness of illness in delusion:

> There is evidence that both in dream states and in insanity the emotional side of the idea may be wanting, and this must have great effect on both memory and consciousness. . . . I have over and over again noticed that people with delusions of a very depressed type do not show the emotional tone which should co-exist with the delusions. (Shaw, 1909, pp. 406–407)

### German Views

A young Gustav Störring (1907) defined delusions as not susceptible to correction and as insightless, regardless of whether the function of judgment was affected (p. 210). Mendel (1907) agreed with this view; when discussing the issue of patterns of improvement from the psychoses, he wrote:

> the dictum of Willis, that "no one can be regarded as cured till he voluntarily confesses his insanity" cannot be accepted in this categorical form. There are sporadic cases which, in spite of a limited residual insanity, may undoubtedly be considered as cured. (p. 147)

*Kraepelin and Bleuler*    The questions of insight and its diagnostic and predictive value do not seem to have interested Kraepelin a great deal. He briefly touched on them under judgement: "what always surprises the observer anew is the quiet complacency with which the most nonsensical ideas can be uttered by them and the most incomprehensive actions carried out" (Kraepelin, 1913/1919, p. 25). But then he added:

> the patients often have a distinct feeling of the profound change which has taken place in them. They complain that they are "dark in the head," not free, often in confusion, no longer clear, and that they have "cloud thoughts" . . . "understanding of the disease disappears fairly rapidly as the maladie progresses in an overwhelming majority of the cases even where in the beginning it was more or less clearly present." (p. 26)

Bleuler was no different. The nearest he came to discussing awareness of illness was in the section on the nature of delusional ideas, but in the end he did not elaborate on his views.

*Jaspers*    Continuing in the tradition of Parant, Karl Jaspers (1948) wrote:

> Patients' *self-observation* is one of the most important sources of knowledge in regard to morbid psychic life; so is their *attentiveness* to their abnormal experience and the *elaboration* of their observations in the form of a psychological judgement so that they can communicate to us something of their inner life. (our italics) (p. 350)

Jaspers observed that in the early stage of their illness patients became perplexed, and he explained this as an understandable reaction. As the illness progressed, patients tried to make sense of their experiences—for example, by elaborating delusional systems.

Jaspers then introduced personality as an explanatory concept; as personality became involved in the illness, the patient's attitude changed—for example, patients appeared indifferent or passive to the most frightening delusions. As we saw above, Shaw believed that this lack of reaction was due to lack of emotions.

Jaspers also observed that transient insight may occur during acute psychoses, but that this soon disappeared. He believed that where insight persisted, the patient was more likely to be suffering from a personality disorder than a psychosis. In patients who recovered from the psychotic state, Jaspers made a distinction between psychoses such as mania and alcoholic hallucinosis, where patients were able to look back on their experiences with complete insight; and a psychosis such as schizophrenia, where they did not show full insight. He described the latter patients as unable to talk freely about their experiences, becoming overtly affected when pressed to do so and occasionally maintaining some features of their illnesses. For chronic psychotic states, he described patients who, from their verbal contents, often appeared to have full insight, yet in fact these verbal contents would turn out to be learned phrases, meaningless to the patients themselves.

Jaspers's concept of insight was defined in terms of the patient's ability to judge what was happening to him or her during the development of psychosis, and the reasons why it was happening. He made a distinction between awareness of illness—that is, experiences of feeling ill or changed—and insight proper—where a correct estimate could be made of the type and severity of the illness. These judgments, however, depended on the intelligence and education of the individual; indeed, because judgments of this nature are an inherent part of the personality make-up, with patients of intelligence below a certain level (e.g., idiocy), it is more appropriate to think of loss of personality rather than loss of awareness as the feature of their lack of self-knowledge.

Jaspers was aware of the difficulty involved in theorizing about insight, and of the extent to which the outsider can hope to understand a patient's attitudes toward his or her illness. In other words, it is easier to assess objective knowledge—that is, the ability of a patient to understand and apply medical knowledge to him or herself—than what Jaspers called the *comprehending appropriation* of it. This latter function, Jaspers stated, is intrinsically linked to the patient's self, and cannot be divorced from knowledge of self-existence itself.

## The Aftermath

*Hartmann, Ogden, and Lewis*    Between the two World Wars, insight gained currency and usage became unclear. George Hartmann (1931), the German psychologist, expressed this neatly:

> Terminological difficulties are a notorious source of confused thinking. . . . The notion of insight as elaborated by the Gestalt psychologists during the last decade is a case in point. . . . Examination of recent usage reveals at least three important meanings of insight . . . insight as general comprehension[14] . . . insight as a personality trait . . . and insight as configurational learning.[15] (pp. 242–243)

The second of these meanings concerns the theme of this book (namely, insight in the psychoses):

Psychiatrists have long sought to discriminate between the functional disorders in psychotic and neurotic cases on the basis of awareness of one's condition. The sufferer from neurosis is maladjusted and knows it; the frankly insane person is said to be relatively oblivious to his abnormality. . . . Insight in this case has fundamentally an egocentric reference. (p. 243)

In 1932, R. M. Ogden replied to Hartmann and criticized his introspective leanings. He also called into question the plausibility of trying to use insight as a clear and simple idea, for questions about insight could not be answered in general. In a claim that fully applies to current empirical work on insight, Ogden (1932) wrote: "The point is that such questions cannot properly be asked outside the framework of a definite set of postulates; and when they are asked the framework will suggest most of the answers as a necessary consequence of the postulates" (p. 356). The same year, Hartmann (1932) retorted, defending the experiential aspects of insight: "My fourth question asked: 'is insight necessarily accompanied by ideas?' Ogden rejects this phrasing as implying a needless loyalty to an outworn creed, but I see no reason why a catholic psychologist of today should hesitate to avail himself of introspective data in the interests of a richer description of the event" (pp. 577–578).

These important exchanges contain the kernel of views to be expressed by Lewis (1934) three years later. In an unreferenced paper, Lewis offers etymological disquisition, gives a summary of Gestalt views, and explores views on the definition of normality. Only half way through the paper is the relevant question asked: "What is complete insight?—a correct attitude towards a morbid change in oneself" (p. 340). After exploring physical causes ("there are numerous instances of grossly defective insight in physical disorder"), Lewis makes the very pertinent observation (lost to later researchers) that

In any mental disorder, whether mild or severe, continued or brief, alien or comprehensible, it is with his whole disordered mind that the patient contemplates his state or his individual symptoms, and in this disorder there are disturbances which are different from the healthy function either in degree, combination or kind. (Lewis, 1934, p. 343)

Lewis believed that during the earlier stage of schizophrenia patients often showed a considerable amount of insight that was "associated with a struggle against the illness that is tragic" (Lewis, 1934, p. 345). Lewis believed that changes in the level of insight had prognostic value, as did the gaining of retrospective insight. He mentioned in this context Targowla's study of Wernicke's autochthonous ideas.[16]

### Conrad

Conrad (1958) carried out long-term observations on schizophrenic patients and described the development and progression of the psychotic state. Although he did not use the term, his conceptualization of awareness of change in the self and the environment owing to mental illness is related to what Jaspers called insight. Conrad named the early stage of the schizophrenic illness the *trema*. During this stage patients found it difficult to express their feelings and experiences; some would talk about fear, tension, anxiety, and anticipation, while others would describe feelings of guilt and helplessness. Conrad believed that the common theme was a feeling of oppression, an awareness that something was not right, and a sense of restriction of one's freedom. During the next stage of the illness, the *apophany*, patients attributed meaning to feelings and experiences; for example, when in the state of anastrophe, patients believed themselves to be the center of the world.

Conrad described further stages during which destructive processes were followed by partial resolution as residual schizophrenic effects persisted, and he postulated that schizophrenia was an illness affecting the higher mental functions that differentiate humans from animals. Thus, it affected the whole self-concept and, in particular, the ability of the individual to effect the normal transition from looking at oneself from within to looking at oneself from the outside—with the eyes of the world.

## Conclusions

The following can be concluded: insight and its derivative insightlessness, including loss of awareness of illness or incapacity to gain it in the first place, are concepts sitting at the incomplete convergence of word, concept, and behavior. This makes life hard for the historian. Before 1850, there is very little on insightlessness in the clinical literature. This is likely to be because questions concerning insight and awareness of illness were meaningless when insanity was defined as the presence of delusions. However, development of concepts such as partial, emotional, and volitional insanity during the second half of the 19th century led to early questioning of the clinical value of evaluating the attitude of patients vis-à-vis their insanity.

Equally important to the development of a concept of insight has been the psychological notions of consciousness, introspection, and self. Whether introduction of the notion of *Verstehen* has been equally useful remains to be seen. Additionally, it is difficult to map out the semantic structure of insight because of the uncertain origins of the concept.

The French and German psychiatric traditions have handled the problem of insight differently. Since there is no single French word to refer to all the mental states and actions pertaining to the German *Einsicht* (insight), the phenomenon has been paraphrased with references to the wider notion of conscience. This has, in general, kept French ideas broader. Having a specific term in English and German is likely to have caused an ontological mirage—that is, resulting in the view that the clinical phenomenon of insight may be circumscribed, specific, and self-subsistent. Further research is required to ascertain these hypotheses.

*Notes*

1. As late as 1875, Prosper Despine discussed in detail two senses of *lucidité*: "In the work of the alienists, the word *lucidity* has been used in two ways; one is a synonym of reason and refers to the moment when the mental faculties become normal . . . the other has been defined by Trélat as the sparing of the intellect in cases where the other mental faculties are diseased" (Despine, 1875, pp. 312–314). Ulysse Trélat (1795–1879) was a creative thinker whose busy political life prevented him from contributing further to psychiatry (Morel, 1988). The work quoted by Despine was *La Folie Lucide*, a rather old-fashioned book, probably written much earlier, where Trélat studied a heterogeneous group of patients whose common denominator was that "in spite of their ill-

ness, they responded exactly to the questions and did not seem insane to the superficial observer" although their behavior betrayed their condition (Trélat, 1861). A few years earlier, in a very popular forensic work, Legrand defined the lucid interval as: "An absolute albeit temporary suspension of the manifestations of insanity. It can be observed in about 25% of manics, less frequently in melancholia, rarely in monomania, never in dementia" (Legrand, 1864, pp. 109–110).

2. Well into the 19th century, see Ernest Martini stating; *"Le symptôme propre et essentiel à la folie, celui qui commence et fini avec elle, est le délire"* (Martini, 1824, p. 3).

3. A typical example was Jules Falret, who wrote:

I firmly believe, both from a theoretical and practical point of view, that there is complete solidarity of the various faculties of the human mind both in the sane and the insane. In reasoning mania *(folie raisonnante)* clinical observation shows that although the moral faculties are predominantly involved there is also involvement of intellect. . . . The fundamental mistake in the work of alienists this century has been to import to the study of the mentally ill the divisions of the mind created by psychologists to study normal individuals. (Falret, 1866, pp. 384–385)

4. Xavier Bichat (1771–1802) developed a viable *tissue* theory that forced changes in the very concept of the localization of disease (see D'istra, 1926; Albury, 1977; Haigh, 1984).

5. Under the name of faculty psychology, the modular view had a distinguished career during the 19th century—for example, in relation to phrenology (Berrios, 1988); it was resuscitated by Marr and later Fodor (1983). For a criticism of the latter's view from a developmental perspective, see Karmiloff-Smith (1992).

6. Unless a Rylean account is offered according to which to have insight is defined as "a disposition to behave in a particular way" (see Ryle, 1949, pp. 116–198).

7. "Experience shows that there exist in us not only a presentation and a judgement, but frequently a third kind of consciousness of the mental act, namely a feeling which refers to this act, pleasure or displeasure which we feel towards this act" (Brentano, 1973, p. 143).

8. *Verstehen* is not a transparent concept. Dilthey defined it in opposition to *explanation* and hence it is supposed to be more mediate and to involve more mental functions than the mere intellectual grasping provided by explanations. "Understanding presupposes experience and experience only becomes knowledge of life if understanding leads us from the narrowness and subjectivity of experience to the whole and the general" (Dilthey, 1976, pp. 187–188).

9. For a recent analysis of a contextualized approach that does not fall into a damaging relativism, see Warnke (1987).

10. This noble Greek term is already present in Heraclitus: τοῦ λογου δ ἐόντοζ ξυνοῦ ζωου σιν οἱ πολλοὶ ὡζ ἰδίαν ἔχοντεζ φρονησιν ("though reason is common to all, men live as though they had a *private understanding*")—Heraclitus, Fr.2, (Kirk & Raven, 1966). On the inconsistent Aristotelian usage of *phronêsis*, see Urmson (1990).

11. *In den späteren Stadien des Irreseins, da wo systematische Wahn-ideen oder ein geistiger Zerfall eingetreten sind, ist der Kranke absolut einsichtslos für seinen krankhaften Zustand* (Krafft-Ebing, 1893, p. 102).

12. Victor Parant was one of the great clinicians of the second half of the century. He also did important work in neuropsychiatry, particularly the mental symptoms of Parkinson's disease (1883, 1892).

13. Echoes of Parant's classification can be found in 20th-century French psychiatry, in a recent tripartite classification of *la reaction consciente du malade à l'égard de son état morbide'* (Deshaies, 1967, pp. 85–88).

14. Here Hartmann made an obscure reference to "the semi-technical employment of the term in the writings of the *Geisteswissenchaften* school (e.g., Erismann)." It is likely that he was referring to a great book by Theodor Erismann (1924).

15. This third meaning referred to Kurt Köhler's usage in the context of Gestalt psychology; see Petermann (1932, p. 33). Elizabeth Bulbrook (1932) wrote on this:

To psychologists familiar with current and recent discussions, it will be unnecessary to dwell upon the revival in periodical and textbook of the term 'insight' . . . some of these meanings are perceptive apprehension, acute observation, understanding, foresight and forethought, rapid learning, an intuitive flash, sudden grasp of illumination, intelligence, sophisticated skill, cognized relations, the felt basis of an attitude, experienced determination, a new perception of a goal, and a new configuration. (p. 410)

16. Lewis is referring here to a book by Targowla and Dublineau (1931). These authors, however, make no mention to Wernicke's work, and the book is on the role of intuition in the formation of delusions in various conditions (Fuentenebro & Berrios, 1995).

*References*

Ackerknecht, E. (1967). *Medicine at the Paris Hospital 1794–1848*. Baltimore: Johns Hopkins Press.

Adelung, T. (1811). *Grammatisch-Kritisches Wörterbuch der hohdeutschen Mundart*. Vienna: Bauer.

Albury, W. R. (1977). Experiment and explanation in the physiology of Bichat and Magendie. *Studies in the History of Biology, 1*, 47–131.

Apel, K. -O. (1987). Dilthey's distinction between "explanation" and "understanding" and the possibility of its "mediation." *Journal of the History of Philosophy, 25*, 131–149.

Baron-Cohen, S. (1995). *Mindblindness*. Cambridge, MA: MIT Press.

Berrios, G. E. (1988). Historical background to abnormal psychology. In E. Miller & J. Cooper (Eds.), *Adult abnormal psychology*, (pp. 26–51). Edinburgh: Churchill Livingstone.

Berrios, G. E. (1992). Phenomenology, psychopathology and Jaspers: A conceptual history. *History of Psychiatry, 3*, 303–327.

Berrios, G. E. (1993). European views on personality disorders: A conceptual history. *Comprehensive Psychiatry, 34*, 14–30.

Berrios, G. E. (1994). Delusions: Selected historical and clinical aspects. In E. M. R. Critchley E.M.R. (Ed.), *The neurological boundaries of reality* (pp. 251–268). London: Farrand Press.

Berrios, G. E., & Gili, M. (1995). The disorders of the will: A conceptual history. *History of Psychiatry, 6*, 87–104.

Bollote, G. (1973). Moreau de Tours 1804–1884. *Confrontations Psychiatriques, 11*, 9–26.

Boring, E. G. (1953). A history of introspection. *Psychological Bulletin, 50*, 169–189.

Brentano, F. (1874/1973). *Psychology from an empirical standpoint* (A. C. Rancurello, D. B. Terrell, & L. L. McAlister, trans.). London: Routledge and Kegan Paul.

Bulbrook, M. E. (1932). An experimental inquiry into the existence and nature of insight. *American Journal of Psychology, 44*, 409–453.

Conrad, K. (1958). *Die beginnende Schizophrenie*. Stuttgart: Thieme.

D'Istria, F. C. (1926). La psychologie de Bichat. *Revue de Metaphysique et de Morale, 23*, 1–38.

Dagonet, M. H. (1881). Conscience et aliénation mentale. *Annales Médico-Psychologiques, 5*, 368–397; 6, 19–32.

Danziger, K. (1980). The history of introspection reconsidered. *Journal of the History of the Behavioral Sciences, 16*, 241–262.

Deshaies, G. (1967). *Psychopathologie générale*. Paris: Presses Universitaires de France.

Despine, P. (1875). *De la folie au point de vue philosophique ou plus spécialement psychologique*. Paris: Savy.

Dilthey, W. (1976). *Selected writings*. Cambridge: Cambridge University Press.

Erismann, T. (1924). *Die Eigenart des Geistigen; Induktive und einsichtige Psychologie*. Leipzig: Quelle & Meyer.

Fabre, Dr. (Ed.) (1840). *Dictionnaire des dictionnaires de medicine français et etrangers*. Paris: Béthune et Plon.

Falret, J. P. (1866). Discussion sur la folie raisonnante. *Annales Médico-Psychologiques, 24*, 382–426.

Fancher, R. E. (1977). Brentano's psychology from an empirical standpoint and Freud's early metapsychology. *Journal of the History of the Behavioral Sciences, 13*, 207–227.

Fodor, J. A. (1983). *The modularity of the mind*. Cambridge, MA: MIT Press.

Fuentenebro, F., & Berrios, G. E. (1995). The predelusional states. *Comprehensive Psychiatry, 36*, 251–259.

Gillett, G. (1995). Insight, delusion and belief. *Philosophy, Psychiatry and Psychology, 1*, 227–236.

Grimm, J. & Grimm, W. (1862). *Deutsches Wörterbuch*, vol. 12. Leipzig: S. Hirzel.

Haigh, E. (1984). Xavier Bichat and the medical theory of the eighteenth century. *Medical History*, Suppl. 4. London: Wellcome Institute for the History of Medicine.

Hartmann, G. W. (1931). The concept and criteria of insight. *Psychological Review, 38*, 242–253.

Hartmann, G. W. (1932). Insight and the context of Gestalt theory. *American Journal of Psychology, 44*, 576–578.

Hutchinson, E. D. (1939). Varieties of insight in humans. *Psychiatry, 2*, 323–332.

Hutchinson, E. D. (1941). The nature of insight. *Psychiatry Journal for the Study of Interpersonal Processes, 4*, 31–43.

Jaspers, K. (1948). *Allgemeine psychopathologie* (5th ed.). Berlin: Springer.

Kageyama, J. (1984). Sur l'histoire de la monomanie. *L'Evolution Psychiatrique, 49*, 155–162.

Karmiloff-Smith, A. (1992). *Beyond modularity*. Cambridge, MA: MIT Press.

Kirk, G. S., & Raven, J. E. (1966). *The presocratic philosophers*. Cambridge: Cambridge University Press.

Kraepelin, E. (1913/1919). *Dementia praecox and paraphrenia* (B. M. Barclay, trans.). Edinburgh: E and S Livingstone.

Krafft-Ebing, R. (1893). *Lehrbuch der Psychiatrie* (5th ed.). Stuttgart: Enke.

Legrand du Saulle, H. (1864). *La folie devant les tribunaux*. Paris: Savy.

Lewis, A. (1934). The psychopathology of insight. *British Journal of Medical Psychology, 14*, 332–348.

Littré, E. (1877). *Dictionnaire de la langue française*, vol. 1. Paris: Librarie Hachette.

Lonergan, B. J. F. (1970). *Insight. A study of human understanding* (3rd ed.). New York: Philosophical Library.

López Moreno, A. (1990). *Comprensión e interpretación en las ciencias del espíritu: Dilhey*. Murcia: El Taller.

López Piñero, J. M. (1983). *Historical origins of the concept of neurosis*. (D. Berrios, trans.). Cambridge: Cambridge University Press.

Lyons, W. (1986). *The disappearance of introspection*. Cambridge, MA: MIT Press.

Makkreel, R. A. (1975). *Dilthey*. Princeton: Princeton University Press.

Marková, I. (1988). The development of self-consciousness: Part I—Baldwin, Mead and Vygotsky. *History and Philosophy of Psychology*, British Psychological Society Newsletter 7 (November), 9–18.

Marková, I., & Berrios, G. E. (1995). Insight in clinical psychiatry revisited. *Comprehensive Psychiatry, 36*, 367–376.

Marková, I. S., & Berrios, G. E. (1992). The meaning of insight in clinical psychiatry. *British Journal of Psychiatry, 160*, 850–860.

Martin-Santos, L. (1955). *Dilthey, Jaspers y la comprensión del enfermo mental*. Madrid: Paz Montalvo.

Martini, E. (1824). *De la folie*. Paris: Migneret.

Maudsley, H. (1885). *Responsibility in mental disease*. London: Kegan Paul & Trench.

Maudsley, H. (1895). *The Pathology of Mind*. London: MacMillan & Co.

McCarthy, T. (1972). The operation called *Verstehen*: Towards a redefinition of the problem. In K. F. Schaffner & R. S. Cohen (Eds.). *Boston studies in the philosophy of science*, vol. 20, *Proceedings of the 1972 Philosophy of Science Section* (pp. 167–193). Dordrecht: Reidel.

Mendel, E. (1907). *Textbook of psychiatry* (W. C. Krauss, Trans.). Philadelphia: Davis.

Moreau de Tours, J. J. (1845). *Du hachisch et de l'aliénation mentale*. Paris: Fortin, Masson et Cie.

Morel, P. (1988). Ulysse Trélat: citoyen contestataire, aliéniste orthodoxe. In U. Trélat, *La Folie Lucide* (pp. V–XXI). Paris: Frénesie Editions.

Müller, Ch. (Ed.). (1973). *Lexicon der Psychiatrie*. Heidelberg: Springer.

Ogden, R. M. (1932). Insight. *American Journal of Psychology, 44*, 350–356.

Parant, V. (1883). La paralysie agitante examinée comme cause de folie. *Annales Médico-Psychologiques, 10*, 45–66.

Parant, V. (1888). *La raison dans la folie*. Paris: Doin.

Parant, V. (1892). Paralysis Agitans. In D. H. Tuke (Ed.), *Dictionary of psychological medicine*. London: Churchill.

Pauleikhoff, B. & Mester, H. (1973). Einsicht. In Müller, *Lexikon der Psychiatrie* (pp. 150–151). Heidelberg: Springer.

Petermann, B. (1932). *The Gestalt theory*. London: Kegan Paul, Trench, Trubner.

Richfield, J. (1954). An analysis of the concept of insight. *Psychoanalytical Quarterly, 23*, 390–408.

Ritter, J. (1972). *Historiches Wörterbuch der Philosophie*. Darmstadt: Wissenschaftliche Buchgesellschaft.

Rose, G. (1878). *Neues Wörterbuch der Französischen und Deutschen Sprache*. Berlin: Schreiter.

Ryle, G. (1949). *The concept of mind*. London: Hutchinson.

Sérieux, P. & Capgras, J. (1909). *Les folies raisonnantes, le délire d'Interprétation*. Paris: Alcan.

Shaw, T. C. (1909). The clinical value of consciousness in disease. *Journal of Mental Science, 55*, 401–410.

SMP (1866). *Société Médico-Psychologique*: Debate on reasoning insanity. *Annales Médico-Psychologiques, 24*, 382–431.

Sternberg, R. J., & Davidson, J. E. (Eds.) (1994). *The nature of insight*. Cambridge, MA: MIT Press.

Störring, G. E. (1907). *Mental pathology in its relation to normal psychology*. London: Swan Sonnenschein.

Targowla, R., & Dublineau, J. (1931). *L'intuition délirante*. Paris: Malone.

Trélat, U. (1861). *La Folie lucide*. Paris: Adrien Delahaye.

Urmson, J. O. (1990). *The Greek philosophical vocabulary*. London: Duckworth.

Warnke, G. (1987). *Gadamer: Hermeneutics, tradition and reason*. Stanford: Stanford University Press.

# 3

K. WILLIAM M. FULFORD

# Completing Kraepelin's Psychopathology

## Insight, Delusion, and the Phenomenology of Illness

Loss of insight, traditionally the essential feature of psychotic mental illness, has an equivocal place in present-day psychiatry. Difficulties of definition have led to mini-milization of its significance in most modern classifications of mental disorders. Yet it remains important to the actual practice of psychiatry, especially in relation to ethical and medicolegal questions.

In this chapter, the philosophical method of linguistic analysis is used to clarify the concept of psychotic loss of insight. *Linguistic analysis* approaches questions of definition indirectly by exploring the ways in which concepts are actually used. The rationale for this analysis is that difficulties in definition often arise from taking a too narrow or too restricted view of the concept in question. But we are generally better at using concepts than at defining them. (Try defining such everyday concepts as time, for instance, or baroque.) Hence, as the philosopher J. L. Austin argued (1956–7/1968; Fulford, 1989a), exploring the ways in which a concept is used may lead to a broader or more complete view of its meaning, and thus may help to resolve difficulties in definition.

## Insight—From Definition to Use

The term *insight* is used with a variety of meanings, nonmedical as well as medical (David, 1990). In nonmedical usage it encompasses everything from mathematical insight (grasping a mathematical conclusion) and Gestalt insight ("seeing" the whole) to human insight (empathic understanding). Medically, *insight* is used to mean insight into pathology. This includes awareness of symptoms, recognition of them as symptoms of illness, understanding of their causal origins, appreciation of their significance (e.g., their seriousness), and compliance with treatment.

An early and seminal attempt to define specifically *psychotic* loss of insight was made by Aubrey Lewis (1934). Insight, he argued, means "a correct attitude to a morbid change in oneself." Loss of insight, so defined, is certainly a feature of conditions traditionally classified as psychotic.

CASE 1*    Mr P. D. Age 48. Bank manager [Diagnosis—psychotic depression]
Presented in casualty with headache, biological symptoms of depression, and the delusion that he had brain cancer. History of attempted suicide. Asking for something to "help him sleep." Refused to believe that he was suffering from depression.

CASE 2    Miss H. M. Age 25. Novice nun [Diagnosis—hypomania]
Brought by superiors for urgent outpatient appointment as they were unable to contain her bizarre and sexually disinhibited behavior. Showed pressure of speech, grandiose delusions (that she was Mary Magdalene), and auditory hallucinations.

CASE 3    Mr S. Age 18. Student [Diagnosis—schizophrenia]
Emergency psychiatric admission from his college. Behaving oddly. Showed thought insertion (Mike Yarwood, a TV presenter, "using his brain"). Complained that people were talking about him.

In each of these cases, the patient had an "incorrect attitude" toward his or her illness. However, as Aubrey Lewis pointed out, an incorrect attitude may also be seen in psychiatric disorders that are not traditionally thought of as psychotic, and even in patients with physical illnesses.

CASE 4    Miss H. Age 30. Secretary. [Diagnosis—hysterical paralysis]
Admitted to neurology ward and transferred to psychiatry under protest. Unable to use right hand (patient right-handed). Paralysis "nonanatomical." History of self-injury. Firmly rejected psychological diagnosis.

CASE 5    Dr A. Age 60. Medical doctor [Diagnosis—acromegaly]
Developed thickening of soft tissues (e.g., lips), skull enlargement, and other features of acromegaly over a period of years but refused to acknowledge that these changes were pathological, even when they were pointed out to him.

CASE 6    Mr V. N. Age 55. Schoolteacher [Diagnosis—visual neglect]
Suffered left-sided stroke. Unable to recognize his paralyzed arm as his own, even when it was placed within his intact visual field.

Moreover, as Aubrey Lewis added, patients with conditions traditionally classified as psychotic may sometimes have relatively good insight.

CASE 7    Mr C. S. Age 27. Unemployed [Diagnosis—chronic schizophrenia]
After a second episode of schizophrenia, responded well to antipsychotic medication. Auditory hallucinations persisted—he heard two female voices talking about him—but

---

*All the patients described in this chapter are based on real cases but with biographical details altered to protect confidentiality.

TABLE 3.1 The Persistent Use of the Psychotic-Nonpsychotic Distinction in *DSM-III* and *ICD-10*, Illustrated by a Two-way Sorting Table of Marbles by Size and Color

| Marble Colors (= particular categories of disorder) | Marble Size (= psychotic-nonpsychotic distinction) | |
|---|---|---|
| | Large | Small |
| Red | + | ++ |
| Green | +++ | |
| Blue | ++ | ++ |
| Yellow | · ++++ | + |
| Orange | ++ | +++ |

Note: That *ICD-9* and its successors, *DSM-III* and *ICD-10*, are equivalent with respect to the psychotic-nonpsychotic distinction can be seen from the following analogy. Suppose you have a bag of marbles, some large and some small; both large and small marbles may be red, green, blue, yellow, or orange. The marbles can be divided up in two ways: either into large and small and then by colors (equivalent to *ICD-9*), or by color and then into large and small (equivalent to *DSM-III* and *ICD-10*). As table 3.1 shows, the large-small distinction (equivalent to the psychotic-nonpsychotic distinction) is equally significant in both classifications.

he described these as "his voices" and recognized them to be symptoms of his illness.

Aubrey Lewis gave a detailed analysis of the elements in his definition—we will return to this in the next section. But his overall conclusion was that since some *nonpsychotic* patients may lack insight, and some *psychotic* patients may show insight, the psychotic versus nonpsychotic distinction is a distinction without a difference and should be abandoned. This has become the official line. Thus, in *ICD-9*, the distinction is retained but grudgingly; the authors of *ICD-9* suggest that it is there only because of its continued wide usage (WHO, 1978). It is ostensibly abandoned in *DSM-III* (APA, 1980) and in *ICD-10* (WHO, 1992).

This could be right. Other distinctions have been dropped on similar grounds—the distinction between endogenous and reactive depression, for example. However, unlike the reactive–endogenous distinction, the psychotic–nonpsychotic distinction has persisted. It remains in everyday psychiatric usage and in academic journals, in expressions such as puerperal psychosis and antipsychotic drug. More remarkably, perhaps, it persists even in our official classifications (Fulford, 1994). In *ICD-9*, it was used as a primary division. But in *DSM-III* and *ICD-10*, notwithstanding the claims of the authors, it is still there, though now as a secondary subdivision of other important categories; affective and organic disorders, in particular, are both subdivided into psychotic and nonpsychotic. As Table 3.1 shows, these two arrangements are strictly equivalent.

From a linguistic analysis perspective, continued use of the psychotic–nonpsychotic distinction suggests that, contrary to Aubrey Lewis, it remains not only a useful distinction but one that is essential to ordinary usage. This can be seen by adapting Wittgenstein's picture of words as tools (Wittgenstein, 1958). Tools are developed to do different jobs. With gardening tools, for example, we have forks, spades, hoes, rakes, and so forth. Someone trying to define a spade might notice that all garden spades have wooden handles and pick this as a definition. If this definition is then applied to spades and forks, it would suggest that the fork–spade distinction is a distinction without a difference. But gardeners will continue to make the distinction precisely because it is the sharp end, not the handle, that is crucial to their use. What is needed, then, is a better definition. Following Austin (1956–7/1968), this new definition depends on a wider or more complete view of the tools in question (looking at the sharp end as well as the handles). And one way to achieve such a new view is to look carefully at how gardeners use their tools.

In the case of psychotic versus nonpsychotic, continued use of the distinction suggests that it is a useful linguistic tool, notwithstanding the difficulties of definition. Hence, what is required is not to abandon the psychotic–nonpsychotic distinction, as Aubrey Lewis proposed, but to find a better definition. If Wittgenstein and Austin are right, we should approach this by way of a more thorough examination of how the concept of psychotic loss of insight is used.

## Features of the Use of Psychotic Loss of Insight

The core use of the concept of psychotic loss of insight is illustrated by cases 1–3 above: psychotic depression, hypomania, and schizophrenia. These conditions are characterized by two kinds of symptom in particular—delusions and hallucinations—together with certain closely related symptoms, such as thought insertion (case 3— some classify thought disorder of this kind with delusion; see Sims, 1988). We will be looking at how these symptoms are defined in more detail later. But a first feature of the use of psychotic loss of insight is simply that it is associated with symptoms of this kind. Particular psychoses are defined by particular psychotic symptoms, together with certain other symptoms. Some of the latter may involve loss of insight of a nonpsychotic kind—for example, the severe cognitive disturbances (memory, attention, orientation, and general IQ) which are the defining characteristics of organic psychoses.

CASE 8   Mrs. D. Age 65. Retired shopkeeper [Diagnosis—dementia]
Brought to casualty by the police. Found wandering and unable to recall her address. Complained that she was being chased by cats. Cognitive function testing showed marked impairment of short- and long-term memory and disorientation for time.

Among psychotic symptoms in general there is a sense in which, as Jaspers (1913/1963) emphasized, delusions are phenomenologically basic. Hallucinations, for instance, are generally defined in the medical textbooks as perceptions in the absence of appropriate stimuli (Harré & Lamb, 1986). However, true or psychotic hallucinations are perceptions in the absence of stimuli that are *delusionally believed to be real*. This difference was recognized in classical phenomenology: hallucinations as such may be normal experiences—for example, hearing the telephone ring as you drop off to sleep. Even in pathological conditions, hallucinations may occur that are recognized to be hallucinatory, as in case 7. The difference is that with fully psychotic hallucinations not only do the patients believe their experiences to be veridical but they may even elaborate a complex argument to protect this belief, a process which is called *delusional elaboration* (Wing, Cooper, & Sartorius, 1974).

CASE 9   Mr D. E. Age 50. Clerk [Diagnosis—delusional elaboration]
Patient reported hearing voices coming from an adjacent room. When shown room to be empty, said the people concerned had jumped out of the window. When shown

that they were on the fourth floor, suggested that a microphone had been used. On finding no microphone, he claimed they were invisible. And so on.

This observation leads to a second feature of psychotic loss of insight. Psychotic disorders, especially as defined by delusions, have a central place in what I have called elsewhere the *map of psychiatry* (Fulford, 1993a). Thus, broadly identifiable as they are with the traditional "mad" or "insane" categories, psychotic disorders have been thought of as illnesses at least since classical times (Kenny, 1969). They are cross-culturally stable (Wing, 1978), and individual psychotic symptoms are identifiable with a degree of reliability at least as good as that of the symptoms of physical illness (Clare, 1979). The centrality of psychotic disorders comes out most clearly, however, in respect to their ethical and medicolegal implications. Insanity is the central case of mental illness as an excuse in law (Butler, 1975; Grubin, 1991). Similarly, although legally sanctioned for any mental disorder (at least in the United Kingdom), involuntary psychiatric treatment is largely confined to psychotic disorders (Sensky, Hughes, & Hirsch, 1991).

It might be thought that the centrality of psychotic disorders is explained by nothing more mysterious than the fact that they are serious disorders. However, this begs the meaning of the word *serious*. Psychotic disorders are sometimes immediately life-threatening (case 1), but often they are not (cases 2 and 3). Recognizing this, philosophers (Flew, 1973; Glover 1970) have argued that the relevant sense of *serious* has to do with the extreme degree of objective falsity of delusional beliefs—the belief that one is already dead, for example, or that one is in two places at once, or that one's body contains a nuclear reactor.

We will be returning to the sense in which delusions are false in the next section. However, even a superficial examination of the use made of the clinical concept of delusion shows that this philosophical criterion—extreme objective falsity—is inconsistent with the clinical psychopathology of delusions themselves. In the first place, delusions, although often obviously false, are not always false. Mr A. B.'s belief in case 1 that he had brain cancer could have been true. Moreover, delusions are sometimes not *objectively* false at all; sometimes they turn out to be true. Sometimes, more remarkably, as in Othello syndrome (Shepherd, 1961; Vauhkonen, 1968), they are known to be true even when the diagnosis is made.

CASE 10   Mr O. S. Age 45. Publican [Diagnosis—Othello syndrome]

> Attended general practitioner's surgery with his wife who was suffering from depression. On questioning, delivered an angry diatribe about his wife being "a tart." Unable to talk about anything else. Offered unlikely evidence (e.g., pattern of cars parked in road). Psychiatric referral confirmed diagnosis even though the doctors concerned knew that Mrs. O. was depressed following the breakup of an affair.

That delusions are not necessarily false factual beliefs is shown more dramatically by the occasional delusion of mental illness (Fulford, 1989b, chap. 10). A delusion of this kind would be logically impossible (i.e., a contradiction in terms) if delusions were by definition objectively false.

CASE 11   Mr. M. I. Age 40. [Diagnosis—delusion of mental illness]

> Brought to casualty after an overdose. Had tried to kill himself because he believed he was mentally ill. Diagnosis of hypochondriacal delusion of mental illness.

TABLE 3.2 Three Logically Significant Features of Psychotic Loss of Insight

1. Psychotic loss of insight is shown typically by *hallucinations, delusions*, and certain forms of *thought disorder* (e.g., thought insertion).
2. Delusions are the *central* symptom of mental illness, in particular in respect of its *ethical* and *medicolegal* significance.
3. Delusions may take the form of *true* as well as *false* factual beliefs, and of *value judgments*, positive and negative.

A third feature of psychotic loss of insight, then, is association with a symptom that can take two remarkably different—indeed, contrary—logical forms: delusions occurring as both true and false factual beliefs. The logical range of delusions (i.e., the range of distinct logical forms that delusions, as symptoms of mental illness, can take) is indeed wider even than this. Cases of the kind just described are unusual, though no less significant conceptually. Delusions, however, may quite commonly not be factual beliefs at all, but value judgments (Fulford, 1991a). Value judgments have quite different logical properties from statements of fact (Fulford, 1989b, chap. 1). Yet evaluative delusions, as well as factual ones, occur commonly in affective psychoses, with positive evaluative delusions in hypomania (case 3) and negative in depression.

CASE 12    Mr. E. D. Age 40. Postman [Diagnosis—evaluative delusion of guilt]
Emergency admission with depressed affect, early morning waking and weight loss. Had forgotten to give his children their pocket money, but believed this to be the "worst sin in the world," himself "worthless as a father," and so on.

The use of the concept of loss of insight with respect to psychotic disorders thus shows three main features, summarized in table 3.2: (1) it is associated characteristically with hallucinations, delusions, and certain forms of thought disorder, such as thought insertion; (2) of these, delusions in particular have a central place in the map of psychiatry, especially with regard to the ethical and medicolegal significances of mental disorders; and (3) delusions, although commonly false factual beliefs, may be true or value judgments, positive or negative.

It is possible, of course, that any one of these features could be muddled, confused, or otherwise mistaken. They could be written off, just as the distinction between psychotic and nonpsychotic disorders was written off by Aubrey Lewis. The linguistic analysis method is neutral on this. But in advance of analysis, as features of the ordinary use of the concept of psychotic loss of insight, these features are there and have to be explained. Hence, any conceptual theory of insight must show either why the concept has the features it has or why these features are merely illusory. Either way, ordinary usage forms the "data" of philosophical analysis. In the next section we will find that conventional accounts of insight fail to explain these data.

## Enlarging the Medical Model

Measured against the "data" of ordinary usage, the standard account of insight as developed by Aubrey Lewis is unsatisfactory, in that it fails to explain the features of insight just outlined. Thus, Aubrey Lewis's account fails to differentiate psychotic from other forms of loss of insight; this was taken by Aubrey Lewis to show that the distinction is otiose. But if the *prima facie* association of psychotic loss of insight with such symptoms as delusions and hallucinations (feature 1) is accepted as a datum for linguistic analysis, then the failure of the standard account in this respect is no less a failure to give an adequate account of these key psychiatric symptoms. For the standard account, by the criterion adopted at the end of the last section, explains neither why these and other psychotic symptoms are intuitively different from nonpsychotic symptoms nor, if there is no real difference, why they should *appear* to be different.

As presented thus far, the standard account has been limited to Aubrey Lewis's preliminary definition that insight is a "correct attitude to a morbid change in oneself." Clearly, then, there are defenses for the standard account still available. Aubrey Lewis elaborated on his definition and subsequent authors have modified the approach in various ways. None of these defenses, however, adequately explains the features of psychotic loss of insight. Thus, in his paper, Aubrey Lewis defined a *correct attitude* cognitively—that is, he took it to involve awareness, knowledge, and correct understanding. This leads to a possible account of the centrality of delusion (feature 2; see Table 3.2) since this symptom, as Aubrey Lewis himself argued, seems almost by definition to involve plain mistake. Other authors, similarly, have based their accounts of the central ethical and medicolegal significance of psychotic disorders on lack of insight in this cognitive sense (Flew, 1973; Glover, 1970; Quinton, 1985). But all of these fail to encompass the use of the clinical concept of delusion of beliefs that are true (feature 3; see Table 3.2). Where this is recognized, the standard defense is to assume that there must be a disturbance of cognitive functioning underlying the formation of these symptoms—true beliefs thus occurring occasionally but by accident. This is implicit, for example, in the definition of *delusion* in the *Oxford Textbook of Psychiatry* not as false but as "unfounded beliefs" (Gelder, Gath, & Mayou, 1983). And in a later paper, Aubrey Lewis developed a theory of the nature of disease as disturbance of part functioning (Lewis, 1955).

This is initially persuasive. As we have seen, some forms of loss of insight—as in dementia—do indeed involve gross impairments of cognitive functioning. In other psychotic disorders there may be more subtle deficits—distractibility in hypomania, for instance, or marked slowing of thought in depression. Moreover, cognitive deficits do excuse—we do not hold the patient with dementia or mental deficiency responsible. And in the bioethics literature, a general account of responsibility has been developed in terms of specific cognitive capacities (Beauchamp & Childress, 1989).

Closer inspection, however, shows that there are difficulties with this account. First, it says nothing substantive about the remarkable logical range of delusions (feature 3). This aspect of their phenomenology is merely epiphenomenal. Second, precisely *because* cognitive impairment is the defining feature of other symptoms, the account must specify a *particular kind* of cognitive impairment if it is to differentiate delusion from other symptoms (feature 1). And no such impairment, notwithstanding recent efforts (Hemsley & Garety, 1986), has yet been demonstrated. Third, precisely *because* cognitive impairment forms the basis for the status of other conditions (dementia and mental deficiency) as legal excuses, a different and specific cognitive impairment would have to underlie the status of delusion as an excuse (feature 2). The bioethical account of rationality, as I have argued elsewhere (Fulford & Hope, 1993), fails on just this point. It works well for conditions like dementia, but it fails to explain the irrationality of the functional psychotic disorders.

The discovery of a cognitive impairment specific to delusion could be around the corner. However, this development would not in itself resolve the difficulty. The whole drift of this account runs counter to the intuitively central place of psychotic disorders in psychiatry (feature 2). In the first place, cognitive impairments, when present, impair delusional belief formation just as they impair the formation of normal beliefs—the best-quality delusions (emotionally charged, elaborate, and well sustained) occurring in the paranoid psychoses in which there are few if any associated symptoms. In the second place, if an impaired cognitive functioning account were on the right lines, given the central place of delusions, we should expect the particular cognitive failure to be transparent. In the third place, as no less an advocate of the impaired functioning account than Boorse (1976) has pointed out, such accounts place other symptoms more naturally at the center. This is because the concept of functioning is attached naturally to body or mental parts and systems, whereas functional psychotic disorders involve, as Boorse put it, a more global disturbance of the person as a whole.

There are thus entrenched difficulties with the standard account. This suggests, from the linguistic analytical perspective outlined above, that the account itself has been framed within a view of the conceptual structure of medicine that is too narrow or restricted. And if we look more closely at the standard account this is what we find. Thus, the standard account is broadly within what has become known as the medical model. This term covers a variety of models (Macklin, 1973), the common feature of which is a more or less tacit assumption that medicine is, at heart, a science. The picture is of a body of factual or objective information that forms the basis for disease theories, to which doctors in particular are expert, and which in their highest elaboration are cast as disturbances in the functioning of body and mental parts and systems. Aubrey Lewis's account, for instance, is all to do with awareness, knowledge, and error; much of the development of his initial definition is in terms of data and objectivity; a *correct attitude* turns out to be that which "approximates to that of the clinician"; and a *morbid change* is a disturbance in "part functioning" (all his terms). The medical model is reflected, similarly, in those theories of psychotic loss of insight that point to some putative impairment of cognitive functioning. But even in the bioethical literature, the fact that judgments of rationality may be heavily value laden is taken to imply that such judgments involve, in Beauchamp and Childress's words (1989), "moral *rather than* medical considerations" (my emphasis).

There is nothing wrong with the medical model as such. Its resources are indeed sufficient to explain important species of loss of insight. But if the model fails to explain specifically *psychotic* loss of insight, then, according to the linguistic analysis approach, we must suspect that it is too restricted. In the case of the medical concepts generally, the very success of medical science is sufficient to explain why we should have got stuck with a too exclusively scientific view. And linguistic analysis, focusing on the actual use of the medical concepts, shows that this is indeed the case. For alongside the descriptive or scientific elements in their meanings, linguistic analysis reveals an evaluative element, not peripherally but woven right through the conceptual structure of the subject (see Fulford, 1989b).

The value element in the concept of mental illness is important in its own right in

## The "Medical" Model

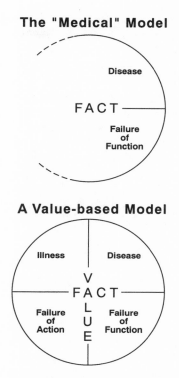

## A Value-based Model

FIGURE 3.1. Diagrammatic representation of the Relationship between the "Medical" Model and a Value-based Analysis of the Medical Concepts

relation to both ethical (Fulford, 1991b; Fulford, Smirnoff, & Snow, 1993) and medicolegal (Fulford, 1993a) aspects of psychiatry. But from the point of view of psychopathology, two elements in particular of this fact + value model stand out as conceptually significant: the patient's *experience of illness* (as distinct from medical knowledge of disease), and the analysis of this experience in terms of incapacity or *failure of intentional action* (as distinct from the analysis of disease in terms of failure of function). We will be looking at these in more detail in the next two sections, when we turn to the characterizations of psychotic loss of insight and of delusion, respectively. But we should note in advance that the analysis does not undermine the importance of science in medicine. It shows only that in the conceptual structure of the subject other elements may be important as well.

### Illness and Insight

The features that mark out an experience as illness, as something wrong with us, have been explored more by sociologists (Parsons, 1951; Lockyer, 1981) than by doctors. A number of such features have been identified; for instance, intensity and duration—a mild, brief pain is unlikely to be experienced as "something wrong." One experiential feature not widely recognized, however, is that illness is characterized in part by a two-way distinction. "Something wrong" is experienced as different both from things that we do and from things that are done or happen to us. For example, paralysis is different both from not moving (i.e., keeping still) and from being prevented from moving; pain (as illness) is different both from hurting oneself and from being hurt; amnesia is different both from not remembering and from being distracted.

This two-way distinction can be shown to be a general feature of the patient's primary experience of illness, as distinct from medical knowledge of disease (Fulford, 1989b, chap. 5). Once recognized, the distinction may seem self-evident, almost trivial. Yet it is sufficient not only to suggest a general account of specifically psychotic loss of insight but also to generate detailed differential diagnostic tables discriminating psychotic symptoms from other symptoms.

Broadly, the account runs thus: if the experience of illness is distinct both from things that we do and from things that are done or happen to us, then psychotic loss of insight could be understood as a *misconstrual across this two-way distinction*. This is quite different from mere lack of awareness of symptoms. It is also different from merely failing to identify an experience as illness. These are both negative accounts of loss of insight. The misconstrual account suggests, rather, a positive relocation of an experience across one or other limb of the two-way distinction by which the experience of illness, all illness, is characterized (Fulford, 1989b, chap. 10).

Thought insertion (illustrated by case 3) provides a case in point (Fulford, 1993b). In terms of the two-way distinction, this is an odd symptom: thinking is in many (though not all) respects like movement, something that we do. Like movement, it may be automatic rather than deliberative. But if thinking runs wholly out of control—as in, say, an obsessional disorder, it ceases to be experienced fully as something that we *do* and becomes something *wrong with us*. On the other hand, if we are merely preoccupied with some genuinely preoccupying experience (bereavement, say), this relative loss of control is experienced as something that is done *to* us. But thought insertion is odder than either of these. Thought insertion is neither our own thoughts running out of control nor our own thoughts being influenced. It is other people's thoughts being thought by us. This is almost paradoxical, then. Certainly it is very difficult to characterize negatively. So much so, indeed, that with the (experientially) closely related epileptic "forced thoughts," the patient more or less readily accepts the doctor's explanation that this is "something wrong" (Lishman, 1987). But a schizophrenic patient with thought insertion, far from accepting such an explanation, actively relocates the experience as something that is being done *to* him.

This active relocation of the experience of thought insertion is summarized in table 3.3 as a differential diagnostic table. We can call this an illness-differential diagnostic table to emphasize the fact that it draws only on the two-way distinction by which the experience of illness (all illness) is (partly) defined. Thus, thought insertion is analyzed along with other kinds of thought in terms of the done by–wrong with–done to distinction, first from the patient's perspective (left side of the table) and then from everyone else's perspective (right side). As can be seen, the psychotic symptom stands out. It is a *done to* experience for the patient, whereas it is a *wrong with* experience for everyone else. The other phenomena listed in the table, by contrast, are the same for both perspectives.

TABLE 3.3  Differential Diagnosis of Thought Insertion Drawing on Illness Theory

| Thoughts in Patient's Mind | Construal | | | | | |
| --- | --- | --- | --- | --- | --- | --- |
| | By Patient | | | By Others | | |
| | Done by | Wrong with | Done to | Done by | Wrong with | Done to |
| Normal | + | | | + | | |
| Epileptic | | + | | | + | |
| Obsessional | | + | | | + | |
| Thought Insertion | | | + | | + | |

Note: The standard medical model, drawing on the elements of disease theory, fails to differentiate thought insertion and other psychotic symptoms from nonpsychotic. In illness theory, psychotic loss of insight emerges as a misconstrual across the two-way distinction (done by, wrong with, done to) by which the primary experience of illness is (partly) defined.

A more complex illness-differential diagnostic table is needed for the more complex symptom of hallucination. This is because whereas thinking is normally something that we do, perception is partly something we do (it is active) and partly something that is done to us (by the environment). But the same principle applies. As can be seen from table 3.4, it is only for true or psychotic hallucinations that there is a discrepancy between the two sides of the table, between the patient's construction of the experience and the construction placed on it by everyone else.

In contrast to the standard account, therefore, the two-way distinction by which the experience of illness is (partly) defined is sufficient to characterize psychotic loss of insight at least as illustrated by symptoms such as thought insertion and hallucination. To this extent, then, it explains, or is at least consistent with, the first feature of the use of the concept of psychotic loss of insight, summarized in table 3.2.

With delusion, rather more is required. We should expect this since delusions underpin all other psychotic symptoms (feature 2 of psychotic loss of insight). As to

TABLE 3.4  Differential Diagnosis of Hallucination Drawing on Illness Theory

| Perception | Construal | | | | | |
| --- | --- | --- | --- | --- | --- | --- |
| | By Patient | | | By Others | | |
| | Done by | Wrong with | Done to | Done by | Wrong with | Done to |
| Normal | + | | + | + | | + |
| Illusion | | | ++ | | | ++ |
| Eye Disease | | ++ | | | ++ | |
| Psychotic Hallucination | + | | + | | ++ | |
| "Normal" Hallucination | ++ | + | | ++ | + | |
| Imagery | ++ | | | ++ | | |

Note: The differential diagnosis of hallucination is more complicated than that of thought insertion because perception is more complicated than thinking in the relevant respect, being part "done by" and part "done to." Nonetheless, the same pattern appears, with true or psychotic hallucinations being differentiated from a range of nonpsychotic perceptual phenomena as a misconstrual across the two-way distinction by which illness is defined. (A more extensive version of this table, including two forms of pseudo-hallucination, is given in Fulford, 1989b, chap. 10.)

content, delusions fit nicely across the two-way distinction. With delusions of guilt, for instance, patients locate the problem as something they have *done*, whereas everyone else locates it as something wrong with them. With delusions of persecution, patients locate the problem as something that is being done *to* them. But classically (Jaspers, 1913/1963), form rather than content is pertinent with delusions. If we want a more complete account of the psychopathology of delusion, then, we have to move from the experience of illness as such to the second main element of our fact + value model; the analysis of this experience in terms of failure of intentional action.

## Delusions and Action Failure

Earlier in this chapter, I showed that accounts of delusion derived from the medical model have been largely in terms of supposed impairment of cognitive function, and we noted that this was a reflection of exclusive focus on the analysis of disease generally in terms of failure of function. In the fact + value model, we have broadened the focus to include the analysis of illness in terms of incapacity or failures of action. This in turn suggests a quite different approach to the analysis of delusion. Specifically, it suggests that we should understand the irrationality of delusional thinking as involving, not, as in the medical model, impaired cognitive functioning, but impaired reasons for action.

To see how this works, we need to look in more detail at the relationship between function and action. Consider a simple action—you wave your hand in the air. We would normally describe this as a simple action of *yours*—something *you* have done; this is the way we generally talk about the things people do in everyday contexts. It carries with it other everyday concepts, such as motive, intention, willing, voluntariness, initiative, and trying. If the circumstances were more medical, however, we might talk about your hand moving in terms of function. A doctor, for example, who carries out a neurological examination might speak of the functioning of your hand and arm.

With simple actions of this kind, either the action way or the function way of talking is entirely appropriate, and we use one or the other depending on context. On a smaller scale, when we talk of the things that our bodies and minds do on the scale of nerves, synapses, speech centers, hearts, livers, and lungs, it is more natural to use function language. This is, of course, the province of science and, hence, of disease theory. It is for this reason, then, that in the medical model, function language has become dominant. But the patient's experience of illness arises in the everyday world, where action language and function language are equally appropriate. The neglect of the patient's experience of illness by the medical model can thus be understood as neglecting action language in favor of function language.

In the case of physical medicine, recognizing the importance of action language alongside function language provides the framework for a more patient-centered practice (Fulford & Hope, 1993). Understanding the patient's actual experience is the basis of both sound medical ethics and good communication (Hope & Fulford, 1993). But in psychological medicine, it has the additional significance of opening up descriptive psychopathology to the rich resources of the concept of action (Fulford, 1989b, chaps. 8–10; Fulford, 1993d).

That action language is important in psychopathology can be seen directly if we look at how psychopathological concepts are defined, even in supposedly scientific classifications. Here we find all those terms ordinarily associated with action, rather than function. For example, in *ICD-9*, the alcoholic is distinguished from the mere drunkard by the fact that he is not acting on his "own initiative"; the hysteric is unaware of his own "motives" (WHO, 1978). Similarly, in *DSM-III*, the hysteric's symptoms are said to be not under "voluntary control," as against those of the malingerer, which are, variously, "purposeful," "intentional," and "voluntary" (APA, 1980). Once we start to think in terms of action as well as function, it comes as no surprise to find terms like *voluntary* and *intentional* being used in the definitions of these conditions. For action language is the language of everyday experience, rather than of scientific disease theory. And it is in everyday experience that the defining symptoms of most psychiatric disorders arise.

Returning now to delusions, it can be seen that if action language is important generally to psychopathology, then *reasons* could be important specifically to the psychopathology of delusions. Thus delusions, uncontentiously, are a form of irrationality, or "unreason." Reasons, equally uncontentiously, are important among those concepts closely associated in ordinary usage with action language. Indeed, reasons may be a characteristic of actions. An arm, for example, has a *purpose* that it serves in functioning, but only people have *reasons* for the things they do, for their actions. As a hypothesis, then, given the analysis of illness as action failure, a fruitful way of exploring delusions would be in terms of defective reasons for action.

I have developed this hypothesis in detail elsewhere (Fulford, 1989b, chap. 10; Fulford, 1993b, 1993c). But it is a potentially fruitful hypothesis in that it helps explain the key psychopathological features of delusions—features that the medical (cognitive-functioning) account fails to explain. Taking these in a different order from Table 3.2, it explains the central place of delusions in the map of psychiatry (see feature 2, Table 3.2). We can see this in a general way in the importance of reasons as part of the language of action already noted; if reasons are important in action, defective reasons will be an important species of action failure, or illness. But the centrality of delusions can be derived more rigorously from the specific sense in which reasons are central to what Austin (1956–7) called the "machinery of action." Thus, other elements of this machinery (such as volition, control, and movement) are merely executive, necessary for successful performance of an action. But reasons are *constitutive*—that is to say, a given action is in part defined by the reasons for which it is done. You wave your hand in the air; this could be the action of hailing a taxi, signaling a bid, calling a waiter, swatting a mosquito, catching a ball, and so on. Which action it is depends not on the movement or how it is performed but on the reasons why it is done. It is, then, the constitutive nature of reasons that places delusions in a central place in the map of psychiatry. For if reasons for action have this central place in the structure of action, so a *failure of reasons* for action (i.e., delusion) will be a central kind of action failure (i.e., illness).

This explains the ethical and medicolegal significance of delusions, an important aspect of feature 2. Recall that psychotic disorders have traditionally been the central case for mental illness as a legal excuse. The essential feature of a legal excuse is a failure of action, as with accident, inadvertence, duress, mistake, and so on (Hart, 1968). It has been something of a mystery, then, when using the standard medical model of delusion, why the deluded should not be held responsible. Accident and inadvertence are not relevant. Some have argued that it is a form of internal duress (Nordenfelt, 1992), but there is no compulsion as such. Nor is it a question of mistake. The deluded may be mistaken; but as Wootton (1959) noted, we would not exonerate the man who has killed someone in the belief that he is being persecuted merely on the grounds that he was mistaken. As a constitutive failure of action, on the other hand, the irrationality of delusions falls automatically within the traditional list. As noted, it is no less than a central kind of failure of action and, hence, of excuse (Fulford, 1993a).

The action-failure account also explains the third feature of delusions—their remarkable logical range. This follows directly from identifying the irrationality of delusions with reasons for action. For just as delusions may take the form of statements of fact or expressions of value, so may reasons. I turn right in my car. Why? Because either this is the way to Oxford (fact) or I want (or ought, etc.) to go to Oxford (value). This correlation is illustrated in figure 3.2. It is no more than a correlation, of course, but as a correlation it is highly significant. Moreover, it leads to an explanation of why true beliefs may be delusions. For the status of a given statement of fact or expression of value as a reason can be shown (Fulford, 1993c) to depend on a background structure of other facts and values, rather than solely on the content of the reason itself. "This is the way to Oxford" is only a reason if, say, I am due to teach a class, which in turn is a reason only if I want (or ought, etc.) to do so" and so on. Hence, if the status of a reason *as* a reason arises from this background structure, the status of a delusion as a *defective* reason arises from defects in this background structure (see also Fulford, 1989b, chap. 10).

In this section I have been able to give only an outline of an action-failure account of delusions. Even set out more completely, however, the account (although explaining more than traditional accounts) raises a number of questions: What is the nature of the proposed defects in the structure of reasons for action? How are these related to the misconstrual by which psychotic loss of insight is characterized existentially? How in turn is this related to the cognitive defects by which other forms of irrationality, as in dementia, are characterized? What is the relationship among all of these, as pathological forms of irrationality and nonpathological forms of irrationality, such as self-deception and weakness of will?

Given that the theory fits the clinical features of the psychopathology of delusions, it has at least a strong *prima facie* plausibility. This is potentially important for, as I have shown elsewhere, it connects the psychopathology of insight to all the resources of that part of the philosophy of mind that has been concerned with the structure of action and intentionality (Fulford, 1993b). Conversely, it connects this part of the philosophy of mind to all the resources of descriptive psychopathology (Fulford, 1991c). This, in turn, opens up the possibility of new models of the structure of psychopathology, significant not only for descriptive psychopathology, diagnosis, and classification but also for the newer sciences of neuroimaging (Harrison, 1991) and artificial intelligence (Park & Young, 1994). In developing our understanding of psychotic symptoms further, then, we will find that philosophy can make a useful contribution to descriptive psychopathology, not supplanting but complementing that of science.

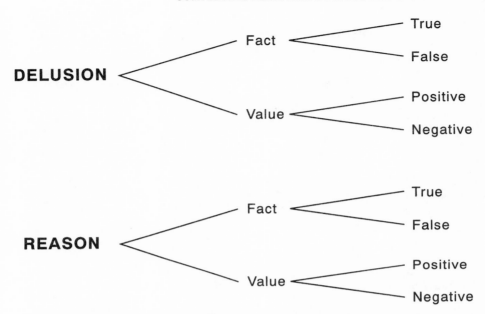

FIGURE 3.2. The Correlation Between the Phenomenological Features of Reasons for Action and Those of Delusions

## Conclusions

The philosophical method of linguistic analysis has been used here to explore the concept of psychotic loss of insight. Linguistic analysis suggests that difficulties of definition often arise from a tendency to take a too narrow or too restricted view of the concepts in question. Applying this to psychotic loss of insight, we have found that the difficulties of definition noted by Aubrey Lewis and his successors have arisen from an attempt to assimilate all forms of insight into an exclusively scientific paradigm of mental illness—the standard medical model encompassing disease concepts defined by objective norms of body and mental functioning. This, in turn, has suggested the need for a broader model of the medical concepts—one in which, alongside and of equal importance with the facts, disease theories and failures of functioning of the standard medical model, are values, the experience of illness, and the analysis of this experience in terms of incapacity or failure of intentional action. Within this more complete picture of the medical concepts, psychotic loss of insight is analyzable as a misconstrual across the two-way distinction (done by, wrong with, done to) by which the primary experience of illness is partly defined. From this simple idea were generated detailed differential diagnostic tables (illness-differential diagnostic tables) for thought insertion and hallucination. The analysis of illness as action failure, in turn, suggested an account of the irrationality of delusions not in terms of impaired cognitive functioning but as impaired reasons for action. Such an account, although tentative and preliminary, explains the central place of delusions in psychiatric phenomenology, in particu-

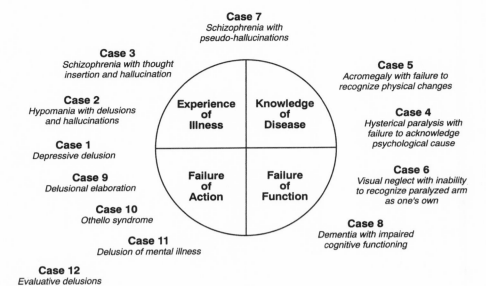

**Case 7**
*Schizophrenia with
pseudo-hallucinations*

**Case 3**
*Schizophrenia with thought
insertion and hallucination*

**Case 5**
*Acromegaly with failure to
recognize physical changes*

**Case 2**
*Hypomania with delusions
and hallucinations*

**Case 4**
*Hysterical paralysis with
failure to acknowledge
psychological cause*

**Case 1**
*Depressive delusion*

Experience
of
Illness

Knowledge
of
Disease

**Case 9**
*Delusional elaboration*

Failure
of
Action

Failure
of
Function

**Case 6**
*Visual neglect with inability
to recognize paralyzed arm
as one's own*

**Case 10**
*Othello syndrome*

**Case 8**
*Dementia with impaired
cognitive functioning*

**Case 11**
*Delusion of mental illness*

**Case 12**
*Evaluative delusions*

FIGURE 3.3. Completing Kraepelin's Phenomenology

lar their central ethical and medicolegal significance. It also explains their remarkable logical range, as true or false factual beliefs and as value judgments.

From the perspective of the conventional medical model, this account of psychotic loss of insight—and the background value theory of the medical concepts within which it is embedded—might seem to undermine the scientific basis of psychiatry. As has been emphasized, however, the effect of linguistic analysis is to give a more comprehensive view of the meaning of a given concept. The genuinely scientific elements of psychiatry are fully encompassed by the view of the medical concepts outlined here. The model does, indeed, suggest that there is more to these concepts than merely judgments of fact (Fulford, 1991a). But this is broadly consistent with aspects of insight noted by recent authors: its complex nature (David, 1990); the importance of the affective aspects of belief (Marková & Berrios, 1992); the links between psychotic phenomena and breakdown of personal identity (the two-way distinction is itself across the boundary between the self and the world; see Stephens & Graham, 1994); and its cultural relativity (Perkins & Moodley, 1993).

So there is no real incompatibility here. As figure 3.3 shows, we need both sides—fact and value, disease and illness, failures of cognitive functioning and failures of reasons for action. The linguistic analysis method, in giving us a more complete picture of the medical concepts, thus complements and extends the scope of traditional descriptive psychopathology. It is in this sense that it completes Kraepelin's phenomenology. Kraepelin reminded us of the need for careful clinical observation and description of the features of particular conditions as a basis for developing scientific psychiatry. Considerable progress has been made in this area by the neo-Kraepelinian development of clear diagnostic criteria; and it is to be expected that developments in computer science and neuroimaging techniques will bring further advances in understanding the neurophysiological basis of psychiatric disorders. Linguistic analysis, as in the account of insight outlined here, subtracts nothing from all this. On the contrary, it adds an understanding of the general features of the experience of illness, thus completing the conceptual picture.

*Acknowledgments*    I am grateful to the editors of this book for their helpful comments on an early draft of this chapter.

## References

American Psychiatric Association (APA). (1980). *Diagnostic and statistical manual of mental disorders* (3rd ed.). Washington, DC: Author.

Austin, J. L. (1956–7/1968). A plea for excuses. *Proceedings of the Aristotelian Society, 57,* 1–30. Reprinted in A. R. White, (Ed.), *The philosophy of action.* Oxford: Oxford University Press.

Beauchamp, T. L., & Childress, J. F. (1989). *Principles of biomedical ethics.* Oxford: Oxford University Press.

Boorse, C. (1976). What a theory of mental health should be. *Journal of Theory Social Behaviour, 6,* 61–84.

Butler, (Chairman). (1975). *Report of the Committee on Mentally Abnormal Offenders.* Comd. 6244. London: HMSO

Clare, A. (1979). The disease concept in psychiatry. In P. Hill, R. Murray, & A. Thorley, *Essentials of postgraduate psychiatry.* New York: Academic Press, Grune & Stratton.

David, A. S. (1990). Insight and psychosis. *British Journal of Psychiatry, 156,* 798–808.

Flew, A. (1973). *Crime or disease?* New York: Barnes and Noble.

Fulford, K. W. M. (1989a). Philosophy and medicine: The Oxford connection. *British Journal of Psychiatry, 157,* 111–115.

Fulford, K. W. M. (1989b). *Moral theory and medical practice.* Cambridge: Cambridge University Press.

Fulford, K. W. M. (1991a). Evaluative delusions: Their significance for philosophy and psychiatry. *British Journal of Psychiatry, 159,* supp. 14, 108–112.

Fulford, K. W. M. (1991b). The concept of disease. In S. Bloch, & P. Chodoff, (Eds). *Psychiatric ethics* (2nd ed., Chap. 6). Oxford: Oxford University Press.

Fulford, K. W. M. (1991c). The potential of medicine as a resource for philosophy. *Theoretical Medicine, 12,* 81–85.

Fulford, K. W. M. (1993a). Value, action, mental illness and the law. In K. Gardner, J. Horden, & S. Shute (Eds.), *Criminal law: Action, value and structure.* Oxford: Oxford University Press.

Fulford, K. W. M. (1993b). Thought insertion and insight: Disease and illness paradigms of psychotic disorder. In M. Spitzer, (Ed.), *Phenomenology, language and schizophrenia.* Springer-Verlag.

Fulford, K. W. M. (1993c). Mental illness and the mind-brain problem: Delusion, belief and Searle's theory of intentionality. *Theoretical Medicine, 14,* 181–194.

Fulford, K. W. M. (1993d). Value, illness and action failure: Framework for a philosophical psychopathology of delusions. In G. Graham & G. L. Stephens (Eds.), *Philosophical psychopathology: A book of readings.* Cambridge, MA: MIT Press.

Fulford, K. W. M. (1994). Closet logics: Hidden conceptual elements in the DSM and ICD classifications of mental disorders. In J. Z. Salder, M. Schwartz, & O. Wiggins (Eds.),

Philosophical perspectives on psychiatric diagnostic classification. Baltimore: Johns Hopkins University Press.

Fulford, K. W. M., & Hope, R. A. (1993). Psychiatric ethics: A bioethical ugly duckling? In G. Raanon (Ed.), *Principles of health care ethics* (Chap. 58). New York: John Wiley.

Fulford, K. W. M., Smirnoff, A. Y. U., & Snow, E. (1993). Concepts of disease and the abuse of psychiatry in the USSR. *British Journal of Psychiatry, 162,* 801–810.

Gelder, M. G., Gath, D., & Mayou, R. (1983). *Oxford textbook of psychiatry.* Oxford: Oxford University Press.

Glover, J. (1970). *Responsibility.* London: Routledge & Kegan Paul.

Grubin, D. H. (1991). Unfit to plead in England and Wales, 1967–88, a survey. *British Journal of Psychiatry, 158,* 140–548.

Harré, R., & Lamb, R. (Eds.). (1986). *The dictionary of physiological and clinical psychology.* Oxford: Basil Blackwell Ltd.

Harrison, P. J. (1991). Are mental states a useful concept? Neurphilosophical influences on phenomenology and psychopathology. *Journal of Nervous and Mental Disease, 179* (6), 309–316.

Hart, H. L. A. (1968). *Punishment and responsibility: Essays in the philosophy of law.* Oxford: Oxford University Press.

Hemsley, D. R., & Garety, P. A. (1986). The formation and maintenance of delusions: A Bayesian analysis. *British Journal of Psychiatry, 149,* 51–56.

Hope, R. A., & Fulford, K. W. M. (1993). Medical education: Patients, principles and practice skills. In G. Raanon (Ed.), *Principles of health care ethics* (Chap. 59). New York: John Wiley.

Jaspers, K. (1913/1963). *General psychopathology* (J. Hoenig & M. W. Hamilton, trans.). Manchester: Manchester University Press.

Kenny, A. J. P. (1969). Mental health in Plato's republic. *Proceedings of the British Academy, 5,* 229–253.

Lewis, A. J. (1934). The psychopathology of insight. *British Journal of Medical Psychology, 14,* 332–348.

Lewis, A. J. (1955). Health as a social concept. *British Journal of Sociology, 4,* 109–124.

Lishman, W. A. (1987), Personal communication.

Lockyer, D. (1981). *Symptoms and illness: The cognitive organisation of disorder.* London: Tavistock Publications.

Macklin, R. (1973). The medical model in psychoanalysis and psychotherapy. *Comprehensive Psychiatry, 14* (1), 49–69.

Marková, I. S., & Berrios, G. E. (1992). The meaning of insight in clinical psychiatry. *British Journal of Psychiatry, 160,* 850–860.

Nordenfelt, L. (1992). *On crime, punishment and psychiatric care.* Stockholm: Almqvist & Wiksell International.

Park, S. B. G., & Young, A. H. (1994). Correctionism and psychiatry: A review. *Philosophy, Psychiatry and Psychology, 1,* 51–58.

Parsons, T. (1951). *The social system.* Glencoe, IL: Free Press.

Perkins, R., & Moodley, P. (1993). The arrogance of insight? *Psychiatric Bulletin, 17,* 233–234.

Quinton, A. (1985). Madness. In A. P. Griffiths (Ed.), *Philosophy and practice* (Chap. 2). Cambridge: Cambridge University Press.

Sensky, T., Hughes, T., & Hirsch, S. (1991). Compulsory psychiatric treatment in the community, Part 1. A controlled study of compulsory community treatment with extended leave under the Mental Health Act: Special characteristics of patients treated and impact of treatment. *British Journal of Psychiatry, 158,* 792–804.

Shepherd, M. (1961). Morbid jealousy: Some clinical and social aspects of a psychiatric syndrome. *Journal of Mental Science, 107,* 687–704.

Sims, A. (1988). *Symptoms in the mind: An introduction to descriptive psychopathology*. London: Bailiere Tindall.

Stephens, G. L., & Graham, G. (1994). Self-consciousness, mental agency, and the clinical psychopathology of thought insertion. *Philosophy, Psychiatry and Psychology, 1*, 1–11.

Vauhkonen, K. (1968). *On the pathogenesis of morbid jealousy, with special reference to the personality traits of and interaction between jealous patients and their spouses*. Copenhagen: Munksgaard.

Wing, J. K. (1978). *Reasoning about madness*. Oxford: Oxford University Press.

Wing, J. K., Cooper, J. E., & Sartorius, N. (1974). *Measurement and classification of psychiatric symptoms*. Cambridge: Cambridge University Press.

Wittgenstein, L. (1958). *Philosophical investigations* (2nd. ed.). (G. E. M., Anscombe, Trans.). Oxford: Basil Blackwell.

Wootton, B. (1959). *Social science and social pathology*. London: George Allen and Unwin.

World Health Organization (WHO). (1978). *Mental disorders: Glossary and guide to their classification in accordance with the ninth revision of the international classification of diseases*. Geneva: Author.

World Health Organization (WHO). (1992). *Mental disorders: Glossary and guide to their classification in accordance with the tenth revision of the international classification of diseases*. Geneva: Author.

# 4

PHILLIPA A. GARETY

# Insight and Delusions

Delusion is a key concept in psychosis, representing the symptom that epitomizes madness. For Karl Jaspers, the German phenomenologist, whose writings have so influenced Anglo-American psychiatry, a delusion "constitutes a transformation of one's total awareness of reality" (Jaspers, 1913/1959). Contemporary definitions of delusion reflect Jasper's views—for example, the *DSM-IV* definition states:

> a false personal belief based upon incorrect inference about external reality that is firmly sustained despite what almost everyone else believes and despite what constitutes incontrovertible and obvious proof or evidence to the contrary. The belief is not one ordinarily accepted by other members of the person's culture or sub-culture. (APA, 1995, p. 783).

A person who is deluded is conventionally regarded as "lacking insight." David (1990) has argued that this concept is composed of three different but overlapping constructs: treatment compliance, both expressed and observed; recognition by the individual that he or she is suffering from an illness and that the illness is mental; and the ability to relabel unusual mental events (e.g., hallucinations and delusions) as pathological. It can be seen that while a deluded person may score poorly on all three components, it is the last of these that makes a definitional link between insight and delusion. A deluded person may comply with treatment and recognize that he or she has an illness and that the illness is mental, but if that person asserts the truth of that delusion, he or she would be inconsistent in labeling the belief as pathological. Marková and Berrios (1992) suggest that psychosis (and, implicitly, delusion) is by definition linked to impaired insight, since "being psychotic means being out of touch with real events and experiences. It is therefore incompatible for such people to have knowledge of, or be aware of, true changes taking place within them and the environment" (p. 857).

The definition of delusion is problematic, however. A number of writers have criticized most elements of the *DSM-IV* and similar definitions for inaccurately reflecting the phenomenon of delusion as seen in the clinic. Thus, the criteria of falsity, fixity, and subcultural relativity have been frequently questioned; even the assumption that delusions are best viewed as *beliefs* has been challenged—see, for example, Sims (1991) and Spitzer (1990, 1992). In this chapter, I wish particularly to consider the proposal that delusions are based upon incorrect inference and how this idea is relevant to the concept of insight. To examine this question, I will describe contemporary theories of delusion, together with relevant recent experimental work, then return to the concept of insight and consider the relationship between it and delusion.

## Theories of Delusion

Although the reasoning of people with delusions has been regarded as faulty, as in the *DSM-IV* definition, which cites "incorrect inference," there have until recently been very few studies of reasoning in deluded people. A number of theories or accounts of delusions, in contrast to the definitions, have instead proposed that the reasoning of the person with delusions is *not* defective, suggesting that motivational factors or perceptual abnormalities play the central causal role. While most of the literature deals with delusions of schizophrenia, there is also some interest in delusions as found in mania and paranoia (or delusional disorder). Useful reviews of this literature can be found in Winters and Neale (1983) and Butler and Braff (1991).

### Motivational Theories

Motivational theories of delusion have a long history. Psychoanalytic theorists dating from Freud (1915/1956) have proposed that delusions are projections of personal inner, unconscious states (e.g., unfulfilled wishes or unresolved conflicts) onto external sources. An early example of such thinking comes from Jaques Lacan (1932). He describes a case of "psychogenic psychosis," in which a 38-year-old woman, Aimée, stabbed a famous actress, saying that the actress had instigated a scandal against her. Lacan describes Aimée's early experiences, personality, and later relationships. He argues that her attack on the actress is an attack on her "externalized ideal," since the freedom and social ease that actresses reputedly possess were the very qualities that Aimée had dreamt of obtaining.

More recent psychoanalytic theories continue to maintain the view that delusions reflect the memories, affects, and fantasies of the individual before the psychosis overcomes the person. For example, Freeman proposes that persecutory delusions are "derived from wish phantasies and conflicts which come to a height immediately before the onset of an acute attack. These wish phantasies . . . existed because anxiety or guilt prevented a satisfactory outlet for instinctual wishes either directly or in sublimated form" (Freeman, 1981, p. 531).

Neale (1988) has drawn on psychoanalytic thinking to provide an account of one type of delusional idea—namely, grandiose delusions in mania. He suggests that unstable self-esteem is the psychological predisposition to such delusions. He hypothesizes that the predisposed person characteristically uses pleasant fantasies as a means of coping with stress. Grandiose delusions occur in response to a stress, whether an external event or negative cognitions, as a means of keeping distressing cognitions out of consciousness, and thus they serve a defensive function. The person with grandiose delusions is seen as motivated to protect a fragile ego from distress and thus unconsciously engages in self-deception. Neale cites some evidence that indirectly supports his theory (Winters & Neale, 1985). While patients with remitted bipolar disorders reported normal self-esteem on ordinary questionnaire assessments, on an opaque test of self-esteem, which is presented as an attribution task, these patients showed a pattern of responses consistent with low self-esteem, similar to the responses of remitted depressives.

Recently, Bentall and colleagues (Bentall, Kaney, & Dewey, 1991; Bentall, 1993) have also proposed a motivational account of persecutory delusions, again drawing on attribution theory. In a series of studies they have found characteristic biases in attributional style in subjects with persecutory delusions: a tendency to blame others for negative outcomes and to credit themselves for positive outcomes, showing an exaggerated "self-serving bias" (see also chap. 6, this volume). The term *self-serving bias* is used by social psychologists to describe the general tendency to attribute positive outcomes to self and negative outcomes to external causes, a mechanism for maintaining self-esteem found in normal individuals. Bentall et al. (1991) suggest that these biases serve a function for the person with persecutory delusions. Using the opaque method of accessing self-esteem developed by Winters and Neale (1985), they found that the patients with persecutory delusions—in contrast to their depressed controls, who reported normal questionnaire-assessed self-esteem on the opaque test—had a pattern of responses that indicated low self-esteem. They conclude that delusions of this sort are motivated by a strong need to avoid the presence of aversive negatively self-referent thoughts in consciousness.

## Perceptual Theories

Perceptual accounts, in which the delusion is viewed as a logical deduction from an altered body sensation or perception, can be found in early psychiatric writings (e.g., Serieux & Capgras, 1909/1988; Dupre & Logre, 1911/1988). Maher (1974, 1988) is one of the chief contemporary proponents of a perceptual theory. He argues that delusions are the result of an entirely normal attempt to account for abnormal perceptual experiences. For example, a person has the anomalous experience of hearing voices in the absence of an obvious cause, which results in a sense of puzzlement; this in turn leads to a search for an explanation, which, because the initial experience is strange, is likely to be abnormal—say, that the voice is being transmitted through an invisible transmitter. The arrival at an explanation, albeit odd, is accompanied by relief, which serves to reinforce the belief. Thus, the delusion is a product of abnormal experience but of normal reasoning. Here, there is no suggestion of motivation playing a part until after the belief is formed, when anxiety reduction may help maintain the delusion.

Maher (1988) cites evidence from a study of normal subjects under anomalous environmental conditions, which suggests that irrational beliefs can be "readily provoked." Building on earlier reports of an association between hearing loss and paranoid delusions in the elderly (Cooper, Kay, Curry, Garside, & Roth, 1974) and in late onset schizophrenia (Kay, Cooper, Garside, & Roth, 1976), Zimbardo, Anderson, & Kabat (1981) propose that a loss of auditory acuity, if unacknowledged, could be interpreted as other people whispering unfavorable things. In an experiment, subjects with hypnotically induced partial deafness scored higher than controls on a questionnaire measure of paranoia. Johnson, Ross, & Mastria (1977) also report a case study in which they argue that a delusion arose from misattributions for unusual experiences.

## Cognitive Accounts

The third group of theories of delusions is cognitive: these propose that reasoning or other cognitive abnormalities are involved in delusion formation. Again, such ideas are not new. In 1911, Dupre and Logre described "misinterpretative delusional states" where they found no error in the sphere of perception but errors of logic: "the problem is not one of registering information, but of appreciating it, recognizing its links with other phenomena and establishing its relative importance and significance, in short, its interpretation" (1911/1988, p. 161).

Garety and colleagues have found evidence of probabilistic reasoning biases in some deluded subjects (Garety, Hemsley, & Wessely, 1991; Huq, Garety, & Hemsley, 1988). These biases were a tendency of subjects to make decisions on the basis of very little information (jumping to conclusions) and to express high levels of certainty (overconfidence). They also were more responsive to disconfirming information than were controls, changing their decisions more rapidly. These biases were present only in a subgroup of deluded people, and were associated with reports of current anomalous experiences (e.g., hallucinations) and lower verbal IQ. The material in the studies was neutral (concerning judgments about jars of colored beads), in a deliberate attempt to investigate judgments that were not personally involving or emotionally loaded, in contrast to the studies of attributional style cited above. These findings, therefore, appeared consistent with a cognitive hypothesis for *some* delusions, and Garety and Hemsley (in press) have suggested that cognitive theories of schizophrenia, such as Hemsley's (1987) account may fit: that some deluded subjects may show excessive attention to stimuli present in the environment and weakened influence of past learning, resulting in inaccurate judgments.

Chapman and Chapman (1988) also posit that a reasoning bias may account for some delusions. They examined the relationship of beliefs to experiences in "psychosis-prone" subjects (as identified by responses to questionnaires), and they found that subjects responded to similar experiences with beliefs that ranged from the normal to the fully delusional. In some cases, Maher's perceptual hypothesis seemed to apply, in that acceptance of the veridicality of an anomalous perceptual experience demanded, or almost demanded, a delusional belief. However, other subjects reported delusions that had no apparent relationship to any unusual experience. Some of these subjects appeared to reason badly when talking about their experiences: they expressed themselves vaguely, became tangential, jumped from one topic to another, and had difficulty finding the right words. They seemed to constrict the information used in reaching a conclusion, ignoring or giving inadequate weight to other experiences, some of which may have contradicted the delusional belief. These informal accounts of people reasoning about their delusions bear some similarity to the findings of reasoning biases by Garety and colleagues.

Frith (1979, 1987, 1992) has written a number of intriguing and influential papers, in which he proposes that particular cognitive neuropsychological deficits may account for the symptoms of schizophrenia. He thus attempts to account not only for delusions but also for other symptoms, such as hallucinations, passivity phenomena, and negative symptoms. Most recently (1992), he has suggested that all of these share a basic underlying dysfunctional cognitive process: abnormalities in metarepresentation. *Metarepresentation* is the cognitive mechanism that enables us to be aware of our goals, our intentions, and the intentions of others. Frith then considers how impairments with respect to the different elements of metarepresentation may relate to specific symptoms. For example, he proposes that an inability to monitor one's own "willed intentions" can lead to delusions of alien control, while an inability to monitor the beliefs and intentions of others can lead (among other symptoms) to paranoid delusions.

A number of cognitive theorists have attempted to provide accounts at both the psychological and the physical level—"linking the mind and brain," as Frith (1992) calls it. Frith has suggested that, for one aspect of metarepresentation—willed actions—the prefrontal cortex plays a vital part; Shallice, Burgess, & Frith (1991) have found frontal deficits in a small group of people with schizophrenia. Butler and Braff (1991), in a review of theories of delusion, also propose that failures of *metathinking* (the ability to think about one's thoughts) may lead to delusions, and they note that this type of executive function is a role of the frontal lobes. Keefe (see chap. 8, this volume) also implicates the frontal cortex in delusions, suggesting that delusions involve a lack of awareness of the division between self and others. He proposes that the frontal cortex is responsible for working memory, the operation of which enables the person to hold in awareness a concept of self.

Ellis and Young (1990) have focused on delusions of misidentification, such as Capgras syndrome, and offer an account in terms of cognitive processes and anatomical pathways. They have considered the routes to face recognition, noting that there is evidence for two independent routes—one which permits the face to be identified and the other which permits a face to be recognized as familiar or unfamiliar. Two different anatomical pathways are thought to underlie these routes. Ellis and Young (1990) suggest that it is the route concerned with feelings of familiarity that is damaged in Capgras syndrome, while the route to face identification remains intact. As a consequence, the patient can identify the face of his wife, but she seems somehow unfamiliar, a different person. He infers that his wife has been replaced by a double.

While I have grouped together a number of theories under the heading "Cognitive Accounts," there are important differences. While some consider that there may be characteristic features of the general reasoning style of people with delusions (e.g., Garety et al., 1991; Chapman & Chapman, 1988), others suggest that the cognitive abnormalities are specific to particular experiences, such as experiencing one's thoughts as withdrawn (Frith, 1992) or feeling that an identifiable face is not familiar (Ellis & Young, 1990). Thus, some find *biases in inference* in some people with delusions, while others argue, in line with Maher (1988), that it is the *experience* rather than the judgments made about experience that is deviant.

## Delusion Maintenance

Most of the theories reviewed above, whether motivational, perceptual, or cognitive, address the question of the *formation* of delusion. However, an important further consideration is the *maintenance* of the delusion. Much of the psychiatric literature has assumed that the definitional fixity of delusion, being "firmly sustained in spite of what constitutes incontrovertible and obvious proof or evidence to the contrary" (*DSM-IV*), is a clear indication of irrationality or faulty reasoning. Others have suggested that it stems from an overriding need: "The delusional content is of vital necessity . . . and without it he would inwardly collapse. . . . In the case of delusion we may see someone irretrievably lost in untruth." (Jaspers, 1913/1959, p. 411).

Models of normal belief formation and maintenance suggest, however, that strong beliefs are generally maintained with little evidential support (Alloy & Tabachnik, 1984). Evidence can be found in normals for perseveration of beliefs in the face of contradictory information and ignoring of relevant information once a strong belief is held (e.g., Lord, Lepper, & Ross, 1979). The "confirmation bias" is also well documented (Ross & Anderson, 1982; Klayman & Ha, 1987). For example, in a classic experiment in which subjects were required to construct a hypothesis, Wason and Johnson-Laird (1972) found that subjects approached the task with a verification method, ignoring alternatives and seeking to confirm only the chosen hypothesis. Sometimes subjects became convinced of the correctness of their theory, so that all attention was funneled on the first decision, and the subject "contradict[ed] himself . . . and denie[d] the facts which confront[ed] him" (p. 239).

While motivational accounts have been offered for these processes in normals, others have argued that cognitive processes also operate, such as a normal tendency to ignore the informational value of nonoccurrences (Ross & Anderson, 1982). Ross and Anderson conclude a review of shortcomings in judgment by asserting that there can be little doubt that our existing beliefs influence the process by which we seek out, store, and interpret relevant information. Indeed, such processes make manageable the innumerable items of information with which each person is presented at every moment. They posit a number of mechanisms underlying these phenomena, including biased search for and interpretation of the evidence and a tendency to search for causal explanations that, once found, tend to buttress and sustain the original belief, even in the face of subsequent challenges. While there has been some debate over the extent to which the documented shortcomings in human judgment are as pervasive as suggested by some theorists, it is now uncontroversial that "human judgment and inference are not always logical and rational and that certain types of errors creep into the process" (Kihlstrom & Hoyt, 1988).

This work, which demonstrates deviations in the inferential performance of normals from rational behavior, especially when a strong belief is already held, has implications for our understanding of delusions. It may be argued that delusional incorrigibility, in particular, is less abnormal than had been assumed. It is possible that the phenomenon represents a quanitative rather than a qualitative difference from normal performance or that maintaining a strong belief in the face of contradictory evidence is not, in itself, at all abnormal. Thus if the process—whether motivational, perceptual, or cognitive—responsible for the formation of the delusion was transient or corrected by some therapeutic means, it is possible for the delusion to be maintained in the absence of any underlying abnormality. However, where such biased or defective causal processes persist, they may clearly also play a role in belief maintenance.

## Theoretical Overview

Theories of delusions thus posit the involvement of a variety of underlying mechanisms, whether motivational, perceptual, or cognitive. Empirical studies of such processes in groups of people with delusions typically find a large variance in responses and that the phenomenon of interest are present in only a subgroup of subjects (e.g., Garety et al., 1991). Delusions appear to be heterogeneous phenomena. In light of this, Garety (1991) has attempted to draw together findings relating to these disparate theories into a tentative multifactorial model of delusion formation and maintenance. In this model, based upon models of belief formation in normals, the delusional belief is seen as a judgment that is made when the individual encounters (or seeks out) some information and interprets it. In all cases, the delusion is seen as a secondary phenomenon: the person's attempt to make sense of events, the self, or experiences. However, it is argued, different types of delusions may then involve different mechanisms. In some cases, expectations and biases arising from personality, self-esteem, and motivation are thought to play a part, while in others, information-processing abnormalities in perceptual and judgmental processes may be considered more prominent. In many cases, these processes may operate as interacting causal mechanisms, although one pathway may exert a stronger influence than another. Garety and Hemsley (1994) suggest that the model may most effectively be used to provide a set of hypotheses for understanding delusions in single cases, once particular abnormal processes have been detected (e.g., Garety, 1992).

## Insight and Delusion

How then do these theories of delusion illuminate our understanding of the concept of insight? There are a number of implications to be drawn.

### Multifactorial View of Insight

The first implication derives from the heterogeneity of delusion and the resultant need for a multifactorial view of delusion formation. Where lack of insight refers to a person's being deluded (i.e., the person's assertion that a given delusional belief is true), we can conclude that the processes involved may be motivational, cognitive, perceptual, or a complex interaction of these. It would be unwise to attempt an explanation based on a single abnormal process for all cases of lack of insight. Marková and Berrios (1992) have observed that different models of insight exist for different broad categories of psychiatric disorders (psychotic, neurotic, and neurological); I would argue that even within more narrowly defined categories, such as schizophrenia, a fine-grained analysis of the processes underlying particular delusions (and hence associated insight) is warranted. Recent work on delusions emphasizes the value of specifying the type of delusion under consideration and also of using single cases to investigate the processes hypothesized to be abnormal.

A related but different point concerns the multidimensional nature of insight. When a person with delusions is found to have poor insight in terms of more than one component of insight as defined by David (1990), there may be different mechanisms involved for particular components. Kirmayer and Corin (see chap. 10, this volume) consider insight from a sociocultural perspective, and they suggest that insight is not a transparent act of self-reflection but a cognitive and social construction of the self, profoundly shaped by cultural beliefs and practices. Thus, with respect to David's three different components of insight, it is quite possible, for example, that a person may reject treatment by doctors or medication for cultural or social reasons, have difficulty in relabeling certain mental phenomena as pathological owing to a cognitive deficit, such as impaired metarepresentative processes, and yet be capable of recognizing that he or she is suffering from a mental illness. Thus, the different components of insight may reflect the action of different causal processes.

### Self-Knowledge in Delusion and Insight

Another implication in the review of theories of delusion concerns the role of self-knowledge in delusion and in insight. Certain cognitive theories, most notably Frith's (1992), proposes that some delusions are the result of a failure of self-knowledge — knowledge of one's own goals and intentions. Insight also involves self-knowledge. Thus, the very cognitive faculty thought to be responsible for the genesis of the delusional symptom may also be employed in identifying particular mental events as categorically different from other mental events, before then determining them to be pathological. Marková and Berrios (1992) make a similar point when they cite Lewis (1934), who stated that it was with the "disordered mind [that] the patient contemplates his state or individual symptoms" (p. 343). Thus, Lewis made an intrinsic connection between the patient's insight and the disease process itself.

Self-knowledge is also relevant to motivational theories of delusions. Neale (1988) and Bentall (1993) suggest that people with grandiose delusions or with persecutory delusions, respectively, may engage unconsciously in self-deception to protect a fragile self-esteem. Such people may lie at an extreme point on a continuum of self-knowledge, such as is discussed in chapter 6 of this volume. The unrealistic view of the self, motivated by a need to protect oneself against perceived threat, leads directly to both the delusions and also to a denial of illness. In such cases, insight and delusions are intricately interwoven.

Other work on delusion may suggest that the faculties employed in self-knowledge are not always specifically impaired, however. For example, more general cognitive biases, such as a tendency to jump to conclusions, resulting from an overemphasis on data immediately present (Garety et al., 1991), do not directly implicate aspects of metarepresentation. The relationships among self-knowledge, delusion, and insight may be seen to differ according to the particular theory of delusions.

### Change in Insight

A final implication of the literature is that insight may be less immutable than is sometimes supposed. In studying delusions in terms of biases in normal cognitive and emotional processes, rather than qualitative differences, the work discussed has led to the conclusion that delusions may be more susceptible to understanding and change than previously thought. A number of small studies of psychological therapies for drug-resistant delusions have produced promising results (e.g., Chadwick & Lowe, 1990; Garety et al., 1994). If such delusions are amenable to change by cognitive approaches, so also may be the associated insight.

Some data indicate that this may be true. In a recent study of cognitive behavioral therapy for psychosis, in which the subjects were selected for being highly deluded at the beginning of therapy (in terms of high levels of conviction, distress, and preoccupation), data were also collected on insight before and after therapy (Garety et al., 1994). The subjects were 11 people with longstanding psychoses (on average 14 years), diagnosed as suffering from schizophrenia (10) or schizoaffective disorder (1). The participants were given up to 20 sessions of cognitive behavioral therapy, and significant improvements were found in terms of reduced delusional conviction and preoccupation, as well as general symptomatology, in comparison to a control group.

Using David's scale (1990), the three components of insight were assessed. Before therapy, the group had a mean total insight score of 8.06 (range 2–14), where 14 is the maximum score, representing complete insight. At the end of therapy, the mean insight score had increased to 10.55 (range 5–14). Compared with the controls, this was not a significant improvement. However, these mean total scores fail to reflect the precise change that occurred. The scores for the individual components are more informative. At the beginning of therapy, the group scored quite well in terms of treatment compliance, 5 subjects scoring the maximum of 4 points on this item and a further 3 scoring 3 points. These scores did not substantially change. Before therapy, 7 of the 11 subjects recognized that they suffered from a mental illness and could give an account of this (scoring 5 or 6 out of a total possible 6 points). There were modest improvements in this component. However, it was in the final component of insight—the recognition that the delusion is part of the illness—that the most substantial changes occurred. Before therapy, 9 of the 11 subjects did not regard their delusion as part of an illness (scoring 0–2 of a possible 4 points; group mean score, 1.04); by the end of therapy only 3 subjects still held this position, and of the remaining 8 subjects, 7 now scored the maximum of 4 points, fully recognizing their delusions as part of their illness (group mean score, 3.0).

Thus, certain aspects of insight appear susceptible to change through psychological therapy. That the changes occurred in our study principally in the third component of insight is perhaps not in itself surprising. It is this aspect, as I noted at the beginning of this chapter, that has a definitional link to delusion. Also, in this group of patients, there may have been a ceiling effect for the other two components: most subjects scored as having good insight before therapy for these aspects. Additionally, these data indicate that, whatever processes were responsible for forming or maintaining the patients' delusions, they did not render them *incapable* of reflecting further on their mental processes, albeit with the guidance of a therapist. The failure in self-knowledge was not absolute, just as their delusions were not immutable.

## Conclusions

A review of the literature on theories of delusion has highlighted both the heterogeneity of delusion and the large number of causal mechanisms for delusions that have been proposed. Clearly, the *DSM-IV* definition oversimplifies matters by asserting that delusions are based on incorrect inference. While all delusions can be seen as a person's attempt to explain and make sense of events, the self, or other experiences, it is probable that different processes underlie different types of delusions. All accounts implicating the involvement of motivational, perceptual, and cognitive processes have some evidential support, and the most promising current work is directed at generating more specific hypotheses for subtypes of delusion.

We have seen how the concept of insight in psychosis is closely linked to the concept of delusion. When a person is said to lack insight, specifically by virtue of being deluded, it follows that accounts of insight should reflect the variety of processes found relevant to delusions. Failures of insight may, therefore, derive from the same range of biased or faulty mechanisms as do the delusions to which they are related. One group of cognitive theories of delusion has a particularly intriguing overlap with notions of insight. Both delusions and insight can be seen as reflecting a failure in self-knowledge. It is apparent that where impairments in the ability to think about one's own mental processes account for a delusion, there may be particularly important implications for insight. Some of the motivational theories similarly invoke mechanisms that may bear a direct relationship to both delusion and insight. Thus, self-deception to preserve a fragile self-esteem may lead to both grandiose delusions and a denial of mental illness. Other theories of delusion, in contrast, do not specifically implicate the processes involved in self-knowledge, such as those that point to more general reasoning biases. In addition, it is important to note that a person may be said to lack insight for reasons quite unconnected to delusions, such as not complying with a medication regime. Clearly, the reasons for this may be entirely independent of the mechanisms underlying delusions.

Delusions are said to be "firmly sustained" in spite of counterevidence. However, the social and cognitive psychological literature has clearly identified a tendency for normals to maintain beliefs in the face of contradictory information, especially when the belief is strongly held. The "confirmation bias" phenomenon is also well documented, where subjects seek confirmatory rather than disconfirmatory evidence when testing a hypothesis. I have argued that the maintenance of delusions may not, therefore, be abnormal, especially if the processes responsible for the original formation of the delusion have been corrected. The same may apply to insight.

There is a growing consensus that delusions may be more susceptible to change by psychotherapeutic means than previously thought. This also has implications for change in insight. I have described how scores on the component of insight directly linked to psychotic symptoms changed in the context of cognitive behavioral therapy for the associated delusions, although these are preliminary and crude data. Such findings, and other studies of change in delusions, offer grounds for greater optimism for change in insight. In future years, we may see insight increasingly as a suitable focus for therapy rather than principally as an outcome predictor.

*References*

Alloy, L. B., & Tabachnik, N. (1984). Assessment of covariation by humans and animals: The joint influence of prior expectations and current situational information. *Psychological Review, 91,* 112–149.

American Psychiatric Association (APA). (1995). *Diagnostic and statistical manual of mental disorders (DSM-IV).* Washington, DC: Author.

Bentall, R. P. (1993). Cognitive biases and abnormal beliefs: Towards a model of persecutory delusions. In A. S. David & J. Cutting (Eds.), *The neuropsychology of schizophrenia.* London: Erlbaum.

Bentall, R. P., Kaney, S., & Dewey, M. E. (1991). Paranoia and social reasoning: An attribution theory analysis. *British Journal of Clinical Psychology, 30,* 13–23.

Butler, R. W., & Braff, D. L. (1991). Delusions: A review and integration. *Schizophrenia Bulletin, 17,* 633–647.

Chadwick, P., & Lowe, F. (1990). The measurement and modification of delusional beliefs. *Journal of Consulting and Clinical Psychology, 58,* 225–232.

Chapman, L. J., & Chapman, J. P. (1988). The genesis of delusions. In T. F. Oltmanns & B. A. Maher (Eds.), *Delusional beliefs,* (chap. 8). New York: John Wiley.

Cooper, A. F., Kay, D. W. K., Curry, A. R., Garside, R. F., & Roth, M. (1974). Hearing loss in paranoid and affective disorders of the elderly. *Lancet, 2,* 851–854.

David, A. (1990). Insight and psychosis. *British Journal of Psychiatry, 156,* 798–808.

Dupre, E., & Logre, J. (1911/1988). Confabulatory delusional states. In M. Shepherd (Ed.), *The clinical roots of the schizophrenia concept* (J. Cutting, Trans.). Cambridge: Cambridge University Press.

Ellis, H. D., & Young, A. W. (1990). Accounting for delusional misidentifications. *British Journal of Psychiatry, 157,* 239–248.

Freeman, J. (1981). On the psychopathology of persecutory delusions. *British Journal of Psychiatry, 139,* 529–532.

Freud, S. (1915/1956). A case of paranoia running counter to the psychoanalytic theory of the disease. In *Collected Papers, Vol. 2.* London: Hogarth Press.

Frith, C. D. (1979). Consciousness, information processing and schizophrenia. *British Journal of Psychiatry, 134,* 225–235.

Frith, C. D. (1987). The positive and negative symptoms of schizophrenia reflect impairments in the perception and initiation of action. *Psychological Medicine, 17,* 631–648.

Frith, C. D. (1992). *The cognitive neuropsychology of schizophrenia.* Hove, East Sussex: Erlbaum.

Garety, P. A. (1991). Reasoning and delusions. *British Journal of Psychiatry, 159* (suppl. 14), 14–18.

Garety, P. A. (1992). Making sense of delusions. *Psychiatry, 55,* 282–291.

Garety, P. A., Hemsley, D. R., & Wessely, S. (1991). Reasoning in deluded schizophrenic and paranoid patients: biases in performance on a probabilistic inference task. *Journal of Nervous & Mental Disease, 170,* 194–201.

Garety, P. A., & Hemsley, D. R. (1994). *Delusions: Investigations into the psychology of delusional reasoning.* Oxford: Oxford University Press.

Garety, P. A., Kuipers, L., Fowler, D., Chamberlain, F., & Dunn, G. (1994). Cognitive behavioural therapy for drug-resistant psychosis. *British Journal of Medical Psychology, 67,* 259–271.

Hemsley, D. R. (1987). An experimental psychological model for schizophrenia. In H. Hafner, W. F. Gattaz, & W. Janzarik (Eds.), *Search for the causes of schizophrenia.* Heidleberg: Springer-Verlag.

Huq, S. F., Garety, P. A., & Hemsley, D. R. (1988). Probabilistic judgements in deluded and non-deluded subjects. *Quarterly Journal of Experimental Psychology, 40A*, 801–812.

Jaspers, K. (1913/1959). *General psychopathology* (J. Hoenig & M. W. Hamilton, Trans.). Manchester: Manchester University Press.

Johnson, W. G., Ross, J. M., & Mastria, M. A. (1977). Delusional behaviour: An attributional analysis of development and modification. *Journal of Abnormal Psychology, 86*, 421–426.

Kay, D. W. K., Cooper, A. F., Garside, R. F., & Roth, M. (1976). The differentiation of paranoid from affective psychoses by patients' premorbid characteristics. *British Journal of Psychiatry, 129*, 207–215.

Kihlstrom, J. F., & Hoyt, I. P. (1988). Hypnosis and the psychology of delusions. In T. F. Oltmanns & B. A. Maher (Eds.), *Delusional beliefs.* New York: John Wiley.

Klayman, J., & Ha, Y. W. (1987). Confirmation, disconfirmation and information in hypothesis testing. *Psychological Review, 94*, 211–228.

Lacan, J. (1932/1988). The case of Aimee, or self-punitive paranoia. In M. Shepherd (Ed.), *The clinical roots of the schizophrenia concept* (J. Cutting, Trans.). Cambridge: Cambridge University Press.

Lewis, A. (1934). The psychopathology of insight. *Journal of Medical Psychology, 14*, 332–348.

Lord, C., Lepper, M. R., & Ross, L. (1979). Biased assimilation and attitude polarisation: the effects of prior theories on subsequently considered evidence. *Journal of Personality & Social Psychology, 37*, 2098–2110.

Maher, B. A. (1974). Delusional thinking and perceptual disorder. *Journal of Individual Psychology, 30*, 98–113.

Maher, B. A. (1988). Anomalous experience and delusional thinking: The logic of explanations. In T. F. Oltmanns & B. A. Maher (Eds.), *Delusional beliefs* (chap. 2). New York: John Wiley.

Marková, I. S., & Berrios, G. E. (1992). The meaning of insight in clinical psychiatry. *British Journal of Psychiatry, 160*, 850–860.

Neale, J. M. (1988). Defensive functions of manic episodes. In T. F. Oltmanns & B. A. Maher (Eds.), *Delusional beliefs.* New York: John Wiley.

Ross, L., & Anderson, C. A. (1982). Shortcomings in the attribution process: On the origins and maintenance of erroneous social assessments. In D. Kahneman, P. Slovic, & A. Tuersky (Eds.), *Judgment under uncertainty: Heuristics and biases.* New York: Cambridge University Press.

Serieux, P., & Capgras, J. (1909/1988). Misinterpretative delusional states. In M. Shepherd (Ed.), *The clinical roots of the schizophrenia concept* (J. Cutting, Trans.). Cambridge: Cambridge University Press.

Shallice, T., Burgess, P. W., & Frith, C. D. (1991). Can the neuropsychological case study approach be applied to schizophrenia? *Psychological Medicine, 21*, 661–673.

Sims, A. (Ed.). (1991). Delusions and awareness of reality. *British Journal of Psychiatry, 159*, (suppl. 14).

Spitzer, M. (1990). On defining delusions. *Comprehensive Psychiatry, 31*, 377–397.

Spitzer, M. (1992). The phenomenology of delusions. *Psychiatric Annals, 22*, 252–259.

Wason, P. C., & Johnson-Laird, P. N. (1972). *Psychology of reasoning: Structure and content.* London: Batsford.

Winters, K. C., & Neale, J. M. (1983). Delusions and delusional thinking in psychotics: A review of the literature. *Clinical Psychology Review, 3*, 227–253.

Winters, K. C., & Neale, J. M. (1985). Mania and low self-esteem. *Journal of Abnormal Psychology, 94*, 252–290.

Zimbardo, P. G., Anderson, S. M., & Kabat, L. G. (1981). Induced hearing deficit generates experimental paranoia. *Science, 212*, 1529–1531.

# 5

JEAN-PAUL C. J. SELTEN
ROBERT J. VAN DEN BOSCH
A. E. S. SIJBEN

# The Subjective Experience
# of Negative Symptoms

There can be little doubt that negative symptoms have serious consequences. They are incapacitating and may lead to long-term hospitalization. Remarkably, however, we know almost nothing about patients' experiences of these symptoms. Our ignorance in these matters is almost total. We do not know which patients are aware of these symptoms and which are not. We do not know to which symptoms awareness or unawareness applies and to what extent patients suffer from these symptoms.

Jaspers was the only classical author who wrote on this topic. In his view there is an inverse relationship between severity of illness and awareness of negative symptoms:

> Below a certain level of psychic differentiation, individuals seem to live purely in their environment and seem to lack all knowledge of themselves. In the case of idiocy, the fully developed acute psychoses and deep dementia, the problem does not even arise as to what attitude the personality adopts. It would be better here not to speak of the absence of any awareness of illness but to talk of a loss of personality, which embraces the missing awareness of illness automatically as a part-element. (1963, p. 421)

It should be pointed out that "deep dementia" is an incorrect translation of the German *tiefer Verblödung*. The translation should be "severe deficit." Of patients with a mild deficit, Jaspers wrote:

> Some patients with a mild degree of illness will talk about how their nature has changed. They are "less excitable, their interest is shallower but they talk much more." They notice that they keep on talking and cannot stop but show no kind of agitation. They sometimes observe that they are staring into the corner for no particular reason and that their general performance is suffering. Some can only say that they feel "a profound change" has

78

taken place. They feel "they are not as flexible as before" and not so excitable. (1963, p. 447).

In first-person accounts, negative symptoms are mentioned only rarely. A notable exception is the French schizophrenic artist Antonin Artaud. His notebooks and private papers contain many exclamations relating to his suffering from negative symptoms. In *The Umbilicus of Limbo* he described a physical state, undoubtedly his own, as:

> a staggering and central fatigue, a kind of gasping fatigue. Movements must be recomposed, a sort of deathlike fatigue, a fatigue of the mind in carrying out the simplest muscular contraction, of unconsciously clinging to something, must be sustained by a constant effort of the will. A fatigue as old as the world, the sense of having to carry one's body around, a feeling of incredible fragility which becomes a shattering pain. (Sontag, 1988, pp. 64–65)

In a letter to George Soulié de Morant, Artaud described his intellectual and related emotional sufferings, which serve to illustrate the insufficiency of our surface descriptions of the negative syndrome state:

> Since the mechanism of the mind has been destroyed in its continuity, I can no longer think except in fragments. When I do think, the major part of the stock of terms and vocabulary which I have personally accumulated is unusable, being rusty and *forgotten* somewhere, but even after the term has appeared, the underlying thought collapses, the contact is suddenly broken, the underlying nervous response no longer corresponds to the thought, the mechanism has broken down—*and I am talking about the times when I am thinking!!!* . . . It seems to me that I have even forgotten *how to think*. Yes, it is the notion of this private intellectual vacuum which I should like to *illuminate* once and for all. It seems to me the dominant characteristic of my condition. . . . The affective or emotional confusion which I mentioned earlier is intimately related to this disappearance, this catastrophe at the higher level. . . . In my case this obscuring, this uprooting of the higher levels of consciousness and thought holds true, unfortunately, for all the circumstances of life, if intellectually my brain has become inoperative, can no longer function, the moments during which this void possesses me, fills me with anguish and sorrow, and makes me feel that my life is wasted, unusable, have an emotional value as well, they are expressed in the soul as a coloration of nothingness, an affect of total despair well designed in my own image, but as for this affect, on the other hand, it is its lack of resonance, its coagulation. . . . (Sontag, 1988, pp. 289–290)*

In recent years, several authors have complained about the neglect of subjective experiences in psychiatric research (e.g., Strauss, 1989; van Praag, 1992). They have argued that a better understanding of the patient is of vital importance for psychiatry, because it not only contributes to a more empathic approach toward the patient but may also prove a necessary tool in understanding the etiology and pathogenesis of mental illness.

These considerations may apply to our study of negative symptoms as well. Patients who are unaware of these symptoms are unlikely to benefit from or even to participate in rehabilitation programs. In addition, because disturbances in self-monitoring have been proposed as being at the core of schizophrenia (Frith, 1987), a better understand-

---

*From *Antonin Artaud: Selected Writings*, S. Sontag, ed., 1988, Berkeley: University of California Press. Reprinted with permission.

ing of altered self-awareness in schizophrenia may provide insights into the pathogenesis of this disease.

## Measurement of Subjective Experiences of Schizophrenic Deficit

Current operationalizations of the schizophrenic defect state usually involve the concept of *negative symptoms* (e.g., Andreasen, 1982; Carpenter, Buchanan, & Kirkpatrick, 1991; Crow, 1985). The concept of negative symptoms has become so influential that one might almost forget that the deficits of schizophrenia have also been operationalized in other ways. The German psychiatrist Huber, for instance, developed the concept of *basic symptoms* (Huber, 1966, 1983; Koehler & Sauer, 1984). As the differences between basic symptoms and negative symptoms may not be immediately apparent, a short discussion of Huber's concept would seem useful.

Huber elaborated on Japsers's distinction between subjective experiences and observable behavior. He defined basic symptoms as patients' complaints about disturbances in their cognitive and emotional functioning. Thus, the assessment of basic symptoms is based on patients' reports. According to Huber, basic symptoms reflect the primary cognitive disorders (basic disorders) in schizophrenia and are most prominent in the so-called pure defect states: residual states without productive (positive) symptomatology. It is not supposed that basic symptoms are specific to schizophrenia, but they are thought to be much more substrate close than are other symptoms. According to Huber, delusions and hallucinations are secondary elaborations of basic symptoms.

The most widely used German-language rating scale to measure basic symptoms is the Frankfurt Complaint Questionnaire (Süllwold & Huber, 1986). Two English-language scales measuring these symptoms are the Subjective Deficit Syndrome Scale, or SDSS (Jaeger, Bitter, Czobor, & Volavka, 1990) and the Scale for the Assessment of Subjective Experience of Deficits in Schizophrenia, or SEDS (Liddle & Barnes, 1988). Since the terms *defect symptoms* and *negative symptoms* are currently being used as synonyms, the titles of these two English-language instruments may convey the impression that the scales are intended to measure the subjective experience of negative symptoms. Actually, they measure mainly basic symptoms and include few items that we would consider as negative symptoms.

The differences between basic symptoms and negative symptoms can be summarized as follows:

1. Basic symptoms are *symptoms* (subjective complaints) in the narrow sense of the word, wheras negative symptoms are actually *signs* (observable abnormalities) that do not need to be perceived by the patient in order to be present. It follows that, in the case of basic symptoms, the issue of awareness does not arise, whereas in the case of negative symptoms, it does.
2. Basic symptoms relate to a larger domain of psychological functioning than do negative symptoms and include complaints about disturbances in physical sensations, perception, autonomic reactions, and tolerance of stress (Koehler & Sauer, 1984). Accordingly, the SDSS and SEDS include several items (e.g., "excessive irritability," "insomnia," "indecisiveness," "decreased patience," "sensitivity to the weather") that do not occur in rating scales of negative symptoms (Fenton & McGlashan, 1992).

The difference between basic symptoms and negative symptoms is highlighted by the recent finding of a higher correlation between basic symptoms and positive symptoms than between basic symptoms and negative symptoms (Peralta, Cuesta, & de Leon, 1992). Similarly, the SDSS was found to be related to depression and a variety of positive symptoms, but not to negative symptoms (Jaeger et al., 1990).

A recent development concerns the subjective experience of attentional deficits. It is well known that many schizophrenic patients complain of attentional and perceptual dysfunctions. These seem to be of a heterogeneous nature. The cognitive problems are probably in part due to a reduced ability to sustain mental effort—that is, a deficit in controlled effort-demanding processing. These energetic deficits of cognition are particularly prominent in patients with negative symptoms (Schmand, 1992). There are anecdotal reports and many autobiographical accounts of attentional deficits, and there have been many studies based on experimental-psychological tasks. However, there are surprisingly few systematically collected data on the subjective experience of attentional problems. In contrast to the objective measurement by cognitive tasks, the subjective experience of cognitive impairment in schizophrenic subjects has received very little attention thus far.

A self-report questionnaire for measuring subjective attention has been described: the Test of Attentional Style (TAS; van den Bosch, van Asma, Rombouts, & Louwerens, 1992; van den Bosch, Rombouts, & van Asma, 1993). The scale contains subscales measuring distractibility, overload, processing capacity, attentional control, and conceptual control. Results showed that various kinds of psychiatric patients experience higher levels of distractibility and of cognitive overload than do normal subjects. These subjective cognitive dysfunctions correlated significantly with symptoms of anxiety and depression, but overload experiences shared most of their variance with positive psychotic symptoms.

A remarkable finding was that negative symptoms did not correlate with any of the subjective cognitive measures. It is well known that many objective attentional dysfunctions are primarily associated with negative symptoms. The authors suggest that the negative findings might be due to the fact that patients with negative symptoms have little awareness of their cognitive deficits, and consequently don't report their problems. Another explanation would be that the self-protective nature of negative symptoms prevents negative cognitive experiences, like sensations of overload or distraction, by reducing information processing.

## Scale for Measuring the Subjective Experience of Negative Symptoms

When Andreasen published the first version of the Scale for the Assessment of Negative Symptoms, or SANS (Andreasen, 1982), it included subjective ratings for the five subscales. The definitions for these subjective items, however, were variable and referred alternately to awareness and complaints. In later versions of the SANS the author discontinued these subjective ratings, "largely because most users did not read the instructions (which indicated that they could not be used in summary scores) and complained that the scale included both subjective and objective ratings" (Andreasen, personal communication, 1988). Systematic studies of the subjective experience of negative symptoms did not follow.

We developed an instrument to measure several aspects of the subjective experience of negative symptoms: awareness, causal attributions, and the severity of related disruption and distress (Selten, Sijben, van den Bosch, Omloo-Visser & Warmerdam, 1993). Our approach to the issue of negative symptom awareness is the comparison of patients' ratings and staff ratings. We developed a self-rating scale based on the items of the SANS (Andreasen, 1989) and called this new instrument the Subjective Experience of Negative Symptoms (SENS). The advantage of this procedure is that definitions of items for patient and staff ratings are identical, and can thus be compared.

Since we expected that many patients would not be able to complete a self-report questionnaire, we decided to elicit self-ratings in a semistructured interview. Thus, questions are preceded by a standardized explanation of the item in everyday language. For instance, the explanation for item 5 (affective nonresponsivity) is as follows:

> People sometimes feel great emotion when something important is happening. We get angry, for instance, or we get excited. At other times we feel little or no emotion at important events. Then these events hardly affect us at all.

After giving this explanation, the interviewer asks the first question—for example, How much emotion do you feel when something important happens? If the patient has not understood the explanation or the question, the interviewer is allowed to clarify the item in his or her own words, basing this explanation on the definition of the item. This procedure is similar to that of the Present State Examination (Wing, Cooper, & Sartorius, 1974).

The patient is asked to compare him or herself with other people of that age who have not been admitted to a psychiatric hospital, and is invited to rate him or herself on a five-point scale. For this purpose, the interviewer hands the patient a card that lists the following five answers to the question "How much?":

1. Very little
2. Little
3. Average
4. A lot
5. Very much.

In the same way, the patient answers questions about frequency with the help of a second card, displaying response categories ranging from 1, Rarely, to 5, Very often. The interviewer then proceeds to ask two more questions about those items that elicit a rating of 1 or 2 (i.e., the patient indicated the presence of the symptom). The purpose of this second, open-ended question is to collect information on the patient's opinions about the cause of negative symptoms. Finally, the interviewer asks the patient whether he or she is bothered or distressed by the symptom. If the patient answers affirmatively, the individual is asked how much he or she is bothered or distressed and is given a third card, listing five answers ranging from 1, Very little, through 3, Quite a lot, to 5, Very much.

This rating procedure has two important advantages over that in which the interviewer decides to what extent the patient is aware of the symptom. First, the latter entails a serious risk of interpretation bias. Second, if the interviewer bases the ratings on the patient's verbal reports, he or she may gain the erroneous impression that

TABLE 5.1.   Stability and Prevalence of SENS Items

|  | K 1 | K 2 | Prevalence % |
|---|---|---|---|
| A. Affective flattening | | | |
| 1. Unchanging facial expression | .65 | .48 | 32 |
| 2. Decreased spontaneous movements. | .25 | .13 | 36 |
| 3. Paucity of expressive gestures | .41 | .51 | 40 |
| 4. Poor eye contact | .71 | .64 | 10 |
| 5. Affective nonresponsivity | .43 | .68 | 18 |
| 6. Lack of vocal inflections | .71 | .45 | 36 |
| 7. Inability to feel | .46 | .47 | 20 |
| B. Alogia | | | |
| 8. Poverty of speech | .71 | .22 | 46 |
| 9. Poverty of content of speech | .28 | .30 | 16 |
| 10. Increased latency of response | .13 | .60 | 18 |
| 11. Absence of thoughts | .69 | .40 | 16 |
| C. Avolition-apathy | | | |
| 12. Poor grooming and hygiene | 1.00 | .65 | 2 |
| 13. Impersistence | .31 | .19 | 34 |
| 14. Physical anergia | .59 | .59 | 36 |
| 15. Lack of motivation | .38 | .57 | 24 |
| 16. Lack of energy | .59 | .47 | 38 |
| D. Anhedonia-Asociality | | | |
| 17a. Decreased recreational interest | .71 | .40 | 26 |
| 17b. Decreased recreational activity | .41 | .12 | 34 |
| 18a. Decreased sexual interest | 1.00 | .54 | 62 |
| 18b. Decreased sexual activity | .89 | .69 | 74 |
| 19. Inability to feel intimacy and closeness | .41 | .17 | 48 |
| 20. Few relationships with friends and peers | .73 | .45 | 52 |
| 21. Asociality | .56 | .26 | 24 |
| 22. Anhedonia | .61 | .29 | 20 |
| E. Attention | | | |
| 23. Impaired social attentiveness | .32 | .31 | 24 |
| 24. Impaired attentiveness | .73 | .72 | 38 |

K 1 are kappas across a period of 5 to 7 days ($n = 30$).
K 2 are kappas across a period of 2 months ($n = 36$).
*Prevalence* is prevalence of reported negative symptoms (ratings of 1 or 2, recoded as 1; first interview, $n = 50$).

patients with poverty of speech experience few symptoms. The results of our rating method are independent of the amount of the patient's spontaneous speech.

## First Findings with SENS

We examined the reliability of self-ratings on the SENS in patients from medium- and long-stay wards of a psychiatric hospital. Inclusion criteria were as follows:

1. A diagnosis of schizophrenia according to *DSM-III-R* criteria (APA, 1987)
2. The presence of at least two of five negative symptoms—that is, flat affect, poverty of speech, apathy, asociality, or poor attention
3. Display of an intellect that is not mentally subnormal—that is, having finished primary school and not having repeated more than one class

4. Absence of major depressive disorder, manic episode, organic mental disorder, or current substance abuse (*DSM-III-R* criteria)

Fifty patients completed the study: 32 men and 18 women, with a mean age of 39.5 years (*SD*-10.8; range 22–63 years). The mean length of illness (number of years since first admission) was 12.3 years (*SD*-8.8); mean length of current admission was 21.5 months (*SD*-24.6); and mean dosage of antipsychotic medication, converted into equivalents of haloperidol, was 19.9 mg (*SD*-34.5).

Thirty-two patients were interviewed on two occasions by the same investigator at intervals of 5 to 7 days (*n* = 12) or 2 months (*n* = 20). Eighteen patients were interviewed by different investigators on two occasions with an interval of 5 to 7 days. Three interviewers participated in the study, which allowed for three possible combinations of two interviewers. We therefore divided the sample into three groups of 6 each. All but 2 patients agreed to have a third interview after 2 months with one of the prior interviewers. Test-retest reliability across intervals of 5 to 7 days and 2 months could thus be calculated for 30 (12 + 18) and 36 (20 + 16) patients, respectively.

In order to obtain an acceptable test-retest reliability, ratings of 1 or 2 (suggesting awareness of the symptom) were recoded 1, and ratings of 3, 4, or 5 were recoded 2. The internal consistency of the scale was determined using the Kuder-Richardson 20 formula for the results of the first interview (*n* = 50). Measures of test-retest reliability were based on Cohen's kappa and on persistence—that is, the percentage of patients reporting the same symptom (by a rating of 1 or 2, recoded as 1) after 2 months. Interviewer variance was estimated with the Wilcoxon matched-pair signed-rank test applied to the differences between average scores on five subscales in 18 patients, who were interviewed by two different interviewers.

Results showed a good internal consistency of the scale (K-R 20 coefficient .76). At the item level, test-retest reliability was fair (see table 5-1). The average values of Cohen's kappa across intervals of 5 to 7 days and 2 months were .56 and .43, respectively.

Persistence over a period of 2 months was high, averaging 67% (range 46–100%). These results are comparable to those obtained with the SANS. As for the internal consistency of the SANS, Andreasen, Flaum, Arndt, Alliger, & Swayze (1991) recently reported a Cronbach's alpha of .80. Kuipers (1992) examined 39 hospitalized schizophrenic patients across intervals of 2 months and found SANS summary scores to be moderately correlated ($r = .66$; $p < .001$).

Self-assessments were independent of the interviewer. Wilcoxon tests, based on five subscales and three pairs of interviewers, showed no significant differences between average scores on subscales. Test-retest reliability of the experience and the rating of disruption and distress (third question) was high. The average percentages of perfect agreement between answers to these questions were 74% and 40%, respectively.

The prevalence of reported negative symptoms varied (Table 5.1). Women reported significantly more disturbances than men regarding relationships with friends and peers ($t = 2.91$, $p < .01$), sexual interest ($t = 3.04$, $p < .005$), recreational activity ($t = 2.52$, $p < .05$) and attentiveness ($t = 2.65$, $p < .05$). Age correlated with the experience of decreased spontaneous movement ($r = .33$, $p < .05$) and lack of motivation ($r = -.32$, $p < .05$). Length of illness and dosage of antipsychotic medication did not correlate significantly with any item.

Six hundred and eighty-seven answers from 102 interviews were available for the analysis of causal attributions. Most answers (66%) to questions about the cause of negative symptoms could reliably (84% agreement between two independent raters) be classified into one or more of the following nine categories (it should be noted that the vast majority of our sample had not participated in psychoeducational programs on schizophrenia):

1. Patients quite often replied that they did not know (17% of all replies).
2. Psychotropic medication was mentioned most frequently as a causal factor (13%).
3. Negative symptoms could be experienced as determined by almost any other negative symptom (10%); e.g., "I can't make friends because when people visit me I have little to say"; "I can't focus my thoughts on sex"; "My voice is monotonous because I have little energy"; "My concentration is bad because I have lost interest in books"; "I do not look people in the eye because I am not interested in them", etc.).
4. Negative symptoms were sometimes attributed to positive symptoms (2%; e.g., "My concentration is continuously hampered by voices" or "The voices take all the energy away").
5. Occasionally, negative symptoms had taken on a meaning within a delusional system (3%; e.g., "I never have emotions because other people are living in me," or, "I am the Holy Ghost, the Angel of the Covenant, in whose image the other angels were created. I have no time for hobbies").
6. Negative symptoms were sometimes experienced as entirely determined by outside factors (10%; e.g., "I do so little because, in this hospital, nothing is organized for me," or "I do nothing because, in this hospital, everything is done for me").
7. Other patients experienced their symptoms as egosyntonic (9%; e.g., "I have always been like that"; "I have always disliked sex").
8. Only 4 patients viewed at least one negative symptom as a direct manifestation of mental disease—that is, not secondary to other symptoms or to medication.
9. Only 1 patient reported the use of active withdrawal as a preventive coping strategy against psychotic relapse ("I avoid talking to people for a longer time. Otherwise my mind gets confused").

Disruption and distress, as assessed at the first interview, were reported most often for "lack of relationships with friends and peers" (38%), "inability to feel intimacy and closeness" (36%), "lack of energy" (34%), and "impaired attentiveness" (32%). The experience of "decreased sexual interest and activity," while very prevalent in this sample, seemed to bother relatively few patients (16%). High ratings for the severity of disruption and distress (ratings of 4, a lot, or 5, very much) were assigned most frequently to "lack of energy" (26%), "impersistence" (20%), "impaired attention" (20%), "inability to feel intimacy and closeness" (20%), "few relationships with friends and peers" (14%), and "physical anergia" (14%).

Recently we completed a study of patients' and psychiatrists' ratings of negative symptoms in a psychiatric hospital setting. Preliminary results from a new sample of 86 patients point, as expected, toward a large discrepancy between subjective and objective ratings. The prevalence of negative symptoms, according to the psychiatrist (SANS ratings of at least 2, mild), and to the patients (SENS ratings of 1 or 2), were on average 62% and 37%, respectively. Agreement between the patients and the psychiatrist on the presence or absence of each negative symptom was generally low, yielding an average value of Cohen's kappa of .13.

Moreover, the results confirm our earlier findings of a small proportion of patients reporting "poor grooming and hygiene" (12%) and of a large proportion reporting "decreased sexual interest and activity" (70%). High ratings for the severity of disruption and distress were assigned again to "lack of energy" (22%), "impersistence" (20%), and "impaired attention" (15%). Causal attributions for negative symptoms followed a pattern roughly similar to that reported above.

## The Experience of Negative Symptoms: Present and Future

The SENS proved to be easy to administer in a 30- to 45-minute interview. It showed a high internal consistency and an acceptable test-retest reliability. The values of Cohen's kappa were acceptable when ratings were dichotomized. It seems, therefore, that patients are able to indicate reliably the presence or absence of negative symptoms, but have difficulty making more subtle distinctions.

The stability of self-ratings in our study was fair, but not very high. How is this to be explained? Firstly, variance in self-ratings may reflect an instability of the negative syndrome. Objective ratings of negative symptoms have been shown to be subject to a certain amount of change (e.g., Addington & Addington, 1991; Kuipers, 1992). In some patients, poor motivation or inability to understand questions may have led to indiscriminate answers. However, it is our impression that these factors were generally of minor importance. Another source of error may be that patients forget the instructions and, more or less systematically, compare themselves with fellow-patients and not with people outside the hospital. Furthermore, some patients may give random answers. Jaspers (1963) already pointed out that some patients with severe deficits do not adopt an attitude toward their illness at all (see quotation above). An alternative explanation is that in certain patients the subjective experience of negative symptoms varies greatly. With this in view, the changes in self-ratings are reliable and valid indicators of an instable subjective experience of negative symptoms. Finally, the instrument might measure other experiences in addition to negative symptoms—fluctuations of mood or side effects of antipsychotic drugs, for instance.

As for the causal attributions of negative symptoms, we are not aware of earlier studies based on a semistructured interview. Other investigations in this area were concerned with patients' concepts of the etiology of positive symptoms (e.g., Angermeyer & Klusmann, 1988). Some results of our study differ markedly from results of studies with a different starting point. Both Thurm and Häfner (1987) and Dittman and Schüttler (1990) asked their patients about the use of preventive strategies against psychotic relapse and found that a substantial proportion of patients (28% and 43%, respectively) considered some form of active withdrawal a useful coping strategy. It is uncertain whether these divergent results are accounted for by sample differences relating to variables such as length of illness or by positive and negative symptomatology. If it is true that the type of question has so much influence on the answers given by patients, then deriving a reliable differentiation between active withdrawal as a coping strategy and negative symptoms arising from other causes will be a difficult task, and the comparative use of various interview techniques should be encouraged.

What do the results of our studies teach us about the insight into negative symptomatology displayed by hospitalized chronic schizophrenic patients? Although definitions of concepts as complex as insight are always beset by shortcomings, a practical definition of insight is needed here. Within the context of our research questions the hierarchical definition of insight, recently proposed by Raven, Mullen, and Clapstick (1992), seems useful. These authors distinguished four levels of insight:

Level 1:  The patient is aware of change in perceptual experiences, cognitive processes, emotions, or behaviors.
Level 2:  The patient has a feeling of disease engendered by these changes.
Level 3:  The patient gives verbal recognition that the changes causing disease are pathological — that is, they amount to an illness.
Level 4:  The patient acts on this in a manner appropriate to his or her intellectual background by seeking treatment, or complying with treatment, from a psychiatrist.

The first question for each SENS item relates to level 1 (awareness), and answers to the second SENS question (causal attributions) provide information about level 3. The preliminary findings from our second study — namely, large discrepancies between subjective and objective ratings — suggest that at least some patients are unaware of negative symptoms and suffer from a disturbance of insight at level 1. The causal attributions reported by our patients suggest that disturbances of insight at level 3 are also very common. We are currently examining variables that might predict poor insight, such as severity of negative symptoms and chronicity.

Unawareness of negative symptoms in schizophrenia requires explanation. The traditional interpretation of unawareness of illness in schizophrenia implies that patients use the defense mechanism of denial — that is, unawareness of illness is a coping mechanism — as a way of avoiding anxiety and pain (e.g., Mayer-Grosz, 1920; McGlashan, Levy, & Carpenter, 1975). A second theory seeks to explain unawareness of illness on the basis of an organically determined inability to become aware of certain deficits — that is, anosognosia (Amador, Strauss, Yale, & Gorman, 1991; Selten, 1990). Historically, the concept of anosognosia has most often been applied to a variety of neurological disorders, for example, unawareness of left hemiplegia after lesion to the right parietal lobe, unawareness of cortical blindness (Anton's syndrome), or hemianopsia. It has been shown that psychodynamic accounts of these unawareness phenomena present insurmountable problems (McGlynn & Schacter, 1989). In view of the fact that schizophrenia is at least in part a brain disease, and in view of some striking resemblances between poor insight in schizophrenia and in certain neurological disorders, the concept of anosognosia seems of great value for research in this area.

A third explanation for unawareness phenomena in schizophrenia focuses on a possible interaction between neural factors and psychological defense mechanisms. Amador et al. (1991) pointed out that some degree of self-deception is a normal and universal phenomenon, essential to the regulation of normal mood, and then proposed that in schizophrenia cerebral damage leads to disinhibition of these cognitive biases. Thus, as a consequence of cerebral damage, an otherwise adaptive distortion of reality assumes abnormal proportions.

In our opinion, both neural factors and defense mechanisms are important to the understanding of poor insight in schizophrenia. Theories that seek to explain unawareness phenomena in schizophrenia on the basis of psychological defense mechanisms alone encounter significant obstacles. These obstacles are similar to those presented by psychodynamic explanations for poor insight into certain neurological disorders:

1. If defense mechanisms played a dominant or single role in the development of unawareness of illness in schizophrenia, one would expect that patients would apply the same mechanisms to all serious deficits and to all traumatic events. Clinical experience teaches that this is often not the case: we know of patients who are fully aware of a life-threatening physical illness or the recent death of loved ones, but remain unaware of their mental illness. Single case studies could shed greater light on these matters.
2. Denial is not a very strong defense mechanism. Denial of illness in serious physical diseases, for instance, usually runs a short course (Martin, 1980). Unawareness of illness in schizophrenia, however, may last for years or may be lifelong (again, single case studies are needed).
3. Finally, with regard to some symptoms of schizophrenia, there is a relative absence of reason for defensive denial. Admitting the presence of some negative symptoms, for instance, should not be too embarrassing. As large numbers of males from our samples readily reported decreased sexual interest and activity, it is unlikely that the underreporting of other negative symptoms was strongly influenced by shame.

Our insight into the nature and mechanisms of insight in our patients is still poor. We believe that the questions raised here should be a major challenge to future research.

*Acknowledgments*   Some of the data presented here were published in: Selten, J.-P. C. J., Sijben, A. E. S., van den Bosch, R. J., Omloo-Visser, H., & Warmerdam, H. (1993). The subjective experience of negative symptoms: A self-rating scale. *Comprehensive Psychiatry, 34,* 192–197.

*References*

Addington, J., & Addington, D. (1991). Positive and negative symptoms of schizophrenia: Their course and relationship over time. *Schizophrenia Research, 5,* 51–60.

Amador, X. F., Strauss, D. H., Yale, S. A., & Gorman, J. M. (1991). Awareness of illness in schizophrenia. *Schizophrenia Bulletin, 17,* 113–132.

American Psychiatric Association. (1987). *Diagnostic and statistical manual of mental disorders* (3rd ed., rev.). Washington, DC: Author.

Andreasen, N. C. (1982). Negative symptoms in schizophrenia: Definition and reliability. *Archives of General Psychiatry, 39,* 784–788.

Andreasen, N. C. (1989). Scale of the assessment of negative symptoms (SANS). *British Journal of Psychiatry, 155* (suppl. 7), 53–58.

Andreasen, N. C., Flaum, M., Arndt, S., Alliger, R., & Swayze, V. W. (1991). Positive and negative symptoms: Assessment and validity. In A. Marneros, N. C. Andreasen, & M. T. Tsuang (Eds.), *Negative versus positive schizophrenia* (pp. 29–51). Berlin: Springer.

Angermeyer, M. C., & Klusmann, D. (1988). The causes of functional psychoses as seen by patients and their relatives. *European Archives of Psychiatry and Neurological Sciences, 238,* 47–54.

Bosch, R. J. van den, Asma, M. J. O. van, Rombouts, R., & Louwerens, J. W. (1992). Coping style and cognitive dysfunction in schizophrenic patients. *British Journal of Psychiatry, 161* (suppl. 18), 123–128.

Bosch, R. J., van den, Rombouts, R. P., & Asma, M. J. O. van (1993). Subjective cognitive dys-function in schizophrenic and depressed patients. *Comprehensive Psychiatry, 34*, 130–136.

Carpenter, W. T., Buchanan, R. W., & Kirkpatrick, B. (1991). The concept of the negative symp-toms of schizophrenia. In J. F. Greden & R. Tandon (Eds.), *Negative schizophrenic symp-toms: Pathophysiology and clinical implications* (pp. 3–20). Washington, DC: American Psychiatric Press.

Crow, T. J. (1985). The two-syndrome concept: Origins and current status. *Schizophrenia Bulletin, 11*, 471–486.

Dittman, J., & Schüttler, R. (1990). Disease consciousness and coping strategies of patients with schizophrenic psychosis. *Acta Psychiatrica Scandinavica, 82*, 318–322.

Fenton, W. S., & McGlashan, T. H. (1992). Testing systems for the assessment of negative symp-toms in schizophrenia. *Archives of General Psychiatry, 49*, 179–184.

Frith, C. D. (1987). The positive and negative symptoms of schizophrenia reflect an impairment in the perception and initiation of action. *Psychological Medicine, 17*, 631–648.

Huber, G. (1966). Reine Defektsyndrome und Basisstadien endogener Psychosen. *Fortschritte der Neurologie Psychiatrie, 34*, 409–426.

Huber, G. (1983). Das Konzept substratnaher Basissymptome und seine Bedeutung für Theorie und Therapie schizophrener Erkrankungen. *Nervenarzt, 54*, 23–32.

Jaeger, J., Bitter, I., Czobor, P., & Volavka, J. (1990). The measurement of subjective experience in schizophrenia: The subjective deficit syndrome scale. *Comprehensive Psychiatry, 31*, 216–226.

Jaspers, K. (1963). *General psychopathology* (J. Honig & M. W. Hamilton, Trans.). Manchester: Manchester University Press.

Koehler, K., & Sauer, H. (1984). Huber's basic symptoms: Another approach to negative psy-chopathology in schizophrenia. *Comprehensive Psychiatry, 25*, 174–182.

Kuipers, T. (1992). *Stille waters: Over de meting en beoordeling van negatieve symptomen*. [Still waters: About the assessment and evaluation of negative symptoms]. Ph.D. thesis. Utrecht: Rijksuniversiteit.

Liddle, P. F., & Barnes, T. R. E. (1988). The subjective experience of deficit in schizophrenia. *Comprehensive Psychiatry, 29*, 157–164.

Martin, M. J. (1980). Psychiatry and medicine. In H. I. Kaplan, A. M. Freedman, & B. J. Sadock (Eds.), *Comprehensive textbook of psychiatry* (3rd ed.). Baltimore: Williams and Wilkins.

Mayer-Grosz, W. (1920). Uber die Stellungnahme zur abgelaufenen akuten Psychose. *Zeitschrift für die gesammelte Neurologie und Psychiatrie, 60*, 160–212.

McGlashan, T. H., Levy, S. T., & Carpenter, W. T. (1975). Integration and sealing over: Clinically distinct recovery styles from schizophrenia. *Archives of General Psychiatry, 32*, 1269–1272.

McGlynn, S. M., & Schacter, D. L. (1989). Unawareness of deficits in neuropsychological syn-dromes. *Journal of Experimental Clinical Neuropsychology, 11*, 143–205.

Peralta, V., Cuesta, M. J., & de Leon, J. (1992). Positive versus negative schizophrenia and basic symptoms. *Comprehensive Psychiatry, 33*, 202–206.

Praag, H. M. van (1992). Reconquest of the subjective. Against the waning of psychiatric diag-nosis. *British Journal of Psychiatry, 160*, 266–271.

Raven, P., Mullen, R., & Clapstick, C. (1992). The meaning of insight (letter). *British Journal of Psychiatry, 161*, 717.

Schmand, B. A. (1992). *The energetics of cognition in psychosis*. Ph.D. thesis. Utrecht: Rijksuniversiteit.

Selten, J.-P. (1990). Schizofrenie en anosognosie. [Schizophrenia and anosognosia]. In J.-P. Selten (Ed.), *Proceedings of the conference Sociale Aspecten van Schizofrenie* (p. 7), The Hague, The Netherlands.

Selten, J.-P., Sijben, A. E. S., Bosch, R. J. van den, Omloo-Visser, H. I., & Warmerdam, H. (1993). The subjective experience of negative symptoms: A self-rating scale. *Comprehensive Psychiatry, 34,* 1–6.

Sontag, S. (Ed.). (1988). *Antonin Artaud: Selected writings.* Berkeley: University of California Press.

Strauss, J. S. (1989). Subjective experiences of schizophrenia: Toward a new dynamic psychiatry II. *Schizophrenia Bulletin, 15,* 179–187.

Süllwold, L., & Huber, G. (1986). *Schizophrene Basisstörungen.* Berlin: Springer.

Thurm, I., & Häfner, H. (1987). Perceived vulnerability, relapse risk and coping in schizophrenia. An explorative study. *European Archives of Psychiatry and Neurological Sciences, 237,* 46–53.

Wing, J. K., Cooper, J. E., & Sartorius, N. (1974). *The measurement and classification of psychiatric symptoms.* Cambridge: Cambridge University Press.

# 6

JUDITH E. KIERSKY

# Insight, Self-Deception, and Psychosis in Mood Disorders

The most widely used clinical assessment of insight takes place during the Mental Status Exam (MSE; Talbott, Hales, & Yudofsky, 1988). When psychiatric patients are interviewed, insight is typically assessed by determining "if the patient realizes that he is ill and the problem is in his own mind" (MacKinnon & Yudofsky, 1986). Much of the empirical work in this area, found primarily in the literature on schizophrenia, has approached the subject of insight from this perspective—that is, narrowly defined as the patient's *perception of illness.*

However, a broader perspective on insight can also be found. Traditionally, a defining feature of mental health has been the capacity for accurate perceptions of the self, the environment, and the future—that is, insight as defined by a global capacity for realistic thinking. Although it has received little empirical validation, this view is strongly held among mental health professionals, particularly those working with the major psychiatric disorders characterized by psychosis. The conventional wisdom with regard to the disorders of mood is consistent with this view. Commonly, mood disorders have been conceptualized as either due to, or characterized by, inaccurate, distorted, and self-punitive thinking (Beck, 1967, 1986; Seligman, et al., 1988). This chapter focuses on insight as it is broadly defined, and examines its role in the psychology of mood, particularly depression. Special attention is given to empirical work on *self-deception,* including its relation to the traditional view of insight in mental health, and to the problem of insight and psychosis.

## Insight, Self-Awareness Phenomena, and Mood

Surprisingly, a considerable body of psychological research points to disparities between the empirical data and our traditional formulation of mental health as defined by good insight and as exhibited in accurate and realistic thinking. Support has grown for the view that, in relation to mood disorders, retention of insight may be characteristic of psychopathology, while inaccurate or distorted perceptions may be associated with normal functioning (see Taylor & Brown, 1988 for a review). In light of these reports, the role that insight plays in the psychology of mood disorders seems to require a more complex model than the traditional view. A complex model would provide a framework for the study of multiple aspects of insight, their differential effects on the psychology of normal versus abnormal functioning, and their differential relations to the variety of mental disorders. These are among the issues that will be examined here.

A recent trend in the study of insight in the major psychiatric disorders has been to attempt to broaden the perspective from that of a focus on the patient's discrete awareness of the illness, to include a view of the patient's realistic (as in consensually validated) awareness of one's self in the environment. To that end, Marková and Berrios (1992) developed an insight scale for use with populations suffering from schizophrenia and depression. They proposed the incorporation of the more narrow concept of insight into the larger domain of self-knowledge. *Self-knowledge* is defined as a dynamic process that includes both the individual's awareness of how the illness affects them and how it affects their interaction with the world.

This attempt to broaden the concept of insight is also seen in studies of *self-awareness phenomena* in schizophrenia. Amador, Strauss, Yale, and Gorman (1991) identified four components common to published reports in this area: (1) awareness of the signs, symptoms, and consequences of illness; (2) general attributions about illness and specific attributions about symptoms and their consequences; (3) self-concept formation; and (4) psychological defensiveness. In mood disorders, and especially depression, although there is a paucity of research focused on the narrow concept of insight into illness, the broader domain of self-awareness phenomena and their relations to mood has been a burgeoning area of interest for over a decade.

The relations of self-awareness phenomena to mood were originally explored in a variety of studies of normal samples. These studies encompass a broad range of content, including studies of causal attributions, judgments of contingencies, expectancies, and self-schema. *Causal attribution* studies attempt to assess how one links an event to its causes. In much of this literature, attributions for the cause of an event are assessed multidimensionally as either internal, global and stable (e.g., based on an individual's abilities); or external, specific and unstable (e.g., based on serendipity or luck). For example, in generating theories about the causes of divorce, individuals are asked to evaluate how their own or their partner's attributes influence the outcome of their marriages (Kunda, 1987). In general, causal attribution studies have focused on viewing oneself in either a favorable or an unfavorable light following a success or failure (Kuiper, 1978; Raps, Reinhard, Peterson, Abramson, & Seligman, 1982; Ross & Fletcher, 1985; Sackeim & Wegner, 1986; Sweeney, Anderson, & Bailey, 1986).

Studies of *judgments of contingencies*, often referred to as illusions of control, attempt to assess the degree to which an outcome is perceived to be dependent on one's own response, as compared to other factors such as chance (e.g., Alloy & Abramson, 1979; Alloy & Clements, 1992; Crocker, 1982; Golin, Terrell, & Johnson, 1977; Miller & Ross, 1975). These studies are quite similar to *expectancy* studies, which investigate the mental representations of response-outcome contingencies—for example, this event is controlled by my skill, therefore it will have a favorable outcome. The focus in these studies is on the individual's judgment of his or her degree of control (e.g., Crocker, 1982; Langer, 1975; Miller & Seligman, 1973, 1976). An example comes from studies of gambling behavior, where subjects believe they are more likely to succeed when they throw the dice than when the dice are thrown by the croupier.

*Self-schema* evaluations often attempt to assess the conceptualizations and perceptions of oneself on a continuum from self-enhancing to self-deprecating (e.g., Alicke, 1985, Brown, 1986; Gotlib, 1983; Vestre & Caufield, 1986). Other terms used in the area of self-schema include positive-negative views of the self, ego fabrication, social perceptions, and optimistic biases.

Across these content areas, research has consistently linked the quality of self-awareness to individual differences in mood. Distortions in self-awareness, as exhibited by overly positive judgments and perceptions, are associated with positive mood states. In contrast, so-called insight, or more realistic and accurate views of the self, have been linked to depressive states. In some special cases, a link has also been seen between depressed mood and negative distortions in self-awareness (see Alloy & Abramson, 1988; Taylor & Brown, 1988, for reviews). What has become increasingly clear is that self-awareness, or insight as more broadly defined, is multidimensional, with various aspects seeming to be differentially related to mood.

The more accurate perceptions, even-handed judgments, and unbiased self-awareness among dysphoric individuals have been termed *depressive realism* (Mischel, 1979). In contrast, the tendency toward overly optimistic and inaccurate perceptions in self-awareness has been referred to as *self-serving biases* (Taylor & Brown, 1988) or as *self-deception* (Fingarette, 1969; Gardiner, 1970; Kiersky, 1992; Sackeim, 1988; Sartre, 1943/1958). Research on self-deception has raised concerns about our traditional formulations of psychological processes—for example, insight as always reflecting healthy thinking, and has raised new conceptions about the role of such processes in mood regulation and mood disorders.

## Research on Self-Deception

### Definition and Operationalization of Terms

The concept of self-deception has been defined as a selective and motivated lack of awareness of psychologically meaningful, self-referential material (Fingarette, 1969; Gardiner, 1970; Sackeim, 1988; Sackeim & Gur, 1978; Sartre, 1943/1958). It has been suggested that self-deception may constitute a pervasive form of optimistic bias in self-awareness (Kiersky, 1992). This differs from the concept of poor insight discussed in the literature on schizophrenia, where poor insight is narrowly defined as a specific lack of awareness of illness and its effects. In self-deception, the lack of awareness is often thought to be global, incorporating broad domains of self-relevant psychological content. Further, some formulations of self-deception emphasize a motivational component, deemphasized in the research on insight in schizophrenia (Sackeim & Gur, 1978).

Sackeim and Gur (1978; Gur & Sackeim, 1979) were the first to operationalize and offer an empirical model of self-deception. They listed four criteria as defining features of the concept (Sackeim & Gur, 1978):

1. The individual has two mental contents, which if expressed as propositions are contradictory (p and not-p).
2. These two mental contents occur simultaneously.
3. The individual is not aware of one of the mental contents.
4. The operation that determines which mental content is and which is not subject to awareness is motivated.

They distinguished between self- and other-deception and developed questionnaires to assess each construct. Other-deception was conceptualized as ordinary, conscious deceit, used to achieve a desired goal, such as impression management.

The original version of the Self-Deception Questionnaire (SDQ; Sackeim & Gur, 1978) contains 20 items based on psychoanalytic themes believed to be universally relevant and psychologically threatening. Sample items include: Have you ever felt hatred toward any of your parents? Do you ever feel attracted to people of the same sex? Do you have sexual fantasies? Have you ever enjoyed your bowel movements? Denial of the applicability of these items to oneself denoted instances of self-deception. Factor analyses of scores on a variety of validity scales designed to assess response biases have found that the SDQ and the Other-Deception Questionnaire (ODQ) provided the best measures of two orthogonal dimensions: self-deception and impression management (Paulhus, 1984; Paulhus & Reid, 1991).

The SDQ has been scored to tap a *denial* component and an *endorsement* component (Kiersky, 1992). Those high on the denial component (e.g., who disclaim having sexual fantasies or hatred toward parents) exhibit self-deception by their extreme disavowal of items applicable to themselves. Those high on the endorsement component (e.g., those who strongly claim to have sexual fantasies or express intense hatred toward parents) exhibit an absence of self-deception and/or a self-denigrating response style. This distinction has been shown to be important to our understanding of self-deception and its relations to the psychology of mood (Kiersky, 1992). Specifically, the use of denial was found to be a stable psychological dimension across both depressed and nondepressed mood states. Further, individuals who were subject to major depressive episodes evidenced abnormally low capacities to employ denial compared to those not vulnerable to depressions. In addition, the tendency to use a self-denigrating style, characterized by high scores on the endorsment dimension, was seen only in patients who reported being in a depressed state. It was not, however, found during periods when patients no longer reported being depressed. The differences in the relations between mood states and these two distinct aspects of self-awareness support the critical need for a complex, multidimensional model when assessing self-deceptive cognitive processes relevant to mental health and illness. These findings are explored further in the following sections.

## Empirical Studies of Self-Deception and Mood

Among college students, level of self-deception (as assessed by the SDQ) has been consistently inversely correlated with self-reported depression (Linden, Paulhus, & Dobson, 1986; Roth & Ingram, 1985; Roth & Rehm, 1980; Sackeim, 1983; Sackeim & Gur, 1979), with general psychopathology (Linden et al., 1986; Sackeim, 1983), and with physical symptoms (Linden et al., 1986). Greater self-deception was consistently associated with fewer or less severe symptoms. To account for these findings, the original hypothesis was that self-deceivers actually experienced the same degree of psychological distress as those who did not deceive themselves, but self-deceivers manifested a tendency to deny or minimize the symptoms (Sackeim & Gur, 1979). It was thought that these individuals were simply lying to themselves about their lack of symptoms. Subsequently, the possibility was raised that self-deception may, in fact, have an adaptive function, such as protecting against depression, and that reports of lesser symptomatology were valid (Sackeim, 1983; Taylor & Brown, 1988). Furthermore, there is initial evidence that individual differences in self-deception are correlated with other measures of self-serving biases, suggesting the possibility of multidimensional and global capacity for biased thinking (Paulhus & Reid, 1991). This global capacity for optimistic, self-serving biases appears to be positively associated with the lack of the manifestation of depressive symptoms.

There are, however, certain caveats. An important limitation of the studies on self-deception and mood has been the reliance on subjective reports of symptoms (Linden, et al., 1986; Roth & Ingram, 1985; Sackeim, 1983; Sackeim & Gur, 1979). In the absence of observer ratings, it has been impossible to determine whether self-deception is associated exclusively with *subjective* evaluations of psychopathology. In clinical samples, subjective versus objective ratings of depressive symptoms are often only modestly correlated (Sayer et al., 1993). There would be stronger support for the view that self-deception mediates the likelihood or severity of psychological distress if associations were also found with observer assessments.

Furthermore, only one study has addressed self-deception in a clinical sample using a control group. Winters and Neale (1985) studied patients following remission from an episode of either mania or depression, as compared to normal individuals. Their data suggested that greater self-deception was characteristic of patients who had recently recovered from a manic episode, with normal individuals and remitted depressives being equivalent. Since patients were evaluated only after remission of the affective episode, the extent to which self-deception was associated with clinical state, or the extent to which it reflected a more persistent process, could not be determined. This is an important issue in establishing whether abnormal levels of self-deception constitute a state versus a trait characteristic, or even some combination of both. Longitudinal studies are needed here.

Recently, the relations between self-deception and depression were explored in a longitudinal study of depressed inpatients (Kiersky, 1992). Self-deception and depression severity were assessed both prior to and following antidepressant treatment in patients, and at equivalent time-points in controls. Depression was measured using the most commonly used observer- and self-rating depression scales, the Hamilton Rating Scale for Depression (HRSD; Hamilton, 1967) and the Beck Depression Inventory

(BDI; Beck, Steer, & Garbin, 1988), respectively. It should be noted that only the HRSD has an item on insight, and there have been virtually no reports on its relations to other factors, dimensions of the phenomenology, or the psychology of depression.

Results of the study indicated that depressed patients exhibited less self-deception than normal individuals. A lack of self-deception was characteristic of both individuals who viewed themselves as depressed (i.e., as measured by the BDI) and individuals who were viewed as depressed by others (i.e., as measured by the HRSD). These findings support suggestions that the negative correlations between self-deception and self-reports of psychological distress (Linden et al., 1986; Roth & Ingram, 1985; Sackeim, 1983) or physical symptoms (Linden et al., 1986) are not simply the result of individuals high in self-deception failing to acknowledge their symptoms. Rather, the findings indicate that self-deception may serve an adaptive function, protecting against the development of depression (Alloy & Abramson, 1979; Greenwald, 1980; Sackeim, 1983; Taylor & Brown, 1988), or that depressive states result in a diminished capacity to self-deceive (Alloy, Abramson, & Viscusi, 1981).

Different aspects of self-deception were also found to be differentially related to subjective versus objective symptom reports. Specifically, patients rated by observers as most symptomatic had the lowest levels of the denial component. On the other hand, patients who strongly endorsed more psychologically threatening material (i.e., a self-denigrating style) rated themselves as most symptomatic. This pattern could not have come about if there was a strong association between the observer and self-report measures of depression. In psychiatric samples, it has been frequently noted that pretreatment correlations between observer rating and self-report depression measures often show only moderate correlations (e.g., Burrows, Davies, & Scoggins, 1972; Fitzgibbon, Cella, & Sweeney, 1988; Sayer et al., 1993; Schnurr, Hoaken, & Jarrett, 1976). These findings suggest that different aspects of self-deception—for example, denial versus endorsement components—may reflect different psychological processes that contribute to the discrepancies between self and observer rating scales.

## State and Trait Abnormalities

Different aspects of self-deception were also uniquely associated with changes in clinical state. The denial component was found to be stable across mood states, both when patients were depressed and when they were not. In contrast, the endorsement component showed change with clinical response, but only when symptoms were assessed by self-report. These findings suggest that in depression, both trait and state abnormalities in self-deception may be found, depending upon which aspect of self-deception is being assessed. Furthermore, the stability of some abnormalities in self-deception appears to be dependent on whether symptoms are subjectively or objectively assessed. This dissociation of the different aspects of self-deception makes it unlikely that the denial versus endorsement components reflect opposite ends of a single psychological dimension. Indeed, it appears that the strong endorsement of psychologically threatening material taps a dimension particularly linked to the phenomenological experience of depression or one that influences the self-report of that experience. In contrast, the absence of denial appears to be a trait particularly characteristic of those prone to depressive episodes.

Conceptually, a lack of denial might be considered a form of depressive realism, reflecting the absence of self-serving biases. The findings in this study support the view that at least some aspects of depressive realism are independent of affective state in patients subject to depression. Hypothetically, frequent strong endorsements of psychologically threatening material may be viewed as reflecting a self-denigrating or self-punitive bias (Alloy & Abramson, 1988; Beck, 1967; Sackeim & Wegner, 1986). Studies of clinical samples have shown that the attributions of depressed patients are often more even-handed than those of controls and/or that the depressed are more likely to manifest self-denigrating biases—for example, a lower threshold for blaming than praising the self (Raps et al., 1982; Rizley, 1978; Sackeim & Wegner, 1986). There has been considerable uncertainty about whether the self-serving biases characteristic of normal functioning, and the even-handed and self-denigrating attributions observed in studies of depressed patients, reflect modulation of the same psychological dimension, perhaps by the severity of depressive symptoms (Beck, 1986; Ruehlman, West, & Pasahow, 1985). The findings in this study suggested that denial is distinct from the strong endorsement of psychologically threatening material, and that they are differentially related to cross-sectional measures of depression and to change in clinical state. Therefore, the even-handed, as compared to the self-denigrating, attributional phenomena seen in depressed patients may also reflect distinct psychological processes.

The findings also highlighted the possibility that seeing abnormal attributions, attitudes, and other cognitive phenomena in depression as state-dependent or state-independent may depend on whether mood is assessed subjectively or objectively. In hindsight, it may not be surprising that findings of state-dependency may be particularly likely when using self-report assessment techniques. A denigrating or negativistic view of the self (Beck, 1967) might have greater influence on self-assessments of symptomatology compared to observer ratings. This issue is of particular concern in interpreting the results of analog studies, where typically the extent of state change is relatively small, there are few objective signs of mood alterations, and assessment is almost always based on self-report (Goodwin & Williams, 1982; Larsen & Sinnett, 1991).

*Prediction of Outcome*

The study also found in depressed patients a positive association between lack of self-deception (as seen specifically in frequent strong endorsements of threatening content) assessed prior to treatment and poor clinical outcome, as well as increased risk of relapse (Kiersky, 1992). It is noteworthy that the denial component did not exhibit consistent relations with clinical outcome, again suggesting that these two aspects of self-deception reflect distinct psychological processes with different implications in predicting outcome. The findings, then, did not support the prediction emanating from a series of studies in the 1950s on anosognosia of illness, in which individuals with so-called denial personalities had better clinical outcomes following somatic treatment for depression (Fink, 1979; Kahn, Pollack, & Fink, 1960; Weinstein, Kahn, Sugerman, & Malitz, 1954). Rather, in this study frequent strong endorsements, possibly reflecting a self-denigrating bias, were associated with poorer outcome. The clinical outcome findings were generally consistent across both subjective and objective symptom evaluations. This, as well as the relations to relapse, underscored the reliability of these phenomena.

These findings on self-deception suggested that a subgroup of patients with mood disorders who strongly endorse psychologically threatening material as characteristic of themselves (e.g., "I have wanted to rape or be raped very much") are particularly likely not to respond to some forms of treatment or, if they respond, to relapse. Since the relations of self-deception to clinical outcome have not been examined across the full range of treatment modalities, generalizability to different forms of treatment is uncertain. Notably, however, there is evidence that patients who, while in a depressed state, manifest certain types of negative biases in thinking—for example, high levels of dysfunctional, self-denigrating, and punitive attitudes—are particularly likely to be nonresponsive to either psychotherapy (Jarrett, Eaves, Grannemann, & Rush, 1991; Keller, 1983; Sotsky et al., 1991) or pharmacology (Peselow, Robins, Block, Barouche, & Fieve, 1990; Sotsky et al., 1991) and/or to have increased risk for relapse (Rush, Weissenburger, & Eaves, 1986; Simons, Murphy, Levine, & Wetzel, 1986). In contrast, individual differences in certain other forms of negative biases, such as in causal attributions (e.g., how unfavorably one views oneself following a success that can be attributed to either luck or skill, versus a failure that can be attributed to the inflexibility of either oneself or one's spouse) among depressed patients do not appear to be predictive of clinical outcome (Cutrona, 1983; Jarrett et al., 1991; Neimeyer & Weiss, 1990; Seligman et al., 1988). Establishing a positive link, then, between dysfunctional attitudes and a lack of self-deception as seen in strong negative endorsements would support the view that high levels of a self-denigrating bias during a depressive episode are predictive of inferior clinical outcome across many treatment modalities. This raises the possibility that high levels of a self-denigrating bias are characteristic of a treatment-resistant subgroup, who might be further distinguished on the basis of phenomenological or historical features and, perhaps, in terms of pathophysiology. Further study in this area is indicated.

Interestingly, in depression, a *lack of self-deception* has been associated with poor clinical outcome. However, in schizophrenia, if any relation is typically thought to exist, it is between a lack of insight and poor outcome. This seeming paradox may suggest that insight and self-deception have complex relations or even different roles in these disorders.

## Insight in Psychotic Depression and Its Relations to Self-Deception

Psychotic depression is most commonly characterized by the presence of delusions of guilt, somatic distress, paranoia, worthlessness, or nihilism. These delusions are almost invariably accompanied by other depressive symptoms, such as sleep and appetite disturbances, impaired concentration, and ruminations. Such patients have a low rate of response when treated with antidepressant medications alone, but respond at higher rates with the addition of antipsychotic medications or when treated with electroconvulsive therapy (Charney & Nelson, 1981). Although open to debate, psychotic depression has been classified as a discrete subtype of major depressive disorder based on these phenomenological and treatment response differences (Charney & Nelson, 1981; Glassman & Roose, 1981; Nelson and Bowers, 1978). This view is further supported by the putative differences reported in patterns of familial aggregation (Leckman et al.,

1984). My view is consistent with this thinking, and one in which psychotic depression has a unique relation to self-awareness phenomena.

Although the nature of delusions, including the dimension of so-called conviction or insight, has been studied in some depth in schizophrenia and related illnesses (e.g., Kendler, Glazer, & Morgenstern, 1983), this has not occurred in delusional depression. Standard self-report instruments for assessing depressive symptoms are noted as being of questionable validity when administered to delusionally depressed patients (Arfwidsson et al., 1974; Prusoff, Klerman, & Paykel, 1972; Snaith, Ahmed, Mehta, & Hamilton, 1971), and none assess insight into illness. The most popular objective rating of depression—the HRSD—does, however, inquire about the patient's awareness of illness. It is notable that of the standard HRSD items, insight has been reported to be among the poorest in terms of inter-rater and test-retest reliabilities, making its utility unclear (Potts, Daniels, Burnam, & Wells, 1990; Rehm & O'Hara, 1985; Williams, 1988). In a recent study of depressed inpatients by Sayer et al. (1993), in which 38% were diagnosed as psychotic, relatively few patients (less than 11%) lacked insight as assessed by observers. This supports the clinical truism that although psychotically depressed patients may lack discrete insight into the nature of their delusional beliefs, they often understand why they are hospitalized and the fact that they are experiencing a depressive episode. Furthermore, in major depression the presence of psychosis may be unrelated to the presence of a more general capacity for insight into or awareness of illness. For example, in the Sayer et al. study, there were no significant differences in insight item scores in the nonpsychotic and the psychotically depressed patient groups.

Of further interest is the finding by Sayer et al. (1993) that patients rated by observers as lacking insight subjectively reported less depressive symptoms. In light of the findings on self-deception, in which the endorsement component of self-deception was associated with less self-reported depressive symptoms, the findings by Sayer et al. are particularly intriguing. They suggest that in mood disorders there are links among poor insight into illness, greater use of self-deception, and subjective report of less symptoms.

Furthermore, similar to the absence of a relation between insight and psychosis in studies of depression by Sayer et al. (1993) and of schizophrenia by Amador et al. (1994), no relation was found by Kiersky (1992) between psychosis and self-deception. This suggests that in depression, nonpsychotic cognitive distortions are phenomenologically distinct from psychotic delusions. Indirectly, this supports the view that, psychologically, delusional depression is a distinct entity in which lack of insight into delusional beliefs is pathological, while in nondelusional depression, poor insight in the form of higher levels of self-deception may contribute to lesser symptomatology. By this account, the view that insight in and of itself is healthy and distortions in and of themselves are pathological is no longer supportable, as has been traditionally held.

## Conclusions

Relations between self-awareness phenomena (e.g., self-deception and insight) and psychopathology are not straightforward. Much of the traditional thinking regarding mental health views self-deception and poor insight as pathological. Emanating from this assumption, many forms of psychotherapy identify the correction of distorted thinking as the active therapeutic agent (e.g., Beck, 1986).

The literature on self-deception challenges these traditional views. Across both clinical and normal populations, greater use of self-deception appears to be characteristic of less depression and better mental health. This relation may be unique to depressive mood states and depressive mood disorders. Indeed, preliminary evidence suggests that, even in remission, manic patients characteristically exhibit more self-deception. Similarly, it is clear that some depressed patients are delusional, where delusions are defined by a lack of insight into unusual mental content. This suggests complex relations among the capacity for self-deception, insight, and various forms of psychopathology.

Further, insight, self-deception, and the variety of self-serving or self-denigrating biases may not be unitary phenomena. We have seen that the subjective experience of depressive states is particularly associated with the extent to which the individual endorses psychologically threatening, even self-denigrating, material. In contrast, denial is uniquely associated with observer assessments of depression.

At yet another level of complexity, self-deception and other self-serving biases in self-awareness appear to be characterized by both state-dependent and state-independent processes. The endorsement, or self-denigrating, component of self-deception has been shown to be associated with change in mood state, and seems to signal in depressed individuals a lack of capacity to recover and remain well following treatment. In contrast, the denial component has been shown to remain stable regardless of mood state, and may reflect a more enduring personality trait. Denial, and possibly other state-independent self-serving processes, may protect the healthy individual from depressive episodes. When deficient, they may leave the individual depression-prone. Whether the lack of denial as a trait characteristic predates the manifestation of illness or this deficit is acquired following the experience of one or more episodes is open to question. However, it appears that self-deception, and denial in particular, has the potential as a vulnerability marker. Individuals low in the denial component may lack a self-regulatory capacity that, in healthy individuals, is protective against depressive mood states.

Overall, in mood states and mood disorders, the self-awareness phenomena discussed here may be seen conceptually as lying on a continuum. At one end are the self-denigrating attributions associated with severe depressive symptoms. Insight or realistic thinking, known as depressive realism, is next, and is associated with mild to moderate depression. High levels of self-deception are found on the opposite end, in which individuals deny the negative and enhance the positive. This is associated with psychological health and the capacity for normal mood regulation. Furthermore, this continuum may be independent of psychotic processes.

It is clear that traditional perspectives equating realistic and even-handed thinking with psychological health are untenable. These perspectives have been contradicted by a large body of data. It is also clear that we are at only the threshold of developing empirically based explanatory models of the interplay between self-awareness phenomena and mood. Such models may prove critical in designing more effective treatments, as we now know that there are intimate relations between the quality of our self-awareness and our moods.

*References*

Alicke, M. D. (1985). Global self-evaluation as determined by the desirability and controllability of trait adjectives. *Journal of Personality and Social Psychology, 49,* 1621–1630.

Alloy, L. B., & Abramson, L. Y. (1979). Judgment of contingency in depressed and nondepressed students: Sadder but wiser? *Journal of Experimental Psychology: General, 108,* 441–485.

Alloy, L. B., & Abramson, L. Y. (1988). Depressive realism: Four theoretical perspectives. In L. B. Alloy (Ed.), *Cognitive processes in depression* (pp. 223–265). New York: Guilford Press.

Alloy, L. B., & Clements, C. M. (1992). Illusion of control: Invulnerability to negative affect and depressive symptoms after laboratory and natural stressor. *Journal of Abnormal Psychology, 101,* 234–245.

Alloy, L. B., Abramson, L. Y., & Viscusi, D. (1981). Induced mood and the illusions of control. *Journal of Personality and Social Psychology, 41,* 1129–1140.

Amador, X. F., Strauss, D. H., Yale, S. A., & Gorman, J. M. (1991). Awareness of illness in schizophrenia. *Schizophrenia Bulletin, 17*(1), 113–132.

Amador, X. F., Andreasen, N. C., Flaum, M., Strauss, D. H., Yale, S. A., Clark, S., & Gorman, J. M. (1994). Awareness of illness in schizophrenia, schizoaffective, and mood disorders. *Archives of General Psychiatry, 51,* 826–836.

Arfwidsson, L., d'Elia, G., Laurell, B., Ottosom, J. O., Perris, C., & Persson, G. (1974). Can self-rating replace doctor's rating in evaluating anti-depressive treatment? *Acta Psychiatrica Scandinavica, 50,* 16–22.

Beck, A. T. (1967). *Depression: Clinical, experimental, and theoretical aspects.* New York: Harper & Row.

Beck, A. T. (1986). Cognitive therapy, behavior therapy, psychoanalysis, and pharmacotherapy: The cognitive continuum. In J. B. W. Williams, & R. L. Spitzer (Eds.), *Psychotherapy research: Where are we and where should we go?* (pp. 114–134). New York: Guilford.

Beck, A. T., Steer, R. A., & Garbin, M. G. (1988). Psychometric properties of the Beck Depression Inventory: Twenty-five years of evaluation. *Clinical Psychology Review, 8,* 77–100.

Brown, J. D. (1986). Evaluations of self and others: Self-enhancement biases in social judgments. *Social Cognition, 4,* 353–376.

Burrows, G. D., Davies, B., & Scoggins, B. A. (1972). Plasma concentration of nortriptyline and clinical response in depressive illness. *The Lancet, 2,* 619–623.

Charney, D. S., & Nelson, J. C. (1981). Delusional and nondelusional unipolar depression: Further evidence for subtypes. *American Journal of Psychiatry, 138*(3), 328–333.

Crocker, J. (1982). Biased questions in judgment of covariation studies. *Personality and Social Psychology Bulletin, 8,* 214–220.

Cutrona, C. E. (1983). Causal attributions and perinatal depression. *Journal of Abnormal Psychology, 92,* 161–172.

Fingarette, H. (1969). *Self-deception.* London: Routledge & Kegan Paul.

Fink, M. (1979). *Convulsive therapy: Theory and practice.* New York: Raven Press.

Fitzgibbon, M. L., Cella, D. F., & Sweeney, J. A. (1988). Redundancy in measures of depression. *Journal of Clinical Psychology, 44,* 372–374.

Gardiner, P. L. (1970). Error, faith, and self-deception. *Proceedings of the Aristotelian Society, 50,* 221–243.

Glassman, A. H., & Roose, S. P. (1981). Delusional Depression: A distinct clinical entity? *Archives of General Psychiatry, 38,* 424–427.

Golin, S., Terrell, F., & Johnson, B. (1977). Depression and the illusion of control. *Journal of Abnormal Psychology, 86,* 440–442.

Goodwin, A. M., & Williams, J. M. (1982). Mood-induction research — Its implications for clinical depression. *Behavioral Research Therapy, 20,* 373–382.

Gotlib, I. H. (1983). Perception and recall of interpersonal feedback: Negative bias in depression. *Cognitive Therapy and Research, 7*, 399–412.

Greenwald, A. G. (1980). The totalitarian ego: Fabrication and revision of personal history. *American Psychologist, 35*, 603–618.

Gur, R. C., & Sackeim, H. A. (1979). Self-deception: A concept in search of a phenomenon. *Journal of Personality and Social Psychology, 37*, 147–169.

Hamilton, M. (1967). Development of a rating scale for primary depressive illness. *British Journal of Social and Clinical Psychology, 6*, 278–296.

Jarrett, R. B., Eaves, G. G., Grannemann, B. D., & Rush, A. J. (1991). Clinical, cognitive, and demographic predictors of response to cognitive therapy for depression: A preliminary report. *Psychiatry Research, 37*, 245–260.

Kahn, R. L., Pollack, M., & Fink, M. (1960). Social attitude (California F Scale) and convulsive therapy. *Journal of Nervous and Mental Disease, 130*, 187–192.

Keller, K. E. (1983). Dysfunctional attitudes and the cognitive therapy for depression. *Cognitive Therapy and Research, 7*(5), 437–444.

Kendler, K. S., Glazer, W. M., & Morgenstern, H. (1983). Dimensions of delusional experience. *American Journal of Psychiatry, 140*(4), 466–469.

Kiersky, J. E. (1992). Self-deception and its relations to affective states. *Social Work Research and Abstracts, 28*(3). University Microfilms No. 3 517-377.

Kuiper, N. A. (1978). Depression and causal attributions for success and failure. *Journal of Personality and Social Psychology, 36*, 236–246.

Kunda, S. (1987). Motivated inference: Self-serving generations and evaluation of causal theories. *Journal of Personality and Social Psychology, 53*(4), 636–647.

Langer, E. J. (1975). The illusion of control. *Journal of Personality and Social Psychology, 132*(2), 311–328.

Larsen, R. J., & Sinnett, L. M. (1991). Meta-analysis of experimental manipulations: Some factors affecting the Velten mood induction procedure. *Personality and Social Psychology Bulletin, 3*, 323–334.

Leckman, J. F., Weissman, M. M., Prusoff, B. A., Caruso, K. A., Merikangas, K. R., Pauls, D. L., & Kidd, K. K. (1984). Subtypes of depression. *Archives of General Psychiatry, 41*, 833–838.

Linden, W., Paulhus, D. L., & Dobson, K. S. (1986). The effects of response styles on the report of psychological and somatic distress. *Journal of Consulting and Clinical Psychology, 54*, 309–313.

MacKinnon, R. A., & Yudofsky, S. C. (1986). *The Psychiatric Evaluation in Clinical Practice.* Philadelphia: J. B. Lippincott Company.

Marková, I. S., & Berrios, G. E. (1992). The assessment of insight in clinical psychiatry: A new scale. *Acta Psychiatrica Scandinavica, 86*, 159–164.

Miller, D. T., & Ross, M. (1975). Self-serving biases in attribution of causality: Fact or fiction? *Psychological Bulletin, 82*, 213–225.

Miller, W. R., & Seligman, M. E. P. (1973). Depression and the perception of reinforcement. *Journal of Abnormal Psychology, 82*, 62–73.

Miller, W. R., & Seligman, M. E. P. (1976). Learned helplessness, depression, and the perception of reinforcement. *Behavior Research and Therapy, 14*, 7–17.

Mischel, W. (1979). On the interface of cognition and personality: Beyond the person-situation debate. *American Psychologist, 34*, 740–754.

Neimeyer, R. A., & Weiss, M. E. (1990). Cognitive and symptomatic predictors of outcome of group therapies for depression. *Journal of Cognitive Psychotherapy, 4*(1), 23–32.

Nelson, J. C., & Bowers, Jr., M. B. (1978). Delusional Unipolar Depression; Description and Drug Response. *Archives of General Psychiatry, 35*, 1321–1328.

Paulhus, D. L. (1984). Two-component models of socially desirable responding. *Journal of Personality and Social Psychology, 46,* 598–609.

Paulhus, D. L., & Reid, D. B. (1991). Enhancement and denial in socially desirable responding. *Journal of Personality and Social Psychology, 60,* 307–317.

Peselow, E. D., Robins C., Block, P., Barouche, F., & Fieve, R. R. (1990). Dysfunctional attitudes in depressed patients before and after clinical treatment and in normal control subjects. *American Journal of Psychiatry, 147*(4), 439–444.

Potts, M. K., Daniels, M., Burnam, M. A., & Wells, K. B. (1990). A structured interview version of the Hamilton Depression Rating Scale: Evidence of reliability and versatility of administration. *Journal of Psychiatric Research, 24,* 335–350.

Prusoff, B. A., Klerman, G. L., & Paykel, E. S. (1972). Concordance between clinical assessments and patients' self-report in depression. *Archives of General Psychiatry, 26,* 546–552.

Raps, C. S., Reinhard, K. E., Peterson, C., Abramson, L. Y., & Seligman, M. E. P. (1982). Attributional style among depressed patients. *Journal of Abnormal Psychology, 91,* 102–108.

Rehm, L. P., & O'Hara, M. W. (1985). Item characteristics of the Hamilton Rating Scale for Depression. *Journal of Psychiatric Research, 19,* 31–41.

Rizley, R. (1978). Depression and distortion in the attribution of causality. *Journal of Abnormal Psychology, 87,* 32–48.

Ross, M., & Fletcher, G. J. O. (1985). Attribution and social perception. In G. Lindzey & E. Aronson (Eds.), *The handbook of social psychology* (pp. 73–122). Reading, MA: Addison-Wesley.

Roth, D. L., & Ingram, R. E. (1985). Factors in the self-deception questionnaire: Associations with depression. *Journal of Personality and Social Psychology, 48,* 243–251.

Roth, D., & Rehm, L. P. (1980). Relationships among self-monitoring processes, memory, and depression. *Cognitive Therapy and Research, 4,* 149–157.

Ruehlman, L. S., West, S. G., & Pasahow, R. J. (1985). Depression and evaluative schemata. *Journal of Personality, 53,* 46–92.

Rush, A. J., Weissenburger, J., & Eaves, G. (1986). Do thinking patterns predict depressive symptoms? *Cognitive Therapy and Research, 10,* 225–236.

Sackeim, H. A. (1983). Self-deception, self-esteem, and depression: The adaptive value of lying to oneself. In J. Masling (Ed.), *Empirical studies of psychoanalytic theories* (pp. 101–157). Hillsdale, NJ: Erlbaum.

Sackeim, H. A. (1988). Self-deception: A synthesis. In J. S. Lockard, & D. L. Paulhus (Eds.), *Self-deception: An adaptive mechanism* (pp. 146–165). New Jersey: Prentice Hall.

Sackeim, H. A., & Gur, R. C. (1978). Self-deception, self-confrontation, and self-consciousness. In G. E. Schwartz, & D. Shapiro (Eds.), *Consciousness and self-regulation* (pp. 139–197). New York: Plenum Press.

Sackeim, H. A., & Gur, R. C. (1979). Self-deception, other deception, and self-reported psychopathology. *Journal of Consulting and Clinical Psychology, 47,* 213–215.

Sackeim, H. A., & Wegner, A. (1986). Attributional patterns in depression and euthymia. *Archives of General Psychiatry, 43,* 553–560.

Sartre, J. P. (1943/1958). Being and nothingness: an essay on phenomenological ontology (H. Barnes, Trans.). London: Methuen.

Sayer, N. A., & Sackeim, H. A., Moeller, J. R., Prudic, J., Devanand, D. P., Coleman, E., & Kiersky, J. E. (1993).The relations between observer-rating and self-report of depressive symptomatology. *Psychological Assessment, 5,* 350–360.

Schnurr, R. Hoaken, P. C. S., & Jarrett, F. J. (1976). Comparison of depression inventories in a clinical population. *Canadian Psychiatric Association Journal, 21,* 473–476.

Seligman, M. E. P., Castellon, C., Cacciola, J., Schulman, P., Luborsky, L., Ollove, M., &

Downing, R. (1988). Explanatory style change during cognitive therapy for unipolar depression. *Journal of Abnormal Psychology, 97*(1), 13–18.

Simons, A. D., Murphy, G. E., Levine, J. L., & Wetzel, R. D. (1986). Cognitive therapy and pharmacotherapy for depression: Sustained improvement over one year. *Archives of General Psychiatry, 43*, 43–48.

Snaith, R. P., Ahmed, S. N., Mehta, S., & Hamilton, M. (1971). Assessment of severity of primary depressive illness. *Psychological Medicine, 1*, 143–149.

Sotsky, S. M., Glass, D. R., Shea, M. T., Pilkonis, P. A., Collins, J. F., Elkin, I., Watkins, J. T., Imber, S. D., Leber, W. R., Moyer, J., & Oliveri, M. E. (1991). Patient predictors of response to psychotherapy and pharmacotherapy: Findings in the NIMH treatment of depression collaborative research program. *American Journal of Psychiatry, 148*, 997–1008.

Sweeney, P. D., Anderson, K., & Bailey, S. (1986). Attributional style in depression: A meta-analytic review. *Journal of Personality and Social Psychology, 50*, 974–991.

Talbott, J. A., Hales, R. E., & Yudofsky, S. C. (1988). *Textbook of Psychiatry*. Washington, DC: American Psychiatric Press.

Taylor, S. E., & Brown, J. D. (1988). Illusion and well-being: A social psychological perspective on mental health. *Psychological Bulletin, 103*, 193–210.

Vestre, N. D., & Caulfield, B. P. (1986). Perception of neutral personality descriptions by depressed and nondepressed subjects. *Cognitive Therapy and Research, 10*, 31–36.

Weinstein, E. A., Kahn, R. L., Sugerman, L. A., & Malitz, S. (1954). Serial administration of the "amytal test" for brain disease: Its diagnostic and prognostic value. *Archives of Neurology and Psychiatry, 71*, 217–226.

Williams, J. B. W. (1988). A structured interview guide for the Hamilton Depression Rating Scale. *Archives of General Psychiatry, 45*, 742–747.

Winters, K. C., & Neale, J. M. (1985). Mania and low self-esteem. *Journal of Abnormal Psychology, 94*, 282–290.

# PART II

# Neuropsychology
## of
## Insight

## 7

WILLIAM B. BARR

# Neurobehavioral Disorders of Awareness and their Relevance to Schizophrenia

Clinicians working in neurological settings have long observed that patients with acquired brain dysfunction may exhibit a range of peculiar disturbances of awareness and insight. Some patients may vehemently deny the presence of severe neurological symptoms while others may develop false beliefs about their immediate environment or those around them. Some of these behaviors have such a bizarre quality that patients may be erroneously diagnosed with a psychotic disorder until the results of a complete neurological workup reveal the presence of an acute brain disturbance. The purpose of this chapter is to describe a number of these unusual neurological conditions and discuss their relevance to our understanding of alterations in awareness and insight in schizophrenia.

This chapter is written from a neurobehavioral perspective. A strong emphasis is placed on case descriptions and research coming from the neurological literature. The first section will include a review of the literature on various neurological syndromes affecting awareness. The term *syndrome* is used loosely in this context to refer to a combination of signs or symptoms that enables one to make inferences about pathological mechanisms underlying the behavior (Benton, 1977). *Anosognosia* is a term that is often used to describe a syndrome where a patient exhibits unawareness of the presence of a particular neurological disorder or a specific symptom. By *unawareness*, we are referring to a lack of knowledge of the symptoms, even when confronted with them. The chapter will include descriptions of anosognosia and a number of neurobehavioral syndromes reflecting unawareness of an acute motor or sensory deficit.

One of the purposes of this chapter is to discuss the neurological aspects of psychosis. Therefore, the chapter will also include descriptions of neurological syndromes featuring the presence of delusions or hallucinations. These syndromes are often characterized by erroneous beliefs about the identity of people or places. The third class of disorders will include a wide range of behavioral disturbances that affect awareness in both a global and a specific manner. These disorders have been well described in the literature and are popularly referred to as part of the frontal lobe syndrome. All of these disturbances are characterized by rather unusual behavior that, if seen in a different context, may be misclassified as symptoms of thought disorder. They also reflect a lack of what is typically termed *insight*. In this context, the term is used to describe a change in attitude resulting in an understanding of the presence of the symptom and the factor that has caused it. A factor that is common to all of these syndromes is that they often result from discrete brain disturbances that can be identified by standard neuroimaging procedures or other neurodiagnostic techniques. It is proposed that, although these syndromes may be varied in their presentation and in the nature of their pathology, they may represent a disturbance of similar cognitive and neuroanatomic mechanisms.

The second section of this chapter will review some of the theories that have been used to describe neurologically based awareness syndromes. Theories developed in the clinical literature have emphasized the role of critical brain regions, such as the right parietal lobe, in the manifestation of various conditions affecting awareness. More recently, a renewal of interest in these phenomena has lead to the development of new theories. Some of the reasons for this renewed interest have included the increasing role of self-awareness in theoretical accounts of consciousness and cognition, as well recognition that deficits in awareness often provide a significant obstacle in the rehabilitation of brain-damaged individuals (Bauer & Addeo, 1993). Perhaps the greatest source of interest in the study of awareness deficits has resulted from developments in the field of neuropsychology. A number of neuropsychological theories have attempted to integrate previous neuroanatomic findings with theories drawn from experimental literature in cognitive psychology.

The recent surge of interest in awareness has also extended to the study of schizophrenia. Many patients with a diagnosis of schizophrenia are known to have poor insight into the details of their illness and its effects on their lives. It has been suggested that awareness of illness has important implications for the diagnosis and treatment of schizophrenia (Amador, Strauss, Yale, & Gorman, 1991). Previously, lack of insight in schizophrenia was studied within a psychodynamic framework where it was conceptualized as a primarily defensive maneuver. More recently, with a growing interest in the study of schizophrenia from a biological perspective, it has been suggested that lack of insight may be a direct result of some of the brain abnormalities that are now known to characterize schizophrenia (Amador et al., 1991). The last section of this chapter will include a brief review of the neuropsychological impairments that have been described in schizophrenic patients. The impairments associated with schizophrenia will be compared and contrasted to those seen as a result of other brain disorders. It will be argued that further understanding of the brain mechanisms responsible for the lack of insight in schizophrenia may lead to a greater understanding of the pathophysiology and etiology of the disorder.

## Neurobehavioral Disturbances of Awareness and Insight

### Anosognosia

For over a century, neurologists have described patients with significant difficulties in motor abilities, vision, language, and various other cognitive functions who are totally unaware of their impairments. Over the years, these phenomena have been variably attributed to the direct effects of focal or diffuse brain dysfunction or to the emergence of psychological defense mechanisms aimed at blocking the presence of these symptoms from consciousness. There have been a number of excellent reviews on these phenomena (Fisher, 1970; McGlynn & Schacter, 1989; Prigatano & Schacter, 1991; Weinstein & Kahn, 1955). This section will briefly describe these syndromes characterized by altered awareness of a variety of primary motor or sensory disturbances. Disorders involving unawareness of aphasic or amnestic deficits will not be covered in this discussion, although the clinical and theoretical importance of these conditions is not denied.

Joseph Francois Félix Babinski is generally regarded as having introduced *anosognosia* to describe a denial of motor impairment (Babinski, 1914). Over the years, there has been some misunderstanding about whether anosognosia refers specifically to a lack of awareness of distinct symptoms such as left hemiplegia or left hemianopsia or a lack of knowledge or failure to recognize one's disease in general. Today, the term is often used synonymously with the terms *unawareness of deficits, lack of insight,* and *imperception of disease* to refer to a rather nonspecific lack of awareness of illness or neuropsychological impairment (McGlynn & Schacter, 1989).

The range of terms used to describe symptoms associated with anosognosia are described in table 7.1. As with most neurobehavioral syndromes, it has been observed that unawareness deficits are rarely seen as "all or none" phenomena, but rather are observed on a continuum of severity. Most of these disorders are seen as the result of focal neurological impairment. They are observed rarely in patients with traditional psychotic conditions such as schizophrenia, though dissociations between neurological and psychotic forms of unawareness have never been reported (David, Owen, & Förstl, 1993).

The vast majority of awareness syndromes described in the classical neurological literature involve a disturbance of the ability to detect an acute impairment in motor function. Lhermitte (1939) separated anosognosia into two components. These include classic anosognosia (denial of the hemiplegia) and *anosodiaphoria* (indifference to the hemiplegia). It is well known that symptoms of classic anosognosia are observed almost exclusively in response to the left hemiplegia resulting from focal lesions in the right cerebral hemisphere. Babinski (1914) specified that the lack of awareness in these patients was observed without the loss of general intellectual capacities. It was also seen specifically for some symptoms and not others. For example, one patient denied the existence of her left-side weakness, though she admitted having difficulties with backache and phlebitis. The clinician is typically unable to convince patients of the deficit, even in cases when they are confronted with situations requiring use of the hemiparetic limb. The patient may even accuse the clinician of attempting to fabricate the so-called impairment. The specificity of the symptoms combined with the rel-

TABLE 7.1    A Variety of Terms Used to Describe Symptoms of Anosognosia

| Term | Description | Reference |
| --- | --- | --- |
| 1. Disorders characterized by denial of motor and somatosensory impairment: | | |
|     A. "Classic" anosognosia | Denial of hemiplegia | Babinski (1914) |
|     B. Hemisomatognosia | Denial of unilateral hemiplegia | Lhermitte (1939) |
|     C. Anosodiaphoria | Indifference to hemiplegia | Babinski (1914) |
|     D. Verbal anosognosia | Denial explicitly in response to inquiry | Frederiks (1985a) |
| 2. Disorders characterized by denial of visual and auditory disorders: | | |
|     A. Anton's syndrome | Denial of cortical blindness Denial of cortical deafness | Anton (1898) |
| 3. Disorders characterized by denial of disorders of higher cognitive functions: | | |
| | Denial of amnesia or aphasia | McGlynn & Schacter (1989) |

ative preservation of intellect suggests that this syndrome is not the result of a generalized cognitive disturbance.

In addition to the disorders characterized by the patient's altered awareness of motor disability, there is a range of awareness syndromes that are the result of diminished ability to detect changes or abnormalities in sensory functions or receptive behavior. One of the major features of these disorders is that they are often confined to a single sensory modality.

There are numerous descriptions of disorders affecting awareness of visual and auditory defects. Unawareness of visual field disturbances (hemianopia) has been described by numerous authors (Critchley, 1953; Teuber, Battersby, & Bender, 1960). Cortical blindness is a condition that usually associated with bilateral occipital lesions (Bergman, 1957). Cortical deafness results from bilateral lesions in primary auditory regions (Goldstein, Brown, & Hollander, 1975; Mott, 1907). In most cases, patients are clearly aware of these acquired deficits (Aldrich, Alessi, Beck, & Gilman, 1987; Teuber et al., 1960). However, Anton's syndrome is a variant of cortical blindness characterized by an unawareness of the deficit (Anton, 1898; David et al, 1993; Förstl, Owen, & David, 1993). Patients with this condition may behave as if they are blind, but deny the condition when queried. For example, we saw one man who failed to respond to visual stimuli in his environment but stated that his vision would be fine if somebody would turn on the overhead lights. Brockman and von Hagen (1946) have described patients who developed paranoid delusions and hallucinations in association with cortical blindness.

### Disorders of Body Awareness

*Anosognosic Behavior Disorder*    Frederiks made an important distinction between *verbal anosognosia* and *anosognosic behavior disorder* (Frederiks, 1985a). While the first refers to the patient's explicit denial of the symptom in response to the examiner's query, the second refers to the patient's unusual reactions to the paralyzed half of the

TABLE 7.2    Disorders of Body Awareness

| Term | Description | Reference |
|---|---|---|
| 1. Anososgnosic Behavior Disorders: | | Fredericks (1985a) |
| A. Misoplegia | A "hatred" of affected limb | Critchley (1953) |
| B. Personification | Tendency to refer to the limb with endearing terms or nicknames | Juba (1949) |
| C. Nosoagnosic overestimation | An overestimation of the strength of weakened limb | Anastasopoulis (1961) |
| D. Kinesthetic hallucinations | A false belief that the limb is moving | Waldenstrom (1939) |
| 2. Body schema disorders: | | |
| A. Phantom limb | Perception of the presence of an amputated limb | Frederiks (1985a) |
| B. Phantom supernumerary limb | A sensation that another limb has evolved elsewhere | Critchley (1953) |
| C. Alien hand syndrome | Loss of volitional control of the contralateral hand | Bogen (1993) |
| D. Autotopagnosia | Loss of the ability to identify or name body parts | Pick (1908) |
| E. Macrosomatognosia | Experience body parts as abnormally large | Fredericks (1985a) |
| F. Microsomatognosia | Experience body parts as abnormally small | |
| G. Autoscopia | Experience of seeing oneself projected in external space | Lukianowicz (1958) |

body. A listing of terms used to describe these disorders is provided in Table 7.2. Frederiks considers verbal anosognosia to be a perceptual disorder while anosognosic behavior disorders are considered to be nonconscious disturbances that solely affect behavior (Frederiks, 1985a).

Anosognosic behavioral disorders may include rather bizarre reactions to the affected limb, characterized by beliefs that the affected body parts are no longer part of the self. Some authors describe these conditions as having a *quasipsychotic quality* (Bisiach, 1988). For example, some patients may develop paranoid delusions about the limb, whereas other patients may refer to their limbs by somewhat endearing terms or even give their limbs a nickname (Juba, 1949). One woman referred to her leg as "Fred" and her arm as "Little Fred" (Cutting, 1978). Some patients are known to confuse temporal elements by stating that their limb is not weak at the time of testing, though they will admit that its function may have been disturbed in the distant past (Weinstein & Kahn, 1955).

*Body Schema Disorders*    There are a range of other conditions involving alterations in body awareness that do not involve an explicit denial of disability. Many authors have combined these conditions with the syndromes described above and referred to them as *body-schema disorders* (Frederiks, 1985a). These are listed in the second half of table 7.2. Some of these disorders are characterized by a misperception of sensory information regarding one half of one's own body (Lhermitte, 1939). The most striking of these conditions are the phenomena that may occur following amputation of a limb or other body part. Patients experiencing a phantom limb may continue to perceive the presence of the missing limb, including pain, temperature, and all of the limb's spatial characteristics following the amputation (Frederiks, 1985b). Other conditions involve perceptual distortions about either the size or the location of various parts of the body.

Another unusual condition occurs when patients feel they do not have volitional control of one of their hands. This condition, known as the *alien hand syndrome*, is usually observed in the hand contralateral to a lesion of the mesial frontal region (Bogen, 1993; Goldberg, Mayer, & Toglia, 1981). The limb often behaves as if it "has a mind of its own." For example, patients have described experiences where the hand begins to unbutton their clothing inappropriately and without their awareness. Some patients may react to this condition by slapping or attempting to restrain the hand. Others may refer to it in third person, in a manner similar to that which is seen in patients exhibiting personification of their hemiplegic limbs.

### Brain Lesions Resulting in Disorders of Awareness

Most syndromes affecting awareness appear to be the result of right hemisphere lesions, though controversial cases of similar phenomena resulting from left hemisphere lesions have been reported (Denny-Brown & Banker, 1954; Olsen & Ruby, 1941; Paterson & Zangwill, 1944). Most authors agree that disorders affecting awareness of left hemiplegia are the result of lesions in the inferoparietal cortex of the right hemisphere (Gerstmann, 1942; Critchley, 1953). Others have emphasized the role of the thalamus and its disconnection from the frontal, temporal, and parietal cortices (Ives & Nielson, 1937; Spillane, 1942; Sandifer, 1946). Nielson proposed that syndromes characterized primarily by unawareness are the result of thalamic disconnection, while syndromes producing experiences of absent limbs are the result of lesions affecting the right thalamoparietal peduncle (Nielson, 1938). Feinberg, Haber, and Leeds (1990) supported these findings and stressed the role of lesions in the right supramarginal gyrus and posterior corona radiata in the expression of verbal asomatognosia.

Lesions resulting in Anton's syndrome typically require damage to the primary sensory region and more extensive disruption of secondary sensory zones that may be responsible for awareness of sensory input (Goldberg & Barr, 1991). Cortical blindness is often the result of bilateral lesions involving the primary visual areas including the striate cortices and geniculocalcarine pathways (Bergman, 1957). However, the visual variant of Anton's syndrome appears to be the result of more widespread lesions extending from primary visual areas to adjacent temporal and parietal association regions (Goldberg & Barr, 1991; Joynt, Honch, Rubin, & Trudell, 1984; Redlich & Dorsey, 1945; Von Monakow, 1905). Lesions resulting in the auditory variant of Anton's syndrome usually involve combined damage to the primary auditory regions and adjacent association areas (Earnest, Monroe, & Yarnell, 1977; Goldberg & Barr, 1991; Mesulam, 1985).

Phantom limbs are usually the result of peripheral nerve alterations resulting from amputation, though it has been suggested that they occur more often in left- than right-side amputees. These phenomena have also been reported following lesions in the parietal cortex (Head & Holmes, 1911; Hécaen, Penfield, Bertrand, & Malmo, 1956). It has been argued that no well-defined anatomical localization can be established for most other body schema disorders, since large, bilateral, diffuse cerebral lesions are often present in these cases (Frederiks, 1985b).

### Neurologically Based Delusions and Hallucinations

*Reduplicative Phenomena*    A number of bizarre delusional syndromes resulting from central nervous system (CNS) disorders have been described. The disorders reviewed in this section are characterized primarily by a derangement in the patient's insight. A listing of these disturbances is provided in table 7.3. A number of disorders have been identified, all characterized by a rather specific tendency to confuse identities. The behaviors exhibited by these patients have been given previous labels such as *misidentification symptoms, reduplicative phenomena,* and *confabulation* (Förstl, Almeida, Owen, Burns, & Howard, 1991; Alexander, Stuss, & Benson, 1979; Stuss, Alexander, Lieberman, & Levine, 1978). Most of these conditions involve delusions about the identities of people, places, or body parts. Weinstein and Kahn (1955) have also described a condition where patients exhibit a reduplication of time and may insist that they are currently children, though it is acknowledged that 60 years have passed since their childhood.

There are a number of conditions that involve striking delusions about the relation between self and others. In 1923, Capgras and Reboul-Lachaux described a 53-year-old woman who exhibited a delusional belief that her family and friends had been replaced by identical doubles (Capgras & Reboul-Lachaux, 1923). What is now termed *Capgras syndrome* has been linked to traditional psychiatric disorders (Berson, 1983), though there is ample evidence that many of the patients exhibit some form of brain abnormality (Alexander et al., 1979). Many cases of Capgras syndrome and its variants have been found to have confusional states resulting from toxic, metabolic, or posttraumatic causes (Morrison & Tarter, 1984; Weston & Whitlock, 1971).

A disorder characterized by fixed delusions about locations is commonly referred known as *reduplicative paramnesia* (Pick, 1903; Benson et al., 1976). In this condition, patients are certain that a particular location has been duplicated. For example, they may admit that they are in a hospital, though they may insist that the hospital has been moved across the street from where they live. The prevalent confusion regarding the location of hospitals in this disorder indicates that some aspect of disorientation or memory impairment related to the patient's condition is a major factor in this syndrome.

Delusional syndromes are also known to occur for perception of one's own body parts. Critchley (1953) has described patients who experience their hemiplegic limb as either peculiar or as not belonging to them. Others may develop the delusion that their limb actually belongs to another person; Gerstmann (1942) gave this behavior the label *somatoparaphrenia*. Patients with this disorder may insist that their arm belongs to somebody else who is in the bed with them. On some occasions, these patients may indicate that the limb belongs to themselves and others simultaneously.

There are numerous theories suggesting that delusional syndromes, especially Capgras syndrome, are the result of purely psychological factors (Berson, 1983). This was the result of many early reports suggesting that most of these patients had histories of psychosis and paranoid tendencies. More recently, the trend has been to describe the disorder in terms of neurobehavioral syndrome. It has now been suggested that neurological disorders can be demonstrated in as many as 40% of the patients with Capgras syndrome (Signer, 1987). Many recent studies show that Capgras syndrome is often the result of closed head injury or focal brain impairment (Silva, Leong, & Luong, 1989;

TABLE 7.3    Neurologically Based Delusions and Hallucinations

| Term | Description | Reference |
| --- | --- | --- |
| 1. Reduplicative phenomena: | | |
| A. Capgras syndrome | Delusional beliefs that other individuals are imposters | Capgras & Reboul-Lachaux (1923) |
| B. Fregoli syndrome | Insistence that others have undergone changes in appearance | Christodoulou (1976) |
| C. Intermetamorphosis | Belief that others have changed both their appearance and identity | Silva, Leong, & Luong (1989) |
| D. Subjective doubles | Patient believes that he/she has been replaced by doubles | Silva, Leong, & Luong (1989) |
| E. Reduplicative paramnesia | Delusional belief about an identity of a location | Benson, Gardner, & Meadows (1976) |
| F. Environmental reduplication | Insistence that the hospital bed is in the patient's home | Ruff & Volpe (1981) |
| G. Somatoparaphrenia | Belief that the patient's hemiplegic limb belongs to someone else | Gerstmann (1942) |
| 2. Delusional Syndromes | | Cummings (1985) |
| A. Simple Delusions | Belief that one is infested, that possessions have been stolen, or that a spouse has been unfaithful | |
| B. Complex Delusions | More detailed beliefs including erotomania, delusional jealousy, or grandiose delusions | |
| 3. Hallucinations | | Penfield & Rasmussen (1950) |
| A. Elementary Hallucinations | Visual phosphemes or clicking sounds | |
| B. "Formed" Hallucinations | Perception of faces or voices | |

Weston & Whitlock, 1971). It appears that many of these cases exhibit focal right-hemisphere lesions. Others have emphasized the combination of posterior and frontal lesions of the right cerebral hemisphere (Alexander et al., 1979).

Brain lesions associated with reduplicative paramnesia are similar in location to those associated with Capgras syndrome (Kapur, Turner, & King, 1988). As with Capgras syndrome, there is evidence of reduplicative paramnesias resulting from head injuries (Hakim, Verma, & Greiffenstein, 1988). Again, many authors have stressed the combination of right parietal and frontal lobe lesions (Benson et al., 1976; Kapur et al., 1988). As described previously, lesions causing perceptual alterations of body parts are located primarily in the right parietal cortex. Nielson (1938) stressed involvement of the right thalamoparietal peduncle in those disorders involving delusional symptoms. It appears that these conditions may also be the result of combined damage to the anterior and parietal systems of the right hemisphere.

## Delusions and Hallucinations

Cummings (1985) has provided an extensive review of other delusional syndromes resulting from neurological illness, ranging from simple to complex delusional states. Simple delusions may involve objects that are merely present in the immediate environment, such as intravenous tubes or other medical equipment. They appear to be the result of conditions affecting cognitive abilities in a fairly global manner, such as the dementia resulting from Alzheimer's disease. Levine and Grek (1984) have described similar phenomena in patients with right-hemisphere lesions superimposed on more generalized cerebral atrophy.

Complex delusions refer to those that are more common in psychiatric disorders, such as those involving Schneiderian first-rank symptoms or the grandiose delusions associated with manic episodes (Cummings, 1985). These delusions also frequently appear in neurological conditions affecting limbic structures and the basal ganglia (Cummings, 1985). More complex neurologically based delusions have also been described in some patients with temporal lobe epilepsy. Here again, phenomenological similarities between schizophrenia and temporal lobe epilepsy have been described (Slater, Beard, & Glitheroe, 1963; Davison & Bagley, 1969).

Hallucinations have also been reported as part of numerous neurological syndromes (Hecaen & Albert, 1978; Brown, 1988). It is well known that elementary hallucinations such as visual phosphemes or clicking sounds may result from lesions of the primary visual and auditory cortices. More complex or formed hallucinations, such as faces or voices, are known to result from lesions of the secondary cortical zones (Penfield & Rasmussen, 1950). These may include the bizarre experience of seeing "little people" (Lilliputian hallucinations) or the perception of animals, faces, or figures (Leroy, 1926; Lhermitte, 1951). Hecaen and colleagues have shown that complex visual hallucinations are equally likely to arise from either the right or left hemisphere, whereas auditory hallucinations are more likely to arise from the left hemisphere (Hecaen & Albert, 1978).

In contrast to the typical response to hallucinations resulting from psychotic disorders, patients with neurologically based hallucinations often know that the images are not real and may respond to the images with amusement or wonder (Brown, 1988). Patients exhibiting acute confusional states with hallucinations have been described following right parietal lobe lesions (Mesulam, Waxman, Geschwind, & Sabin, 1976; Peroutka, Sohmer, Kumar, Folstein, & Robinson, 1982). Lhermitte (1939) stressed upper brain stem pathology as the disturbance leading to peduncular hallucinations. Some authors have suggested that psychic phenomena resulting from brain tumors are not perceived as foreign to the patient. Instead, they appear to be more closely related to the patient's "wishes, anxieties, and neurotic complexes" (Mulder, Bickford, & Dodge, 1957).

## Disorders of Awareness Following Frontal Lobe Damage

Damage to prefrontal cortex (both dorsolateral and orbitofrontal) is known to produce a massive, devastating cognitive disturbance, of which the patient may be completely oblivious. The lack of patients' awareness of their impairment has been noted by numerous authors (Luria, 1980; Hecaen & Albert, 1978; Stuss & Benson, 1986; Gold-berg, Antin, Bilder, Gerstman, Hughes, & Mattis, 1989). This lack of awareness usually takes two forms, which may be seen simultaneously in the same patient. The first form is usually characterized by general apathy or a lack of concern. The second form involves a lack of awareness of specific deficits or errors that are seen in the patient's performance on a specific task. The first phenomenon has been labeled by Zaidel (1987) as an impairment in *global* error monitoring, while the second is seen as a deficit in *local* error monitoring. The parallels between these terms and the general and specific uses of the term anosognosia are obvious.

Patients with massive damage to prefrontal systems are notorious for their general lack of concern about their conditions and their implications for their lives. (Luria, 1980; Blumer & Benson, 1975; Goldberg et al., 1989). Such apathy and profound dis-regard for the severity of their situation sets frontal lobe patients apart from virtually every other category of brain-damaged populations. This particular set of behaviors is often associated with the orbitofrontal syndrome, known for the generally euphoric, unconcerned, happy-go-lucky attitude that is completely out of line with the severity of the patient's disability (Goldberg et al., 1989). This implausible attitude is often com-bined with patients' abilities to describe details regarding the changes in their lives that have resulted from their acquired brain impairment.

The terms *positive* and *negative* symptoms are well known in the field of schizo-phrenia (Crow, 1980; Andreasen, 1982a). It is important to remember that these terms originated in Hughlings-Jackson's classifications of symptoms resulting from epilepsy and other neurological syndromes (Taylor, 1932). Like schizophrenia and epilepsy, the classical descriptions of frontal lobe syndromes have been based on descriptions of pro-ductive or positive in contrast to deficit or negative symptoms. Perseveration, stereo-typic behavior, imitative behavior (echopraxia and echolalia), and field-dependent behavior are all positive symptoms that have been described in patients with prefrontal pathology (Luria, 1980; Stuss & Benson,1984; Goldberg & Costa, 1986). Local error monitoring is a phenomenon where the patient may exhibit one of these positive symp-toms and yet be totally unaware of its occurrence. Local error monitoring is also known to occur in situations where the patient actually knows the correct answer.

A common technique of eliciting perseveration in frontal lobe patients is to ask them to draw simple geometric forms following a rapid sequence of verbal commands (Luria, 1980; Goldberg & Tucker, 1979). Early in the sequence, patients are able to draw the correct forms, but as the sequence continues, these symbols become degraded by the properties of intervening stimuli and graphical perseverations develop (Goldberg & Tucker, 1979). These patients may continue to perseverate, completely unperturbed by their errors. This indifference to errors cannot be attributed to lack of knowledge of what the correct response should be, since earlier in the sequence the patients were drawing the same forms correctly. It can also be demonstrated that they can again draw the forms correctly as soon as the intervals between the verbal instructions in the sequence are increased.

A similar dissociation between the preserved knowledge of correct responses and the inability to use this knowledge to monitor one's own output can be demonstrated in frontal lobe patients' field-dependent behavior. Field-dependent motor behavior can be elicited by the *competing programs* technique, first described by Luria (1980). In this technique, two hand postures are introduced (e.g., one finger or two fingers). Patients are instructed to watch the examiner and do the opposite hand posture ("When I raise one finger, you raise two; when I raise two fingers, you raise one"). Patients with frontal lobe dysfunction will often give correct responses initially, but will then will slip into numerous echopraxic imitations of the examiner's postures. Their echopraxic imitation will often be accompanied by correct verbalizations such that, in response to the examiner's fist, they will say, "I know I am supposed to raise only one finger" but they will in fact raise two fingers. Here, too, the patient's indifference to his or her errors cannot be attributed to lack of knowledge of the correct response, since the patient could do the task correctly early in the sequence, can verbalize the correct response even as his or her actual motor output becomes echopraxic, and will be able to resume the correct response as soon as the interval between instructions is increased. This appears to be a genuine instance of an error-monitoring breakdown, in spite of the relatively intact knowledge of the correct response. In Prigatano and Schacter's (1991) terminology, the patient would be described as having intact objective awareness, but disturbed subjective awareness.

Perseveration can be conceptualized as an impairment of behavioral plasticity, or the ability to switch from one cognitive element to another. Field-dependent behavior, on the other hand, can be conceptualized as an impairment of behavioral stability, or the ability to maintain a stable cognitive set in the face of environmental distractors (Goldberg, 1990). These two types of impairment appear to be the fundamental components of the so-called executive syndrome caused by prefrontal dysfunction. Both are characterized by the patient's impaired awareness of his or her own errors in on-line situations, even when the knowledge of correct responses can be elicited (Goldberg & Barr, 1991).

## Theoretical Approaches to Disorders of Awareness and Insight

Many theories have been offered to explain disorders of awareness and insight resulting from cerebral lesions. The majority are extensions of observations initially made in the classic clinical literature. Some theories propose specific awareness functions that are disturbed as a result of focal brain lesions. Others argue that unawareness is merely the result of global intellectual impairment (Sandifer, 1946; Schilder, 1935). More recently, a number of neuropsychological theories have been proposed to explain disorders of awareness. These theories are distinguished from their predecessors by a reliance on explicit cognitive models. While this review is purposely biased toward theories emphasizing neuroanatomic and cognitive explanations of awareness syndromes, it is acknowledged that motivational factors play a significant role in many patients' abilities to acknowledge and recover from their neurological dysfunction.

### Neurobehavioral Theories

Most of the classical neurological literature has emphasized a link between awareness syndromes and disturbances of the right inferotemporal cortex and its connections to the thalamus and the frontal lobes. Many authors have described these syndromes as resulting from a disorder of an internal representation of the body, a construct that is usually termed as either the *body schema* or *body image* (Head & Holmes, 1911; Critchley, 1953; Fisher, 1970). Most theories consider the body schema to be a flexible entity that enables one to assess and adapt to changes in stimulation. It has been argued that lesions affecting the right parietal lobe essentially disconnect these representations from consciousness. Schilder (1935) labeled this process *organic repression*. Geschwind (1965) argued that awareness syndromes resulted from a disconnection of right-hemisphere body awareness mechanisms from left-hemisphere language regions. Some theories have emphasized a failure to integrate and synthesize polysensory input from the other side of the body (Denny-Brown & Chambers, 1958). Other theories have emphasized disturbances of the parietal cortex and its role of integrating exteroceptive and interoceptive stimuli (Mesulam, 1985).

Although no systematic neuroanatomical reviews have been conducted, several authors have commented that disorders affecting awareness of primary visual and auditory functions are most likely a result of widespread cerebral lesions extending from the primary sensory areas to adjacent parietal and temporal association cortices (Joynt et al., 1984; Von Monakow, 1905; Earnest et al., 1977). It has been argued that these phenomena are the result of a combined disturbance of the brain regions responsible for a particular sensory function and those regions responsible for providing feedback about the integrity of that function (Goldberg & Barr, 1991).

Some argument has resulted from what has been considered an integral link between awareness syndromes and disturbances of the nondominant right hemisphere. It is first argued that this link is not necessary, since comparable behavioral disturbances can be observed following left-hemisphere lesions (Denny-Brown & Banker, 1954). In a study of 100 consecutive patients with hemiplegia, Nathanson, Bergman, and Gordon (1952) reported that 28 showed evidence of denial of the disturbance. In these 28 patients, right-hemisphere lesions outnumbered left-hemisphere lesions by a ratio of 3:1. Anosognosia was found in 14% of the right-hemiplegics studied by Cutting (1978). Taken together, these results indicate that there is no absolute relationship between denial and left hemiplegia, though it is clear that the overwhelming majority of cases fit this pattern. Some authors have argued that the lack of left-hemisphere impaired patients with awareness disturbances is merely the result of a link between the left-hemisphere and disorders of language (Weinstein & Kahn, 1955). It is argued that a comparable number of left- and right-hemisphere lesion patients would exhibit awareness syndromes, except for the fact that the patients with left-hemisphere lesions are unable to communicate their symptoms verbally as a result of difficulties with language.

Alternatively, it has been proposed that the right-hemisphere bias is a result of that hemisphere's preferential role in arousal and attention (Heilman, Watson, & Valenstein, 1993; Mesulam, 1985). Heilman and colleagues have proposed that sensory inattention results from the subject's inability to be aroused to multimodal stimuli (Heilman et al., 1993). Lesions of the right parietal lobe may thus impair the subject's ability to determine the significance of a stimulus or detect changes in the internal or external environment. Mesulam proposed that the posterior regions of the right hemisphere are part of an integrated network responsible for attention and integration of sensory input (Mesulam, 1985). He argued that the right hemisphere may have a greater influence on the reticular activating system. Deficits in attentional tone would therefore be expected to be more substantial after right- than left-hemisphere lesions. Goldberg and Costa (1981) provided an outline of neuroanatomical evidence suggesting that the right hemisphere is characterized by greater areas of association cortex and a predominately interregional pattern of connections, when compared to the left. The authors hypothesize that these anatomic features enable the right hemisphere to be preferentially involved in tasks requiring intermodal integration and detection of novelty. It is possible that the link between right-hemisphere disturbances and awareness syndromes is the result of disorders in awareness mechanisms responsible for the ability to discern novelty or changes in motor, sensory, or higher-order cognitive functions.

A theoretical conception of the frontal lobe's role in awareness has been outlined by Stuss and Benson (1986). These authors provide a hierarchical model of frontal lobe functioning where a mechanism of *self-awareness* is considered the highest level of activity. In this model, the self-awareness mechanism is the means by which an individual monitors overall brain functioning and interacts with the environment. This mechanism is distinguished from other frontal executive functions involved in planning and sequencing complex behavior. Stuss and Benson argue that frontal lobe functions direct more basic fixed functional systems originating from more posterior-basal brain regions (Stuss & Benson, 1987). These operations include cognitive processes such as attention, memory, language, and perception. It can be argued that anosognosia and other hemi-awareness syndromes may be the result of a disturbance in the relationship between the self-awareness system and one or more of these posterior-basal operations. Likewise, the disorders of local error monitoring described in this chapter may be the result of a disturbance in the relationship between the self-awareness system and more hierarchically based executive systems.

The functions of cognitive self-monitoring and comparison of the outcome of one's cognitive operations with the objective at hand have been mentioned often in the literature as important elements of the executive controls provided by the prefrontal cortex (Luria, 1980; Stuss & Benson, 1987; Goldberg & Bilder, 1987). Goldberg and Barr (1991) propose that the breakdown of these controls impairs the very machinery of self-awareness, which accounts for the cognitive manifestations described above, both in the small frame of specific, local error self-detection and in the large, global frame of insight into the consequences of one's condition for one's life. In a recent study comparing patients with and without anosognosia who were matched for lesion location, it was found that the anosognosic group had significantly more deficits on frontal lobe tasks (Starkstein, Fedoroff, Price, Leiguarda, & Robinson, 1993).

As mentioned, most of the reduplicative phenomena described in this chapter have been linked to right-hemisphere disturbances. Many authors have emphasized the sensory nature of these disorders. It has been argued that Capgras syndrome may be linked to disturbances in facial recognition while reduplicative paramnesia may be linked to some form of topographic disorientation (Ellis & Young, 1990; Benson et al., 1976). The link between these disorders and right-hemisphere lesions may thus be a result of the right hemisphere's alleged role in nonverbal functions, such as facial recognition and spatial orientation. Most authors have argued that frontal lobe dysfunction also plays a major role in the manifestation of these symptoms. In most instances, the disorders are alleged to be the result of primary sensory impairment, combined with a disorder in problem solving or higher-order cognitive functioning resulting from frontal lobe dysfunction. Benson and Stuss provide numerous examples of the role that frontal lobe dysfunction plays in disorders such as Capgras syndrome and reduplicative paramnesia (Benson & Stuss, 1990; Stuss, 1991).

One of the common features of most awareness and delusional syndromes is that they both almost necessarily result from a disturbance of primary sensory or higher-cognitive functions associated with functions of the right posterior cortex and its connections to more anterior-based frontal systems. Numerous authors have recognized that simple alterations in awareness of hemiplegia or a hemisensory impairment may result from damage to the right parietal lobe (Gerstmann, 1942), while denial of these impairments are more likely to be the result of conditions involving damage to the connections between the parietal lobe and thalamic projections (Nielsen, 1938). In a similar vein, Cummings has indicated that simple delusions may result from damage to posterior brain regions, while more complex delusions are the result of conditions involving damage to more frontally based systems involving the basal ganglia (Cummings, 1985).

## Neuropsychological Theories

Most neuropsychological theories of awareness disturbances have emphasized the role of a theoretical error-monitoring system (Goldberg & Barr, 1991). In a very basic way, the process of error monitoring rests on the three components represented in figure 7.1. These include: (1) an internal representation of a desired output; (2) feedback regarding the output; and (3) a comparison between the desired output and feedback regarding the actual output. This is simply the same three-stage loop that has formed the basic elements of neural cybernetics and early cognitive theories of behavior (Bernstein, 1967; Miller, Galanter, & Pribram, 1960). It can also be applied as the basis for understanding mechanisms underlying the awareness of neurological deficits. Breakdowns of different elements and their combinations of this three-stage mechanism may account for different types of awareness disturbances (Goldberg & Barr, 1991). Most neuropsychological theories of unawareness are examples of a disturbance of one or more components of this three-stage mechanism, either implicitly or explicitly.

In most existing theories, anosognosia results from a disturbance of a feed-forward mechanism responsible for generating the desired output, and/or a breakdown of a feedback or comparator mechanism. In the earliest theories, it was proposed that alterations in awareness resulted from a disruption of a *body schema* mechanism located in the right parietal lobe. It is suggested that this body schema is a representational system that includes both intentional and sensory aspects of body awareness. Other theories use the concept of *corollary discharge* to explain unawareness as a result of a failure in mechanisms responsible for generating the efferent command and/or the mechanism responsible for processing the reafferent signal (von Holst, 1954; Teuber, 1961). Hécaen used this model to explain a number of conditions resulting from a disturbance of intentional and/or proprioceptive mechanisms (Hécaen & Albert, 1978). Heilman (1991) proposes that anosognosia is induced by either a defect in intentional free-forward mechanisms or systems responsible for monitoring or comparatory functions.

Bisiach and Berti (1987) provide a comprehensive model consisting of a sensory transducer that produces a representational network of the desired output. Some disorders, characterized by neglect or denial, may result from an inability to form the

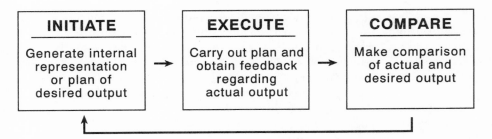

FIGURE 7.1 Schematic Representation of the Tripartite Loop Responsible for the Initiation, Execution, and Modification of Complex Behavior (after Bernstein, 1967; Miller, Galanter, and Pribram, 1960)

required representations, while other conditions, such as the anosognosic behavioral disorders, may be a result of an inappropriate utilization of these representations (Bisiach & Berti, 1987; Bisiach & Geminiani, 1991). McGlynn and Schacter (1989) propose a model of awareness that includes what they term a *conscious awareness system* (CAS). This system is responsible for detecting significant changes in certain output from various perceptual, memory, and knowledge modules. It is proposed that the anatomic location of the CAS is in the inferior parietal lobes. A disconnection of the CAS from these various modules thus leads to disorders of awareness for a particular cognitive or sensory domain. The CAS can also be disconnected from an executive system similar to those described in other models. Like other models, different disorders of awareness can result, depending on whether the disturbance affects anterior or posterior brain systems. Shallice (1988) advances a similar model, stressing the role of a hypothetical supervisory attentional system controlling lower level perceptual systems. As mentioned previously, a self-awareness system involving the frontal lobes is also crucial to the model proposed by Stuss and Benson (1987; Stuss, 1991).

It has been suggested that syndromes resulting from damage to awareness mechanisms themselves are seen following lesions of the prefrontal and related upper brain stem systems (Goldberg & Barr, 1991). Frontal syndromes are characterized not only by massive cognitive deficits but also by a profound lack of awareness of and concern for these deficits. These authors believe that at least some disorders of awareness associated with the lesions of the right hemisphere are best explained by the premorbid selectivity of the subject's awareness (and lack of awareness) of particular sensory or cognitive functions. A similar explanation for other examples of awareness disturbances has been provided by Levine (1990). Empirical support for this hypothesis has been provided more recently (Wagner & Cushman, 1994). Finally, Goldberg and Barr (1991) argue that the lack of awareness associated with conditions such as cortical blindness or cortical deafness can be understood best in terms of the postmorbid disruption of the sensory basis of internal cognitive representations, a feedback or comparator mechanism, or both. According to this hypothesis, unawareness of impairment may be particularly frequent following combined damage to anterior and posterior right-hemisphere systems, since it may disrupt various stages of the neural cybernetic loop for functions in which awareness is already lacking.

Gary Goldberg (1987) has provided important contributions to the understanding of the neuroanatomic basis of intentional and monitoring functions. Using the cytoarchitectonic patterns described by Sanides (1969), he has made a distinction between medial and lateral premotor systems. The *medial* system is associated with the development of intentional states and a bias for receiving interoceptive information. The *lateral* system, in contrast, is associated with a responsive mode and a sensitivity to exteroceptive stimuli. Goldberg argues that the interplay between these two systems is critical to the organism's ongoing behavior and response to the environment. He suggests that the alien hand syndrome is a result of purposeful action occurring independently of conscious volition. This behavior is explained in terms of the lateral system operating in isolation from the medial system. It is clear that this conceptualization can also be used to explain the experiences associated with phantom phenomena. It also provides an updated and more specific anatomic basis for the numerous components of the intention and monitoring deficits seen in other disorders of awareness.

## Disorders of Awareness and Insight in Schizophrenia

It is well known that patients with schizophrenia often exhibit poor insight, or a lack of awareness of their illness. Rapaport (1951) stated that major psychoses are characterized "impressively by lack of awareness of the illness, hallucinations, delusions, and kindred phenomena." David (1990) has proposed that insight, in reference to psychosis, has three recognizable components: recognition that one has a disease, compliance with treatment, and the ability to categorize unusual mental events as pathological. Amador and colleagues make further distinctions and argue that deficits in awareness are of diagnostic significance and are useful in guiding treatment decisions (Amador et al., 1991). All are in agreement that the etiology of unawareness in schizophrenia is poorly understood. It has been proposed that models provided by neuropsychological studies of awareness phenomena may be useful for understanding the mechanisms underlying these disturbances in schizophrenia (David, 1990; Amador et al., 1991).

This section will outline some of the disorders of awareness that have been described in patients with schizophrenia. These disorders will be compared and contrasted with those seen in the neurological conditions described in this chapter. In many ways, the disorders of awareness seen in these two groups may seem very different, since it is clear that acute disturbances such as hemiplegia and cortical blindness are not seen in patients with schizophrenia. However, it will be demonstrated that there are a number of unusual conditions observed in schizophrenia that are analogous to the disorders of awareness observed in patients with focal brain impairment. It is argued that the disturbances of awareness observed in both groups may be the result of similar underlying neuropsychological mechanisms.

### Types of Unawareness in Schizophrenia

Neurologists at the turn of the century became interested in disturbances of awareness regardless of whether the etiology was thought to be psychiatric or neurological in origin. Carl Wernicke, the German neurologist who remains famous for some of the ear-

TABLE 7.4    Classification of Unawareness Syndromes with Wernicke's (1900) Classification Terms

| 1. Somatopsychoses: | 2. Allopsychoses |
|---|---|
| A. Anosognosia | A. Reduplicative phenomena |
| B. Anosognosic behavioral disorders | B. Delusional syndromes |
| C. Body schema disorders | C. Hallucinations |
| D. Somatoparaphrenia | |

liest descriptions of sensory aphasia, made a distinction between disorders of awareness resulting from a patient's response to stimuli originating from the body and those resulting from a disturbed response to stimuli in the external world (Wernicke, 1900). He classified these disturbances as representing different forms of psychosis. He used the term *somatopsychosis* to refer to the class of symptoms resulting from altered awareness of the body and interoceptive stimuli and *allopsychosis* to refer to a disturbance of one's responses to exteroceptive stimuli. These terms receive little use in modern-day neurology and psychiatry, though they do provide a useful manner for grouping the range of awareness disturbances seen in both neurological and psychiatric populations. The various disorders of awareness described in this chapter are divided into these categories in table 7.4.

Karl Kleist, a student of Wernicke's, extended the use of his mentor's terms to describe similar phenomena in schizophrenic patients (Kleist, 1960). Kleist's descriptions included a woman with somatopsychosis who reported that "her bowels were taken out, her blood burnt, her uterus completely filled, her breasts were as heavy as millstones, and her head had disappeared" (p. 250). These ideas were accompanied by abnormal bodily sensations. Kleist attributed the symptoms to a combination of misinterpreted somatosensory perceptions and a paralogical disturbance of thought. His descriptions also included a man who "felt himself mistaken for other men, thought he was given other names, and finally was in doubt of his own identity" (p. 250). He compares these symptoms of allopsychosis to those seen in neurological patients with focal lesions of the cingulate gyrus or insular cortex. We will review a body of literature describing additional forms of somatopsychoses and allopsychoses in patients with a diagnosis of schizophrenia.

SOMATOPSYCHOSES IN SCHIZOPHRENIA: *Altered Awareness of Motor and Sensory Functions.*    Although patients with schizophrenia do not exhibit severe neurological impairments such as hemiplegia, they do exhibit a number of unusual symptoms affecting motor functioning that are clearly similar to what is described among the somatopsychoses. A number of these conditions involve changes in awareness of voluntary and involuntary motor behaviors (Cutting, 1985). Some patients report that their movements seem somewhat alien to them, as if they are passive agents of some external force. McGhie and Chapman (1961) describe patients who perceive altered awareness of seemingly automatic movements such as sitting down. These authors have also described unusual conditions where patients automatically begin to imitate movements of others in their immediate environment (Chapman & McGhie, 1964). Arieti (1974) described a number of features of the volitional nature of movements and behavior, and argued that an understanding of the disturbance of these mechanisms may be important for understanding the schizophrenic process. Others have suggested that experiences of involuntary movements may be intrinsic to schizophrenia, whether or not the patients have been treated with neuroleptic medication (Owens, Johnstone, & Frith, 1982).

Most of the recent literature on motor behavior in schizophrenia has focused on the development of abnormal involuntary movements associated with neuroleptic administration. Tardive dyskinesia (TD) is a syndrome characterized by involuntary choreo-athetoid movements with occasional tics, grimaces, and dystonia. Prevalence studies have indicated that TD occurs in 20% of patients receiving chronic administration of neuroleptic medication (Kane et al., 1985). In spite of the socially debilitating nature of these obvious and unusual features, there are a number of studies indicating that schizophrenic patients are relatively unaware of these symptoms (Alexopoulos, 1979; Rosen, Mukherjee, Olarte, Varia, & Cardenas, 1982; Myslobodsky, 1986; Caracci, Mukherjee, Roth, & Decina, 1990; MacPherson & Collis, 1992).

Myslobodsky (1986) argued that the lack of awareness of TD was so striking that he proposed that it may be a result of an anosognosia stemming from right-hemisphere-based cognitive deficits. Alexopoulos (1979) reported that outpatients with TD rarely complained about their abnormal movements. Others have demonstrated that awareness of these movements may vary, depending on their location, with lack of awareness greater for orofacial than limb-kinetic movements (Rosen et al., 1982). Smith, Kucharski, Oswald, & Waterman (1979) found that patients were able to describe symptoms of TD in others, but not in themselves. Caracci and colleagues (1990) demonstrated that verbal and visual feedback resulted in an immediate increase in patients' awareness of the symptoms, though the patients were not able to sustain the increased level of awareness in a two-week follow-up testing. Another study found unawareness of TD in association with cognitive impairment and negative symptoms characteristic of the defect state of schizophrenia (MacPherson & Collis, 1992).

As with hemiplegia, there is no evidence to suggest that patients with schizophrenia experience or deny acute disturbances in sensory functions. There is, however, ample evidence to suggest that patients with schizophrenia exhibit a number of unusual body sensations or positive symptoms that are more analogous to what is seen in conditions such as the phantom limb phenomena. Unusual sensory experiences, somatic distortions, and a loss of body image are well-known symptoms of schizophrenia (Bleuler, 1950). Experiences of bodily sensations induced by external forces are included among Schneider's first-rank symptoms.

Body-image disturbances and somatic delusions are reported in 14 to 31% of the psychotic patients surveyed in various studies (Lukianowicz, 1967; Cutting, 1980). Lukianowicz (1967) classified these disturbances as those affecting a patient's perception of body shape, size, mass, or position in space. He reported that, in a sample of schizophrenic patients, 61% experienced changes in the shape of their body image, 17% experienced changes in size, and 22% experienced changes in their perceived position in space. He argued that these experiences are the result of a misinterpretation and elaboration of normal body sensations.

Some schizophrenic patients develop delusions that parts of their body are in the process of being mutilated or destroyed. Some authors regard these symptoms as one of the earliest signs of the deterioration and poor outcome associated with the illness (Fenichel, 1945; Hamilton, 1976). It has been suggested that these distortions result from patients' attempts to turn their interest from the outside world to the body (Fenichel, 1945; Szasz, 1957). Arieti (1974) found that somatic delusions most often involve the head, face, eyes, or hands—parts of the body that are often used as organs of communication. Bychowski (1943) recognized that disintegration of the body image in schizophrenia may be the result of combined psychological and somatic factors.

There have been numerous experimental studies examining features of body-image distortion in schizophrenic samples. In empirical studies, schizophrenic subjects have been shown to have impairments in body-image boundaries and in estimation of the size of body parts (Cleveland, Fisher, Reitman, & Rothaus, 1962; Fisher & Cleveland, 1958; Weckowicz & Sommer, 1960). They have also demonstrated higher scores on measures of subjective body distortion (Fisher, 1970). Other investigators have obtained reports of unusual body experiences in schizophrenic patients via use of a question- naire technique (Chapman, Chapman, & Raulin, 1978). In a summary of research using various experimental and questionnaire methods, it was reported that schizo- phrenic subjects were generally "more expansive" than nonpsychotic subjects in their judgments and measures of body image (Reitman & Cleveland, 1964).

ALLOPSYCHOSES IN SCHIZOPHRENIA: *Delusions and Hallucinations.*    Delusions and hallucinations are well-known symptoms that form the core features of schizo- phrenia. Cutting (1980) reported that "abnormal beliefs" were observed in 90% of a sample of psychotic inpatients. An inability to recognize the erroneous nature and implausibility of the delusional belief is one of the key features of schizophrenia. As with patients with frontal lobe dysfunction, it has been observed that schizophrenic patients are able to detect erroneous and implausible beliefs held by others, but not in themselves (Brown, 1973). Most theoretical approaches to the etiology of delusions have considered these phenomena to be the result of primary disorders of attention, perception, or consciousness (Cutting, 1985). One view is that delusions are the result of a normal or expectable interpretation of an abnormal sensory experience (Maher, 1974). Other theories have stressed the opposite, with abnormal logic used to interpret otherwise normal perceptual experiences (Arieti, 1974).

It was previously thought that complex delusional disorders such as Capgras syn- drome were seen only in patients with functional psychotic disorders like schizophrenia (Berson, 1983). It had been suggested that the disturbance could be the result of a num- ber of psychological mechanisms, such as depersonalization, wish fulfillment, inability to face ambivalent feelings, incestuous wishes, or homoeroticism (Todd, 1957; Berson, 1983). A weaker association exists between schizophrenia and other misidentification syndromes, such as reduplicative paramnesia. Förstl and colleagues reported that, in a sample of 260 patients exhibiting misidentification syndromes, delusions regarding the self and others were associated with schizophrenia while reduplicative paramnesia was seen more frequently in patients with neurological disorders (Förstl et al., 1991). One of the primary features of the misidentification syndromes is that patients are able to accept and simultaneously maintain the duplicity of the "truth" and their delusions. A similar phenomenon, labeled the *double awareness phase*, has been described in psychotic patients recovering from delusions (Sacks, Carpenter, & Strauss, 1974).

Hallucinations are one of the major symptoms of schizophrenia. They were reported in 52% of the psychiatric patients studied in Cutting's (1985) sample. Thirty percent of these patients experienced auditory hallucinations, while only 18% experienced visual hallucinations. The majority of these symptoms involve the perception of verbalizations in the form of a human voice. Most appear to be neutral in content and in the third person (e.g., "He is an idiot"). Schneider's symptoms of thought broadcasting and thought insertion are among the most common types of hallucinations (Mellor, 1970). Since these are subjective phenomena, it is clear from patients' reports that they are aware of their existence. One study demonstrated that subjects can report on specific features of these symptoms in a very reliable manner (Junginger & Frame, 1985).

It is often suggested that hallucinations are more detailed and complex in schizophrenia than in those resulting from neurological causes. The major focus in the study of awareness of hallucinations is not in the patient's ability to detect them but in their ability to interpret the source or reality of the experience. Amador and colleagues have developed a scale that evaluates precisely this aspect of awareness (Amador, Strauss, Yale, Gorman, & Endicott, 1993). When used to study hallucinations, the patient's capacity to identify the source of the perception is assessed. More recently, they have reported that nearly 40% of a sample of 221 patients with DSM-III-R diagnoses of schizophrenia were unable to accomplish this (Amador, Flaum, Andreasen, Strauss, Yale, Clark, & Gorman, 1994). As with delusions, there are numerous theories suggesting that hallucinations are the result of a combination of faulty perceptual and interpretive processes.

## Frontal Lobe Impairment in Schizophrenia

Many authors have noted the similarities between symptoms observed in schizophrenia and those seen in neurological patients with frontal lobe dysfunction (Kraepelin, 1919; Kleist, 1960). Parallels between clusters of schizophrenic symptoms and their relations to the dorsolateral and orbital syndromes associated with frontal lobe dysfunction have been recognized by many authors (Levin, 1984; Muller, 1985; Goldberg & Costa, 1986). The frontal lobe model of schizophrenia has received support from studies using neuropsychological tests sensitive to frontal lobe dysfunction (Flor-Henry & Yeudall, 1979; Kolb & Whishaw, 1983; Malmo, 1974). The evidence for selective frontal lobe dysfunction comes from observations that the magnitude and pattern of performance decrements seen in schizophrenic groups is similar to the patterns observed in groups of patients with known frontal lobe pathology. It has not been adequately determined, however, whether these results reflect selective frontal lobe damage or may be secondary to generalized, nonspecific structural and/or biochemical damage (Goldberg, 1986; Bilder & Goldberg, 1987).

Productive symptoms such as perseveration and field-dependent behavior have been described in patients with schizophrenia (Goldberg & Costa, 1986). Most authors have noted that these symptoms are almost identical to those seen in patients with massive frontal lobe damage. As with what is seen in frontal lobe patients, schizophrenic patients appear to be relatively unaware of their impairments in executive functioning. This level of unawareness is similar to the defect in local error monitoring that is seen in patients with frontal lobe disturbance (Zaidel, 1987; Goldberg & Barr, 1991).

Bilder and Goldberg (1987) demonstrated that a variety of motor perseverations could be elicited in drawings from a sample of chronic schizophrenic patients. In many of these cases, patients would perseverate elements of previous drawings despite the fact that they could repeat the correct instructions. They appeared to be completely oblivious to the errors in their performance. Perseverations are also commonly observed in schizophrenic speech (Bleuler, 1950; Freeman & Gathercole, 1966; Chaika, 1982). It has been suggested that these symptoms are the result of a disturbance of language monitoring mechanisms resulting from frontal lobe disturbance (Barr, Bilder, Goldberg, Kaplan, & Mukherjee, 1989; McGrath, 1990). It is interesting to note that, in spite of these peculiarities, patients often fail to notice anything odd in their speech (Chaika, 1974; Amador et al., 1994).

*Echolalia*, or the automatic repetition of others, is the most commonly discussed symptom of field dependence in schizophrenia, though its existence is actually rare (Andreasen, 1982b). Echopraxia is a condition where patients automatically imitate the actions of others. It is similar to the imitative behavior that has been described in patients with frontal lobe impairments (Lhermitte, 1986). Echophraxia has been described in detail in schizophrenic subjects (Chapman & McGhie, 1964). One of the features of this behavior is that the patients feel that the behavior is not under their volition, even in cases where they are told not to do it. The symptom is not characterized by a lack of awareness but rather by an acute awareness of the tendency or "pull" toward performing the act. This awareness may even precede the onset of manifest behavior. One of their patients reported, "I was sitting with a friend, and suddenly he changed and I told him 'don't move or I'll have to move too.'" Patients are often critical of the behavior, though they cannot refrain from doing it (Dromard, 1905).

It is clear that other forms of unawareness in schizophrenia are also similar to the impairments observed in frontal lobe patients. The fact that patients are able to detect delusions and symptoms of TD in others but not in themselves is comparable to the difficulties in error monitoring that have been described in frontal lobe patients (Konow & Pribram, 1970). David's (1990) dimension of recognition of illness and Amador and colleagues' (1991) concept of incorrect attributions about illness are both analogous to the apathy, lack of unconcern, and impairment in global error monitoring seen in frontal lobe patients (Zaidel, 1987; Goldberg & Barr, 1991). Furthermore, the ability to relabel unusual events and unawareness of deficit described by these authors is analogous to the local error-monitoring deficits seen in frontal lobe patients. A recent study examining the relationship between neuropsychological test performance and unawareness found that patients' awareness of schizophrenic illness, as measured by a standardized questionnaire, was correlated with performance on tests of frontal lobe functions (Young, Davila, & Scher, 1993). These findings suggest that at least some components of unawareness in schizophrenia may be related to frontal lobe dysfunction.

## Neuroanatomical Approaches to Awareness Disturbances in Schizophrenia

The theories provided in the preceding review have suggested that the majority of disorders of awareness and insight resulting from neurological disorders involve a combined disturbance of right posterior and frontal brain mechanisms. It has been suggested that combined dysfunction in these brain regions results in disruptions of body-image representations or simultaneous impairment in perception and problem-solving behaviors. Other theories have suggested that a disturbance of these brain regions interferes with mechanisms responsible for planning and monitoring ongoing behavior. These theories have been used to explain a wide range of awareness disturbances, including anosognosia, body schema disorders, delusions, and hallucinations. The following review of the recent neuroanatomic literature will examine whether it is possible to explain disturbances of awareness in schizophrenia in terms of a disruption of similar neuroanatomic and cognitive mechanisms.

## Lateralized Brain Dysfunction

The majority of disorders of awareness in neurological populations are the result of disturbances of the right cerebral hemisphere. Most of the information about lateralized brain dysfunction in schizophrenia has pointed to the presence of left-hemisphere abnormalities. Hypotheses regarding a left-hemisphere disturbance in schizophrenia were initially developed following reports linking delusions and schizophrenia-like symptoms to patients with psychosis and left temporal lobe epilepsy (TLE) (Flor-Henry, 1969). This finding was supported by subsequent results demonstrating lateralized electrophysiological abnormalities in schizophrenic samples (Flor-Henry, Koles, Howath, & Burton, 1979; Gruzelier, 1973). Postmortem studies have provided neuropathological evidence of a greater degree of morphologic abnormalities in various left-hemisphere regions (Brown et al., 1986; Jeste & Lohr, 1989; Crow et al., 1989). Lateralized abnormalities in mesiotemporal regions have also been reported in imaging studies using positron emission tomography (PET) and magnetic resonance (MR) imaging (Kling, Metter, Riege, & Kull, 1987; Wiesel et al., 1987; Johnstone et al., 1989; Suddath et al., 1989; Bogerts et al., 1990). The pattern of structural brain impairment in schizophrenic brains is similar to what is observed in the brains of patients with TLE originating from the left hemisphere (Barr et al., 1993).

A theory of right-hemisphere dysfunction in schizophrenia has been proposed by Cutting (1985). He characterizes the brain impairment in schizophrenia in terms of a hemispheric imbalance where dysfunctional right-hemisphere mechanisms lead to an overactivation of the left hemisphere. In Cutting's (1985) view, right-hemisphere dysfunction is responsible for the perceptual distortions and body-image disturbances seen in schizophrenic subjects. This dysfunction is also responsible for deficits in processing and expressing emotions. Cummings (1985) has argued that right posterior lesions result in abnormal perceptual input into the limbic system, resulting in the development of delusions and hallucinations. Conversely, disorders affecting the left hemisphere disrupt connections between perisylvian language regions and the limbic system, resulting in paranoid delusions and other symptoms characteristic of schizophrenia.

Both Cutting and Cummings assume that it is possible for the heterogeneity of schizophrenic symptoms to be a reflection of the diversity of damage to their underlying brain systems (Cummings, 1985; Cutting, 1985). Symptoms characterized by perceptual alterations or disorders of body awareness may reflect relative dysfunction in the posterior regions of the right hemisphere. Conversely, paranoid delusions and other

more verbal symptoms of formal thought disorder may be linked to a relative disturbance in left-hemisphere mechanisms.

Numerous studies of interictal psychosis observed in patients with epilepsy have
demonstrated a higher incidence of delusions and schizophrenia-like symptoms in
patients with seizures originating from the left temporal lobe (Trimble, 1991). Some
authors have noted an association between left temporal lobe seizures and a greater prevalence of Schneiderian first-rank symptoms (Stevens, 1982; Toone, Garralda, & Ron,
1982; Perez, Trimble, Murray, & Reider, 1985). It has been suggested that this relationship is a result of the primarily verbal nature of the symptoms (Cummings, 1985; Stevens,
1988). Direct evidence to support a relationship between body-image distortions and
right-hemisphere impairment in schizophrenia is not available at present.

## Regional Brain Abnormalities

Most neurobehavioral theories of unawareness and body schema disorders have
stressed a major role for the right inferior parietal lobe (Mesulam, 1985). However, the
evidence for parietal lobe impairment in schizophrenia has been considered minimal
and speculative (Zec & Weinberger, 1986). Mesulam and Geschwind (1978), citing
both behavioral and anatomic evidence, suggested that the right inferior parietal lobe
may be responsible for the attentional impairment that is associated with schizophrenia. They argue that disruptions of parietal lobe connections to various frontal and tem-
porolimbic areas may lead to a failure to respond to motivationally relevant information. Functional evidence for a parietal lobe abnormality has been seen in some
electrophysiological and imaging studies, though the findings are limited to the left
parietal lobe (Morihisa, Duffy, & Wyatt, 1983; Liddle, Friston, Frith, Jones, Hirsch, &
Frackowiak, 1992).

Other hypotheses regarding parietal lobe abnormalities in schizophrenia have been
examined in experimental studies. Some authors have suggested that schizophrenia
may be characterized by a disorder in proprioception, a function that is usually attributed to the parietal lobes. Meehl (1962) proposed that an integrative deficit in kines-
thesis may underlie neural predisposition to schizophrenia. Rado (1953) hypothesized
that a defect in proprioception may underlie the body-image impairment. These theories were tested empirically by Erwin and Rosenbaum (1979) in a comparison to
patients with known brain impairment. Results from this study demonstrated that schizophrenic subjects and those with focal parietal lobe impairment showed comparable
disturbances in proprioceptive functions and disordered body image, but observations
of sensory tactile dysfunction were limited to the parietal lobe group.

There is substantially more evidence to support hypotheses of frontal lobe dysfunction in schizophrenia. Theories of frontal lobe dysfunction have received support from
the results of neurophysiological studies showing patterns of frontal lobe abnormalities
on measures of cerebral metabolism (PET) (Buchsbaum et al., 1982; Farkas, Reivich,
Alavi & Greenberg, 1980), topographic electroencephalography (EEG) (Morihisa &
McAnulty, 1985), and regional cerebral blood flow (rCBF) both under resting conditions and with activation during the performance of complex cognitive tasks (Franzen
& Ingvar, 1975a, 1975b; Berman, Zec, & Weinberger, 1986; Weinberger, Berman, &
Zec, 1986). The evidence for selective frontal lobe dysfunction in these studies comes

from the observation that the magnitude and pattern of performance decrements on these tests in schizophrenic groups appear similar to patterns observed in groups of patients with known frontal lobe pathology.

It is important to understand that the above-described neurophysiological and neuropsychological studies are by their nature capable of providing functional but not structural information. These studies clearly indicate that a selective prefrontal dysfunction is present in schizophrenia, but this does not automatically imply that a selective structural-biochemical lesion is present. The relationship between a structural and functional impairment may be rather complex, and it would be a misconception to expect a simple relationship between these two aspects of the disorder (Goldberg, 1986; Goldberg & Bilder, 1987).

More recent studies examining the pathophysiology of schizophrenia have focused on abnormalities in mesiotemporal-limbic regions. The results of postmortem neuropathological studies have found abnormalities in various mesiotemporal structures including the hippocampus and amygdala (Bogerts, Meertz, & Schonfeld-Bausch, 1985; Falkai & Bogerts, 1986; Altshuler, Casanova, Goldberg, & Kleinman, 1990). These findings have been reinforced by the results of quantitative MR imaging studies finding volume reductions in similar structures (Suddath et al., 1989; DeLisi, Dauphinias, & Gershon, 1988; Bogerts et al., 1990). A number of authors have proposed a link between the symptoms observed in schizophrenia and a disorder of limbic mechanisms (Stevens, 1973; Bogerts, 1989; Gray, Feldon, Rawlins, Hemsley, & Smith, 1991; Bilder & Degreef, 1991).

### Neuropsychological Models of Awareness in Schizophrenia

The cybernetic model, and its emphasis on intention and monitoring systems, has recently been applied to a number of the behavioral phenomena observed in schizophrenia. Frith (1992) has proposed that schizophrenia can be conceptualized as a disturbance in metarepresentation, which he argues plays a major role in awareness. In this model, self-awareness plays a central role in the manifestation of numerous symptoms associated with schizophrenia. Frith's model of self-awareness consists of metarepresentations including awareness of one's goals, awareness of intentions, and awareness of the intentions of others. He hypothesizes that unawareness of goals leads to disorders in willed action, or what may be otherwise classified as negative symptoms such as inertia or apathy. Lack of awareness of intentions leads to disorders of self-monitoring and abnormalities in the experience of action, such as the disorders of movement described in this chapter. Erroneous inferences about the intentions of others leads to paranoid delusions and delusions of reference. Hallucinations are the result of failing to recognize the self-initiated nature of certain actions or inner speech, misattributing their origin to some external agent. Most positive symptoms are thus explained as "an impairment in the ability to distinguish between changes due to our own actions and changes due to external events" (Frith, 1992, p. 81).

Most neurobehavioral theories of hallucinations and delusions have stressed a disturbance in perceptual input. The advantage of Frith's model is its reliance on output rather than input mechanisms. In most theories, input mechanisms have been related to posterior brain systems, including the parietal lobe, while output functions have been attributed to more anterior systems, including the frontal cortex. Frith argues that a disturbance of brain systems underlying willed action, such as the dorsolateral pre-frontal cortex, supplementary motor area, and anterior cingulate gyrus, are responsible for many of the positive symptoms observed in schizophrenia. The role of the monitor has been identified with the hippocampal system (Frith & Done, 1988). Goldberg (1985, 1987) has proposed that these structures form a medial frontal system responsi-ble for mediation of volitional behaviors. It has been argued that a disruption of this medial system is responsible for many of the abnormal behavioral phenomena that are observed in schizophrenia (Frith, 1992; Bilder & Szeszko, in press). Gray and col-leagues have proposed a similar model emphasizing subiculo-accumbens projections and their role in monitoring mechanisms (Gray et al., 1991). In this model, schizo-phrenia is characterized as a failure of monitoring mechanisms responsible for inte-grating representations of past input with ongoing motor or perceptual programs.

## Conclusions

This chapter reviewed a variety of unusual conditions affecting patients' awareness of neu-rological deficits. These included unawareness of left-sided motor or sensory deficits, body schema disturbances, and syndromes characterized by delusions or hallucinations. Many past theories have explained these phenomena as a combined impairment in per-ceptual and problem-solving mechanisms linked to right inferior parietal and frontal sys-tems in the right cerebral hemisphere. A number of disorders in self-awareness or error monitoring have been described following focal damage to the frontal cortex. It has been proposed that these disorders are the result of an inability to monitor ongoing behavior. More recent models have emphasized the role of intention and self-monitoring in a wider range of neurobehavioral disturbances affecting awareness.

There are many similarities between the disturbances of awareness seen in schizo-phrenia and those seen as a result of known neurological impairment. This is most apparent for the many disturbances of body awareness and delusional disorders result-ing from right parietal lobe dysfunction. These have been described in the classical lit-erature in neurology and psychiatry as either the somatopsychoses or the allopsychoses. Other forms of unawareness in schizophrenia are similar to what is observed in patients with frontal lobe impairments or with seizures originating from the left temporal lobe. Recent theories have implicated the role of willed action and self-monitoring in disor-ders of awareness and many of the cognitive impairments and core symptoms of schiz-ophrenia. It has been suggested that these symptoms are the result of a disturbance of a medial frontal system involving the anterior hippocampus, cingulate gyrus, supple-mentary motor area, and dorsolateral prefrontal cortex.

It is clear that there are numerous advantages to using neurological models for understanding the symptoms associated with schizophrenia. The biggest advantage is that one is able to compare behaviors resulting from a known neurological basis to sim-ilar behaviors where the neurological basis is only inferred. This enables the develop-ment of speculations on the brain systems underlying various symptoms. For example, it may be possible to speculate that schizophrenic patients exhibiting disturbances of body awareness or somatic delusions may exhibit a different pattern of brain distur-bance than those presenting with paranoid delusions. One may hypothesize that the patient with somatic delusions might exhibit a disturbance in brain systems involving the right parietal lobe, while the patient with paranoid delusions may have a disturbance involving the left mesiotemporal-limbic system. It is thus possible that neurological models may provide a means for classifying various disorders of awareness. Further application of neurobehavioral models of awareness, emphasizing the roles of intention and self-monitoring functions, is recommended for future studies of awareness in schizophrenia.

*Acknowledgments*    This work was supported in part by the Mental Health Clinical Research Center grant for the Study of Schizophrenia (MH-41960) at Hillside Hospital, Long Island Jewish Medical Center.

*References*

Aldrich, M. S., Alessi, A. G., Beck, R. W., & Gilman, S. (1987). Cortical blindness: Etiology, diagnosis, and prognosis. *Annals of Neurology, 21*, 149–158.

Alexander, M. P., Stuss, D. T., & Benson, D. F. (1979). Capgras syndrome: A reduplicative phenomenon. *Neurology, 29*, 334–339.

Alexopoulos, G. (1979). Lack of complaints in schizophrenics with tardive dyskinesia. *Journal of Nervous and Mental Disease, 167*, 125–127.

Altshuler, L. L., Casanova, M. F., Goldberg, T. E., & Kleinman, J. E. (1990). The hippocampus and parahippocampal gyrus in schizophrenic, suicide, and control brains. *Archives of General Psychiatry, 47*, 1029–1034.

Amador, X. F., Flaum, M. F., Andreasen, N. C., Strauss, D. H., Yale, S. A., Clark, S. C. & Gorman, J. M. (1994). Awareness of illness in schizophrenia and schizoaffective and mood disorders. *Archives of General Psychiatry, 51*, 826–836.

Amador, X. F., Strauss, D. H., Yale, S. A., & Gorman, J. M. (1991). Awareness of illness in schizophrenia. *Schizophrenia Bulletin, 17*, 113–132.

Amador, X. F., Strauss, D. H., Yale, S. A., Gorman, J. M., & Endicott, J. (1993). The assessment of insight in psychosis. *American Journal of Psychiatry, 150*, 873–879.

Anastasopoulis, G. K. (1961). Die nosoagnositische Überschätzung. *Psychiatrie Neurologie, 141*, 228–241.

Andreasen, N. C. (1982a). Negative symptoms in schizophrenia. *Archives of General Psychiatry, 39*, 784–788.

Andreasen, N. C. (1982b). The relationship between schizophrenic language and the aphasias. In F. A. Henn & H. A. Nasrallah (Eds.), *Schizophrenia as a brain disease*. New York: Oxford University Press.

Anton, G. (1898). Ueber Herderkrankungen des Gehirnes, welche von Patienten selbst nicht wahrgenommen werden. *Wiener Klinische Wochenschrift, 11*, 227–229.

Arieti, S. (1974). *Interpretation of schizophrenia* (2nd ed.). New York: Basic Books.

Babinski, M. J. (1914). Contibution a l'etude des troubles menaux dans l'hemiplegie organique cerebrale (Anosognosie). *Revue Neurologique, 12*, 845–848.

Barr, W. B., Ashtari M., Degreef, G., Bogerts, B., Bilder, R. M., Schaul, N., & Lieberman, J. A. (1993). Brain morphometric comparison of first episode schizophrenia and temporal lobe epilepsy. *Schizophrenia Research, 9*(S), 192.

Barr, W. B., Bilder, R. M., Goldberg, E., Kaplan, E., & Mukherjee, S. (1989). The neuropsychology of schizophrenic speech. *Journal of Communication Disorders, 22*, 327–349.

Bauer, R. M., & Addeo, R. R. (1993). There is no denying the importance of awareness. *Contemporary Psychology, 38,* 1041–1043.

Benson, D. F., Gardner, H., & Meadows, J. C. (1976). Reduplicative paramnesia. *Neurology, 26,* 147–151.

Benson, D. F., & Stuss, D. T. (1990). Frontal lobe influences on delusions: A clinical perspective. *Schizophrenia Bulletin, 16,* 403–411.

Benton, A. L. (1977). Reflections on the Gerstmann syndrome. *Brain and Language, 4,* 45–62.

Bergman, P. S. (1957). Cerebral blindness. *Archives of Neurological Psychiatry, 78,* 569–584.

Berman, K. F., Zec, R. F., & Weinberger, D. R. (1986). Physiological dysfunction of dorsolateral prefrontal cortex in schizophrenia: II. Role of medication status, attention, and mental effort. *Archives of General Psychiatry, 43,* 124–135.

Bernstein, N. A. (1967). *Coordination and regulation of movements.* New York: Pergamon Press.

Berson, R. J. (1983). Capgras syndrome. *American Journal of Psychiatry, 140,* 969–978.

Bilder, R. M., & Degreef, G. (1991). Morphologic markers of neurodevelopmental paths to schizophrenia. In S. A. Mednick, T. D. Cannon, C. E. Barr, & J. M. LaFosse (Eds.), *Developmental neuropathology of schizophrenia* (pp. 167–190. New York: Plenum.

Bilder, R. M., & Goldberg, E. (1987) Motor perseverations in schizophrenia. *Archives of Clinical Neuropsychology, 2,* 195–214.

Bilder, R. M., & Szeszko, P. R. (in press). Structural neuroimaging and neuropsychological impairments. In C. Pantelis, H. E. Nelson, & T. R. E. Barnes (Eds.), *The neuropsychology of schizophrenia.* Sussex, UK: John Wiley.

Bisiach E. (1988). Language without thought. In L. Weiskrantz (Ed.), *Thought without language.* Oxford: Oxford University Press.

Bisiach, E., & Berti, A. (1987). Dyschiria: An attempt at its systemic explanation. In M. Jeannerod (Ed.), *Consciousness in contemporary science* (pp. 101–120). New York: Oxford University Press.

Bisiach, E., & Geminiani, G. (1987). Anosognosia related to hemiplegia and hemainopia. In G. P. Prigatano & D. L. Schacter (Eds.), *Awareness of deficit after brain injury: Clinical and theoretical issues* (pp. 17–39). New York: Oxford University Press.

Bleuler, E. (1950). *Dementia praecox or the group of schizophrenias.* New York: International Universities Press.

Blumer, D., & Benson, D. F. (1975). Personality changes with frontal and temporal lobe lesions. In D. F. Stuss & D. Blumer (Eds.), *Psychiatric aspects of neurological disease* (pp. 151–160). New York: Grune & Stratton.

Bogen, J. E. (1993). The callosal syndromes. In K. M. Heilman & E. Valenstein (Eds.), *Clinical neuropsychology,* 3rd ed. (pp. 337–408). New York: Oxford University Press.

Bogerts, B. (1989) Limbic and paralimbic pathology in schizophrenia: Interaction with age- and stress-related factors. In S. C. Schulz & C. A. Tamminga (Eds.), *Schizophrenia: Scientific progress* (pp. 216–226). New York: Oxford University Press.

Bogerts, B., Ashtari, M., Degreef, G., Alvir, J. M., Bilder, R. M., & Lieberman, J. (1990). Reduced temporal limbic structure volumes on magnetic resonance images in first episode schizophrenia. *Psychiatry Research: Neuroimaging, 35,* 1–13.

Bogerts, B., Meertz, E., & Schonfeldt-Bausch, R. (1985). Basal ganglia and limbic system pathology in schizophrenia: A morphometric study of brain volume and shrinkage. *Archives of General Psychiatry, 42,* 784–791.

Brockman, N. W., & von Hagen, K. O. (1946). Denial of blindness (Anton's syndrome). *Bulletin of the Los Angeles Neurological Society, 11,* 178–180.

Brown, J. W. (1988). *The life of the mind: Selected papers.* Hillsdale, NJ: Erlbaum.

Brown, R. (1973). Schizophrenia, language, and reality. *American Psychologist, 28,* 395–403.

Brown, R., Colter, N., Corsellis, J. A. N., Crow, T. J., Frith, C. D., Jagoe, R., Johnstone, E. C.,

& Marsh, L. (1986). Postmortem evidence of structural brain changes in schizophrenia. *Archives of General Psychiatry, 43*, 36–42.

Buchsbaum, M. S., Ingvar, D. S., Kessler, R., Waters, R. N., Cappalletti, J., van Kammen, D. P., King, A. C., Johnson, J. L., Manning, R. G., Flynn, R. W., Mann, L. S., Bunney, W. E., & Sokoloff, L. (1982). Cerebral glucography with emission tomography. Use in normal subjects and in patients with schizophrenia. *Archives of General Psychiatry, 39*, 251–259.

Bychowski, G. (1943). Disorders of the body-image in the clinical pictures of psychosis. *Journal of Nervous and Mental Disease, 97*, 310–335.

Capgras, J., & Reboul-Lachaux, J. (1923). L'illusion des "sosies" dans un délire systématisé chronique. *Bulletin de la Société Clinique de Médecine Mentale, 11*, 6–16.

Caracci, G., Mukherjee, S., Roth, S. D., & Decina P. (1990). Subjective awareness of abnormal involuntary movements in chronic schizophrenia patients. *American Journal of Psychiatry, 147*, 295–298.

Chaika, E. (1974). A linguist looks as "schizophrenic" language. *Brain and Language, 1*, 257–276.

Chaika, E. (1982). A unified explanation for the diverse structural deviations reported for adult schizophrenics with disrupted speech. *Journal of Communication Diseases, 15*, 167–189.

Chapman, L. J., Chapman, J. P., & Raulin, M. L. (1978). Body-image aberration in schizophrenia. *Journal of Abnormal Psychology, 85*, 374–382.

Chapman, J., & McGhie, A. (1964). Echopraxia in schizophrenia. *British Journal of Psychiatry, 110*, 365–374.

Christodoulou, G. N. (1976). Delusional hyper-identification of the Fregoli type. *Acta Psychiatrica Scandinavica, 54*, 304–404.

Cleveland, S. E., Fisher, S., Reitman, E. E., & Rothaus, P. (1962). Perception of body size in schizophrenia. *Archives of General Psychiatry, 7*, 277–285.

Critchley, M. (1953). *The parietal lobes*. London: E. Arnold.

Crow, T. J. (1980). Molecular pathology of schizophrenia: More than one disease process? *British Medical Journal, 280 i*, 66–68.

Crow, T. J., Ball, J., Bloom, S. R., Brown, R., Bruton, C. J., Colter, N., Frith, C. D., Johnstone, E. C., Owens, D. G. C., & Roberts, G. W. (1989). Schizophrenia as an anomaly of development of cerebral asymmetry. *Archives of General Psychiatry, 46*, 1145–1150.

Cummings, J. L. (1985). Organic delusions: Phenomenology, Anatomical Correlations, and Review. *British Journal of Psychiatry, 146*, 184–197.

Cutting, J. (1978). Study of anosognosia. *Journal of Neurology, Neurosurgery, and Psychiatry, 41*, 548–555.

Cutting, J. (1980). Physical illness and psychosis. *British Journal of Psychiatry, 136*, 109–119.

Cutting, J. (1985). *The psychology of schizophrenia*. Edinburgh: Churchill Livingstone.

David, A. S. (1990). Insight and psychosis. *British Journal of Psychiatry, 156*, 798–808.

David. A. S., Owen, A. M., & Förstl, H. (1993). An annotated summary and translation of "On the self-awareness of focal brain diseases by the patient in cortical blindness and cortical deafness" by Gabriel Anton (1899). *Cognitive Neuropsychology, 10*, 263–272.

Davison, K., & Bagley, C. R. (1969). Schizophrenia-like psychoses associated with organic disorders of the central nervous system: A review. In R. N. Hetherington (Ed.), *Current problems in neuropsychiatry* (pp. 113–184). Kent, England: Headley Bros., Ltd.

DeLisi, L. E., Dauphinias, I. D., & Gershon, E. S. (1988). Perinatal complications and reduced size of brain limbic structures in familial schizophrenia. *Schizophrenia Bulletin, 13*, 185–191.

Denny-Brown, D., & Banker, B. Q. (1954). Amorphosynthesis from left parietal lesion. *Archives of Neurological Psychiatry, 71*, 302–313.

Denny-Brown, D., & Chambers, R. A. (1958). The parietal lobe and behavior. *Research Publications—Association for Research in Nervous and Mental Disease, 36*, 35–117.

Dromard, G. (1905). Etude psychologique et clinique sur l'échopraxie. *Journal of Psychology* (Paris) 2, 385–403.

Earnest, M. P., Monroe, P. A., & Yarnell, P. R. (1977). Cortical deafness: Demonstration of the pathologic anatomy by CT scan. *Neurology, 27,* 1172–1175.

Ellis, H. D., & Young, A. W. (1990). Accounting for delusional misidentifications. *British Journal of Psychiatry, 157,* 239–248.

Erwin, B. J., & Rosenbaum, G. (1979). Parietal lobe syndrome and schizophrenia: Comparison of neuropsychological deficits. *Journal of Abnormal Psychology, 88,* 234–241.

Falkai, P., & Bogerts, B. (1986). Cell loss in the hippocampus of schizophrenics. *European Archives of Psychiatry and Neurological Sciences, 236,* 154–161.

Farkas, T., Reivich, M., Alavi, A., Greenberg, Fowler, J. S., MacGregor, R. R., Christman, D. R., & Wolf, A. P. (1980). The application of [18F]2-deoxy-2-fluoro-D-glucose and positron emission tomography in the study of psychiatric conditions. In J. V. Possonneau, R. A. Hawkins, W. E. Lust, & F. A. Welsh ( Eds.), *Cerebral metabolism and neural functions,* pp. 403–404. Baltimore: Williams and Wilkins.

Feinberg, T. E., Haber, L. D., & Leeds, N. E. (1990). Verbal asomatognosia. *Neurology, 40,* 1391–1394.

Fenichel, O. (1945). *The psychoanalytic theory of neurosis.* New York: Norton.

Fisher, S. (1970). *Body experience in fantasy and behavior.* New York: Appleton-Century-Crofts.

Fisher, S., & Cleveland, S. E. (1958). *Body image and personality.* Princeton: Van Nostrand.

Flor-Henry, P. (1969). Psychoses and temporal lobe epilepsy: A controlled investigation. *Epilepsia, 10,* 363–395.

Flor-Henry, P., Koles, Z. J., Howarth, B. G., & Burton, L. (1979). Neurophysiological studies of schizophrenia, mania and depression. In J. Gruzelier & P. Flor-Henry (Eds.), *Hemisphere asymmetries of function in psychopathology,* pp. 189–222. New York: Elsevier.

Flor-Henry, P., & Yeudall, L. T. (1979). Neuropsychological investigation of schizophrenia and manic-depressive psychoses. In J. Gruzelier & P. Flor-Henry (Eds.), *Hemisphere asymmetries of function in psychopathology,* pp. 341–362. New York: Elsevier.

Förstl, H., Almeida, O. P., Owen, A. M., Burns, A. & Howard, R. (1991). Psychiatric, neurological and medical aspects of misidentification syndromes: A review of 260 cases. *Psychological Medicine, 21,* 905–910.

Förstl, H., Owen, A. M., & David, A. S. (1993). Gabriel Anton and "Anton's syndrome": On focal diseases of the brain which are not perceived by the patient. *Neuropsychiatry, Neuropsychology, and Behavioral Neurology, 6,* 1–8.

Franzen, G., & Ingvar, D. H. (1975a). Abnormal distribution of cerebral activity in chronic schizophrenia. *Journal of Psychiatric Research, 12,* 209–214.

Franzen, G., & Ingvar, D. H. (1975b). Absence of activation in frontal structures during psychological testing of chronic schizophrenics. *Journal of Neurology, Neurosurgery, and Psychiatry, 38,* 1027–1032.

Frederiks, J. A. M. (1985a). Disorders of the body schema. In J. A. M. Frederiks (Ed.), *Handbook of clinical neurology: 1 (45): Clinical neuropsychology,* pp. 373–393. Amsterdam: Elsevier.

Frederiks, J. A. M. (1985b). Phantom limb and phantom limb pain. In J. A. M. Frederiks (Ed.), *Handbook of clinical neurology: 1 (45): Clinical neuropsychology,* pp. 394–404. Amsterdam: Elsevier.

Freeman, T., & Gathercole, C. E. (1966). Perseveration—The clinical symptoms in chronic schizophrenia and organic dementia. *British Journal of Psychiatry, 112,* 27–32.

Frith, C. D. (1992). *The cognitive neuropsychology of schizophrenia.* Hove: Erlbaum.

Frith, C. D., & Done, D. J. (1988). Towards a neuropsychology of schizophrenia. *British Journal of Psychiatry, 153,* 437–443.

Gertsmann, J. (1942). Problem of interpretation of disease and of impaired body territories with organic lesions. *Archives of Neurological Psychiatry, 48*, 890–913.

Geschwind, N. (1965). Disconnection syndromes in animals and man. *Brain, 88*, 237–294, 585–644.

Goldberg, E. (1986). Varieties of perseveration: A comparison of two taxonomies. *Journal of Clinical Experimental Neuropsychology, 8*, 710–726.

Goldberg, E. (1990). Higher cortical functions in humans: The gradiental approach. In E. Goldberg (Ed.), *Contemporary neuropsychology and the legacy of Luria*. Hillsdale, NJ: Erlbaum.

Goldberg, E., & Barr, W. B. (1991). Three possible mechanisms of unawareness of deficit. In G. P. Prigatano & D. L. Schacter (Eds.), *Awareness of deficit after brain injury: Clinical and theoretical issues* (pp. 152–175). New York: Oxford University Press.

Goldberg, E., & Bilder, R. M. (1987). The frontal lobes and hierarchical organization of cognitive control. In E. Perecman (Ed.), *The frontal lobes revisited*. New York: IRBN Press.

Goldberg, E., Antin, S. P., Bilder, R. M., Gerstman, L. J., Hughes, J. E. O., Antin, S. P., & Mattis, S. (1989). A reticulo-frontal disconnection syndrome. *Cortex, 25*, 687–695.

Goldberg, E., & Costa, L. D. (1981). Hemisphere differences in the acquisition and use of descriptive systems. *Brain and Language, 14*, 144–173.

Goldberg, E., & Costa, L. (1986). Qualitative indices in neuropsychological assessment: Executive deficit following prefrontal lesions. In K. Adams & I. Grant (Eds.), *Neuropsychological assessment in neuropsychiatric disorders*. New York: Oxford University Press.

Goldberg, E., & Tucker, D. (1979). Motor perseveration and long-term memory for visual forms. *Journal of Clinical Neuropsychology, 1*, 273–288.

Goldberg, G., Mayer, N. H., & Toglia, J. U. (1981) Medial frontal cortex infarction and the alien hand sign. *Archives of Neurology, 38*, 683–686.

Goldberg, G. (1985). Supplementary motor area: Review and hypotheses. *Behavioral & Brain Sciences, 8*, 567–588.

Goldberg, G. (1987). From intent to action: Evolution and function of the premotor systems of the frontal lobe. In E. Perecman (Ed.), *The frontal lobes revisited*. New York: IRBN Press.

Goldstein, M. N., Brown, M., & Hollander, J. (1975). Auditory agnosia and cortical deafness: Analysis of a case with three-year follow-up. *Brain and Language, 2*, 324–332.

Gray, J. A., Feldon, J., Rawlins, J. N. P., Helmsley, D. R., & Smith, A. D. (1991). The neuropsychology of schizophrenia. *Behavioral & Brain Sciences, 14*, 1–84.

Gruzelier, J. H. (1973). Bilateral asymmetry of skin conductance orienting activity and levels in schizophrenics. *Biological Psychiatry, 1*, 21–41.

Hakim, H., Verma, N. P., & Greiffenstein, M. F. (1988). Pathogenesis of reduplicative paramnesia. *Journal of Neurology, Neurosurgery, and Psychiatry, 51*, 839–841.

Hamilton, M. (Ed.) (1976). *Fish's schizophrenia*. Bristol: John Wright and Sons.

Head, H., & Holmes, G. (1911). Sensory disturbances from cerebral lesions. *Brain, 34*, 102–254.

Hecaen, H., Penfield, W., Bertrand, C., & Malmo, R. (1956). The syndrome of apractognosia due to lesions of the minor cerebral hemisphere. *Archives of Neurological Psychiatry, 75*, 400–434.

Hecaen, H., & Albert, M. L. (1978). *Human neuropsychology*. New York: John Wiley.

Heilman, K. M. (1991). Anosognosia: Possible neuropsychological mechanisms. In G. P. Prigatano & D. L. Schacter (Eds.), *Awareness of deficit after brain injury: Clinical and theoretical issues* (pp. 53–62). New York: Oxford University Press.

Heilman, K. M., Watson, R. T., & Valenstein, R. (1993). Neglect and related disorders. In K. M. Heilman & E. Valenstein (Eds.), *Clinical neuropsychology*, 3rd ed. (pp. 279–336). New York: Oxford University Press.

Ives, E. R., & Nielsen, M. D. (1937). Disturbance of body scheme: Delusion of absence of part of body in two cases with autopsy verification of the lesions. *Bulletin of the Los Angeles Neurological Society, 2,* 120–125.

Jeste, D. V., & Lohr, J. B. (1989). Hippocampal and pathologic findings in schizophrenia: A morphometric study. *Archives of General Psychiatry, 46,* 1019–1024.

Johnstone, E. C., Owens, D. G. C., Crow, T. J., Frith, C. D., Alexandropolous, K., Bydder, G. M., & Colter, N. (1989). Temporal lobe structure as determined by nuclear magnetic resonance in schizophrenia and bipolar affective disorder. *Journal of Neurology, Neurosurgery and Psychiatry, 52,* 736–741.

Joynt, R. J., Honch, G. W., Rubin, A. J., & Trudell, R. G. (1985). Occipital lobe syndromes. In J. A. M. Frederiks (Ed.), *Handbook of clinical neurology: 1 (45): Clinical neuropsychology,* pp. 49–62. Amsterdam: Elsevier.

Juba, A. (1949). Beitrag zur Struktur der ein- und doppelseitiger Körperschemastörungen - Fingeragnosie, atypische Anosognosien. *Monatsschrift fur Psychiatrie und Neurologie, 118,* 11–29.

Junginger, J., & Frame, C. L. (1985). Self-report of the frequency and phenomenology of verbal hallucinations. *Journal of Nervous and Mental Disease, 173,* 149–155.

Kane, J. M., Woerner, M., Lieberman, J., Weinhold, P., Florio, W., Rubinstein, M., Rotrosen, J., Mukherjee, S., Bergmann, K., & Schooler, N. R. (1985). The prevalence of tardive dyskinesia. *Psychopharmacology Bulletin, 21,* 136–139.

Kapur, N., Turner, A., & King, C. (1988). Reduplicative paramnesia: Possible anatomical and neuropsychological mechanisms. *Journal of Neurology, Neurosurgery, and Psychiatry, 51,* 579–581.

Kleist, K. (1960). Schizophrenic symptoms and cerebral pathology. *Journal of Mental Science, 106,* 246–255.

Kling, A. S., Metter, E. J., Riege, W. H., & Kull, D. E. (1986). Comparison of PET measurement of local brain glucose metabolism and CAT measurement of brain atrophy in chronic schizophrenia and depression. *American Journal of Psychiatry, 143,* 175–180.

Kolb, B., & Whishaw, I. Q. (1983). Performance of schizophrenic patients on tests sensitive to left or right frontal, temporal, and parietal function in neurological patients. *Journal of Nervous and Mental Disease, 171,* 435–443.

Konow, A., & Pribram, K. H. (1970). Error recognition and utilization produced by injury to the frontal cortex in man. *Neuropsychologia, 8,* 489–491.

Kraepelin, E. (1919). *Dementia praecox and paraphrenia.* Edinburgh: E. & S. Livingstone.

Leroy, E. (1926). *Les visions du demi sommeil.* Paris: Alcan.

Levin, S. (1984). Frontal lobe dysfunction in schizophrenia - II. Impairments of psychological and brain functions. *Journal of Psychiatric Research, 18,* 27–55.

Levine, D. N. (1990). Unawareness of visual and sensorimotor defects: A hypothesis. *Brain and Cognition, 13,* 233–281.

Levine, D. N., & Grek, A. (1984). The anatomic basis of delusions after right cerebral infarction. *Neurology, 34,* 577–582.

Lhermitte, J. (1939). *L'image de notre corps.* Paris. Nouvelle Revue Critique.

Lhermitte, J. (1951). *Les hallucinations.* Paris: Doin.

Lhermitte, F. (1986). Human autonomy and the frontal lobes, I. Imitation and utilization behavior: A neuropsychological study of 75 patients. *Annals of Neurology, 19,* 326–334.

Liddle, P. F., Friston, K. J., Frith, C. D., Hirsch, S. R., Jones, T., Hirsch, S. R., & Frackowiak, R. S. J. (1992). Patterns of cerebral blood flow in schizophrenia. *British Journal of Psychiatry, 160,* 179–186.

Lukianowicz, N. (1958). Autoscopic phenomena. *Archives of Neurological Psychiatry, 80,* 199–220.

Lukianowicz, N. (1967). "Body image" disturbances in psychiatric disorders. *British Journal of Psychiatry, 113,* 31–47.

Luria, A. R. (1980). *Higher cortical functions in man* (2nd ed.). New York: Basic Books.

MacPherson, R., & Collis, R. (1992). Tardive dyskinesia: Patients' lack of awareness of movement disorder. *British Journal of Psychiatry, 160,* 110–112.

Maher, B. (1974). Delusional thinking and perceptual disorder. *Journal of Individual Psychology, 30,* 98–113.

Malmo, H. P. (1974). On frontal lobe functions: Psychiatric patient controls. *Cortex, 10,* 231.

McGhie, A., & Chapman, J. (1961). Disorders of attention and perception in early schizophrenia. *British Journal of Medical Psychology, 34,* 103–115.

McGlynn, S. M., & Schacter, D. L. (1989). Unawareness of deficits in neuropsychological syndromes. *Journal of Clinical Experimental Neuropsychology, 11,* 143–205.

McGrath, J. (1991). Ordering thoughts on thought disorder. *British Journal of Psychiatry, 158,* 307–316.

Meehl, P. E. (1962). Schizotaxia, schizotypy, and schizophrenia. *American Psychologist, 17,* 827–837.

Mellor, C. S. (1970). First rank symptoms of schizophrenia. *British Journal of Psychiatry, 117,* 15–23.

Mesulam, M. (1985). Patterns in behavioral neuroanatomy: Association areas, the limbic system, and hemispheric specialization. In M. Mesulam (Ed.), *Principles of behavioral neurology,* pp. xx–xx. Philadelphia: F.A. Davis.

Mesulam, M., & Geschwind, N. (1978). On the possible role of neocortex and its limbic connections in the process of attention and schizophrenia: Clinical cases of inattention in man and experimental anatomy in monkey. *Journal of Psychiatric Research, 14,* 249–259.

Mesulam, M., Waxman, S. G., Geschwind, N., & Sabin, T. D. (1976). Acute confusional states with right middle cerebral artery infarctions. *Journal of Neurology, Neurosurgery, and Psychiatry, 39,* 84–89.

Miller, G. A., Galanter, E., & Pribram, K. H. (1960). *Plans and the structure of behavior.* New York: Holt, Reinhart, and Winston.

Morihisa, J. M., Duffy, F. H., & Wyatt, R. J. (1983). Brain electrical activity mapping (BEAM) in schizophrenic patients. *Archives of General Psychiatry, 40,* 719–723.

Morihisa, J. M., & McAnulty, G. B. (1985). Structure and function: Brain electrical activity mapping and computed tomography in schizophrenia. *Biological Psychiatry, 20,* 3–19.

Morrison, R. L., & Tarter, R. E. (1984). Neuropsychological findings relating to Capgras syndrome. *Biological Psychiatry, 19,* 1119–1128.

Mott, F. W. (1907). Bilateral lesion of the auditory cortical centre: Complete deafness and aphasia. *British Medical Journal, 2,* 310–315.

Mulder, D. W., Bickford, R. G., & Dodge, H. W. (1957). Hallucinatory epilepsy: Complex hallucinations as focal seizures. *American Journal of Psychiatry, 113,* 1100.

Muller, H. F. (1985). Prefrontal cortex dysfunction as a common factor in psychosis. *Acta Psychiatrica Scandinavica, 71,* 431–440.

Myslobodsky, M. S. (1986). Anosognosia in tardive dyskinesia: "Tardive dysmentia" or "tardive dementia"? *Schizophrenia Bulletin, 12,* 1–8.

Nathanson, M., Bergman, P. S., & Gordon, G. G. (1952). Denial of illness: Its occurrence in one hundred consecutive cases of hemiplegia. *Archives of Neurological Psychiatry, 68,* 380–387.

Nielsen, J. M. (1938). Disturbances of the body scheme. Their physiologic mechanism. *Bulletin of the Los Angeles Neurological Society, 3,* 127–135.

Olsen, C. W., & Ruby, C. (1941). Anosognosia and autotopognosia. *Archives of Neurological Psychiatry, 46,* 340–344.

Owens, D. G. C., Johnstone, F. C., & Frith, C. D. (1982). Spontaneous involuntary disorders of movement. *Archives of General Psychiatry, 39*, 452–461.

Paterson, A., & Zangwill, O. L. (1944) Disorders of visual space perception associated with lesions of the right cerebral hemisphere. *Brain, 67*, 331–358.

Penfield, W., & Rasmussen, T. (1950). *The cerebral cortex of man.* New York: MacMillan.

Perez, M. M., Trimble, M. R., Murray, N. M. F., & Reider, I. (1985). Epileptic psychosis: An evaluation PSE profiles. *British Journal of Psychiatry, 146*, 155–163.

Peroutka, S. J., Sohmer, B. H., Kumar, A. J., Folstein, M., & Robinson, R. G. (1982). Hallucinations and delusions following a right temporoparieto-occipital infarction. *Johns Hopkins Medical Journal, 151*, 181–185.

Pick, A. (1903). Clinical studies: III. On reduplicative paramnesia. *Brain, 26*, 260–267.

Pick, A. (1908). *Überstörungen der Orientierung am eigenen Körper.* Berlin: Karger.

Prigatano, G. P., & Schacter, D. L. (Eds.). (1991). *Awareness of deficit after brain injury: Clinical and theoretical issues.* New York: Oxford University Press.

Rado, S. (1953). Dynamics and classification of disordered behavior. *American Journal of Psychiatry, 110*, 406–416.

Rapaport, D. (1951). Toward a theory of thinking. In D. Rapaport (Ed.), *Organization and pathology of thought* (pp. 689–730). New York: Columbia University Press.

Redlich, F., & Dorsey, J. F. (1945). Denial of blindness by patients with cerebral disease. *Archives of Neurological Psychiatry, 53*, 407–417.

Reitman, E. E., & Cleveland, S. E. (1964). Changes in body image following sensory deprivation in schizophrenia and control groups. *Journal of Abnormal Social Psychology, 68*, 168–176.

Rosen, A. M., Mukherjee, S., Olarte, S. Vria, V., & Cardenas, C. (1982). Perception of tardive dyskinesia in outpatients receiving maintenance neuroleptics. *American Journal of Psychiatry, 139*, 372–373.

Ruff, R. L., and Volpe, B. T. (1981). Environmental reduplication associated with right frontal and parietal lobe injury. *Journal of Neurology, Neurosurgery, and Psychiatry, 44*, 382–386.

Sacks, M. H., Carpenter, W. T., & Strauss, J. S. (1974). Recovery from delusions: Three phases documented by patients' interpretation of research procedures. *Archives of General Psychiatry, 30*, 117–120.

Sandifer, P. H. (1946). Anosognosia and disorders of body scheme. *Brain, 69*, 122–137.

Sanides, F. (1969). Comparative architectonics of the neocortex of mammals and their evolutionaly significance. *Annals of NY Academy of Science, 167*, 404–423.

Scheibel, A. B., & Kovelman, J. A. (1981). Disorientation of the hippocampal pyramidal cell and its processes in the schizophrenic patient. *Biological Psychiatry, 16*, 101–102.

Schilder, P. (1935). *The image and appearance of the human body.* London: Kegan Paul, Trench, Trubner.

Silva, J. A., Leong, G. B., & Luong, M. T. (1989). Split body and self: An unusual case of misidentification. *Canadian Journal of Psychiatry, 34*, 728–730.

Signer, S. F. (1987). Capgras syndrome: The delusion of substitution. *Journal of Clinical Psychiatry, 48*, 147–150.

Shallice, T. (1988). *From neuropsychology to mental structure.* Cambridge: Cambridge University Press.

Slater, E., Beard, A. W., & Glitheroe, E. (1963). The schizophrenia-like psychoses of epilepsy. *British Journal of Psychiatry, 109*, 95–150.

Smith, J. W., Kucharski, L. T., Oswald, W. T., & Waterman, L. J. (1979). A systematic investigation of tardive dyskinesia in inpatients. *American Journal of Psychiatry, 136*, 918–922.

Spillane, J. D. (1942). Disturbances of the body scheme. Anosognosia and finger agnosia. *Lancet, I*, 42–44.

Starkstein, S. E., Fedoroff, J. P., Price, T. R., Leiguarda, R., & Robinson, R. G. (1993). Neuropsychological deficits in patients with anosognosia. *Neuropsychiatry, Neuropsychology & Behavioral Neurology, 6*, 43–48.

Stevens, J. R. (1973). An anatomy of schizophrenia. *Archives of General Psychiatry, 29*, 177–189.

Stevens, J. R. (1982). Risk factors for psychopathology in individuals with epilepsy. In W. P. Koella & M. R. Trimble (Eds.), *Temporal lobe epilepsy, mania, schizophrenia and the limbic system*. Basel: Karger.

Stevens, J. R. (1988). Psychiatric aspects of epilepsy. *Journal of Clinical Psychiatry, 49*, 49–57.

Stuss, D. T. (1991). Disturbance of self-awareness after frontal system damage. In G. P. Prigatano & D. L. Schacter (Eds.), *Awareness of deficit after brain injury: Clinical and theoretical issues*, pp. 63–83. New York: Oxford University Press.

Stuss, D. T., Alexander, M. P., Lieberman, A., & Levine, H. (1978). An extraordinary form of confabulation. *Neurology, 28*, 1166–1172.

Stuss, D. T., & Benson, D. F. (1984). Neuropsychological studies of the frontal lobes. *Psychological Bulletin, 95*, 3–28.

Stuss, D. T., & Benson, D. F. (1986). *The frontal lobes*. New York: Raven Press.

Stuss, D. T., & Benson, D. F. (1987). In E. Perecman (Ed.), *The frontal lobes revisited*. New York: IRBN Press.

Suddath, R. L., Casanova, M. F., Goldberg, T. E., Daniel, D. G., Kelsoe, J., & Weinberger, D. R. (1989). Temporal lobe pathology in schizophrenia: A quantitative magnetic resonance imaging study. *American Journal of Psychiatry, 146*, 464–472.

Szasz, T. (1957). The psychology of bodily feelings in schizophrenia. *Psychosomatic Medicine, 19*, 11–16.

Taylor, J. (Ed.). (1932). *Selected writings of John Hughlings Jackson*. London: Hodder and Stoughton.

Teuber, H. L. (1961). Perception. In J. Field, H. W. Magoun, & V. E. Hall (Eds.), *Handbook of physiology-neurophysiology, III*, pp. 1595–1668. Washington, DC: American Physiological Society.

Teuber, H. L., Battersby, W. S., & Bender, M. B. (1960). *Visual field defects after penetrating missile wounds of the brain*. Cambridge, MA: Harvard University Press.

Todd, J. (1957). The syndrome of Capgras. *Psychiatric Quarterly, 31*, 250–265.

Toone, B. K., Garralda, M. E., & Ron, M. A. (1982). The psychoses of epilepsy and the functional psychoses. *British Journal of Psychiatry, 141*, 256–261.

Trimble, M. R. (1991). *The psychoses of epilepsy*. New York: Raven Press.

von Holst, E. (1954). Relations between the central nervous system and the peripheral organs. *British Journal of Animal Behavior, 2*, 89–94.

Von Monakow, C. (1905). *Gehirnpathologie* (2nd ed.). Vienna: Alfred Holder.

Wagner, M. T., & Cushman, L. A. (1994). Neuroanatomic and neuropsychological predictors of unawareness of cognitive deficit in the vascular population. *Archives of Clinical Neuropsychology, 9*, 57–69.

Waldenström, J. (1939). On anosognosia. *Acta Psychiatrica, 14*, 215–220.

Weckowicz, T. E., & Sommer, R. (1960). Body image and self-concept in schizophrenia. *Journal of Mental Science, 106*, 17–39.

Weinberger, D. R., Berman, K. F., & Zec, R. F. (1986). Physiological dysfunction of dorsolateral prefrontal cortex in schizophrenia: I. Regional cerebral blood flow (rCBF) evidence. *Archives of General Psychiatry, 43*, 114–124.

Weinstein, E. A., & Kahn, R. L. (1955). *Denial of illness: Symbolic and physiological aspects*. Springfield, IL: Charles C. Thomas.

Wiesel, F. A., Wik, G., Sjognen, G., Blomqvist, G., Grutz, T., & Stone-Elander, S. Regional brain glucose metabolism in drug-free schizophrenics and clinical correlates. *Acta Psychiatrica Scandinavica, 76,* 628–641.

Wernicke, C. (1900). *Grundriss der Psychiatrie in Klinischen Vorlesungen.* Leipzig: Thieme.

Weston, M. J., & Whitlock, F. A. (1971). The Capgras syndrome following head injury. *British Journal of Psychiatry, 119,* 25–31.

Young, D. A., Davila, R., & Scher, H. (1993). Unawareness of illness and neuropsychological performance in chronic schizophrenia. *Schizophrenia Research, 10,* 117–124.

Zaidel, E. (1987). Hemispheric monitoring. In D. Ottoson (Ed.), *Duality and unity of the brain* (pp. 247–281). London: Macmillan.

Zec, R. F., & Weinberger, D. R. (1986). Brain areas implicated in schizophrenia: A selective overview. In H. A. Nasrallah & D. R. Weinberger (Eds.), *Handbook of schizophrenia: 1. The neurology of schizophrenia,* pp. 175–206. New York: Elsevier.

# 8

RICHARD S. E. KEEFE

# The Neurobiology of Disturbances of the Self

## Autonoetic Agnosia in Schizophrenia

### Phenomenology of Autonoetic Agnosia in Schizophrenia

The characteristics that embody the self are so broad that it is difficult to reach consensus on a circumscribed definition of self. According to *Webster's American Collegiate Dictionary*, the definition of the self is "the union of elements (as body, emotions, thoughts, and sensations) that constitute the individuality and identity of a person." In this sense, individuality refers to the quality or state of being indivisible, as well as having a separate and distinct existence from others. Thus, one of the primary features of the self is an embodiment of what is internal, as distinguished from what is external to it.

Kraepelin, Bleuler, and Schneider, among many others, characterized schizophrenia as a brain disorder that is manifested as a disturbance of the self. While many psychiatric disorders involved disturbances of the self, in schizophrenia is found the most severe symptoms of confusion between what is part of the self and what is part of the world of external stimuli. Many of the symptoms of schizophrenia suggest that patients have a cognitive deficit in the ability to maintain the distinction between mental events that originate within the limits of their own central nervous systems and those that occur outside of their bodies and are perceived through sensory awareness. These symptoms are referred to as manifestations of *autonoetic agnosia*, meaning literally a "deficit in the ability to identify self-generated mental events." These symptoms include poor insight, hallucinations, and various forms of delusions, such as thought insertion, thought withdrawal, thought broadcasting, delusions of control, and delusions of "made" actions, impulses, and feelings (Schneider, 1959), which are found in schizophrenia more frequently than in other major psychiatric disorders (Carpenter &

Strauss, 1974). While these types of delusions are no longer individually considered as criteria for schizophrenia by the standard diagnostic manual in American psychiatry, the DSM (American Psychiatric Association, 1987), their importance in making a diagnosis of schizophrenia has not been diminished, as the presence of any of these symptoms (grouped together as "bizarre delusions" in DSM-III-R and DSM-IV) are key in making a diagnosis of schizophrenia. In this section I will describe the symptoms of schizophrenia that may reflect a severe disturbance in maintaining the distinction between internally generated and externally generated mental events.

### Hallucinations

Hallucinations are the result of the misinterpretation of an internally generated mental event as having originated in the perceptual realm (Heilbrun, 1980; Bentall, 1990). Although the arguments in this chapter could be applied to hallucinations in any of the five sensory modalities, auditory and visual hallucinations will receive the most attention, as these are the most common hallucinatory experiences of schizophrenic patients. The generation of auditory and visual images is a part of normal, everyday cognitive experience. People without psychiatric disorders may vividly remember particular visual scenes from times long past, or recall words spoken to them, or music played, as though the event were occurring in the present moment. It is also within normal experience to generate visual images or auditory images through fantasy and imagination, that have never been directly experienced. There is a high degree of variability among normal individuals in the vividness of their images (Johnson, 1991). However, it is not within normal experience to interpret these images, no matter how vivid, as having been perceived through external stimulation. This type of misinterpretation, which results in the experience of hallucination, has been found in 70% of patients with schizophrenia (Sartorius, Shapiro, & Jablensky, 1974).

### Delusions

Many of the delusions found in patients with schizophrenia could be argued to involve a severe misunderstanding of the self. Grandiose delusions and religious delusions, for instance, may reflect patients' severe absence of awareness of who they are, how they fit into society, and the general consensus of what is true. However, in this chapter I will focus on a more specific disturbance of the self—that is, the firm belief of some patients with schizophrenia that self-generated, internally mediated events are physically affected by forces outside of the self. The most notable of these delusions have been described as the first-rank symptoms of schizophrenia by Kurt Schneider (1959). Among these delusions are the following:

1. *Thought insertion* involves the experience, and the usually subsequent belief, that alien thoughts, generated by another person or agency, have been literally placed inside the head of the experiencer, resulting in there being more thoughts than were inside one's head previously.
2. *Thought withdrawal* involves the opposite phenomenon, whereby the individual experiences an outside force removing thoughts from one's head, resulting in fewer thoughts than previously held.

3. *Thought broadcasting* involves the belief that one's thoughts are being broadcast into the atmosphere so that other people can hear them.
4. *Delusion of control* involves the belief that one's body movements are not of one's own volition; rather these movements are experienced as having been generated from an agency outside of the self. The same type of delusional interpretation can be present in the form of "made" impulses, actions, and feelings.

## Lack of insight

Insight, defined here as "the ability to view oneself, including one's mental operations, as if from the view of an outside observer," is very frequently impaired in schizophrenia (Amador, Strauss, Yale, & Gorman, 1991). Schizophrenic patients may lack not only insight about the severity of their symptoms but also the general ability to take an observer's perspective about themselves. Since insight involves the capacity of individuals to view themselves accurately in the context of the external world, and to move without confusion between internal and external perspectives, lack of insight is considered part of the manifestation of autonoetic agnosia in schizophrenia that will be discussed in this chapter. Patients with autonoetic agnosia may not be able to move flexibly between internal and external perspectives owing to an inability to maintain the distinction between externally generated mental events and internally generated events.

All of these symptoms—hallucinations, delusions, and lack of insight—involve a disruption of the normal mental flow of consciousness, resulting in a disturbance in the correct identification of internally generated events and externally generated events as such. In each symptom, there is a clear disturbance of consciousness—the misinterpretation of an internal event, generated and maintained by the nervous system of the experiencer, as having originated outside of the self. These mental events can be misinterpreted via the perceptual realm, as in hallucinations, or through the realm of cognition, as in thought insertion, delusions of control, and poor insight.

Previous conceptualizations of the disruption of distinction between internally generated mental events and externally generated perceptions in schizophrenia have been viewed largely in the context of psychodynamic thought. The assumption in these theories was that once the self was developed, it could not be *un*developed. Thus, schizophrenia was viewed as the result of a *lack* of proper development of self-other distinctions (Tausk 1919/1948), and was suggested to have been a result of early child-parent interactions (Freud, 1915/1963, 1924/1963; Fenichel, 1945). These theories of the schizophrenogenic parent have been discarded owing to lack of evidence (Ricks & Berry, 1970), as well as a clearly more convincing argument in favor of biological factors such as genetic etiological factors (Kety, Rosenthal, & Wender, 1975), and obstetric complications (DeLisi, Dauphinais, & Gerson, 1988). Data from various sources support the abandonment of theories positing interpersonal development as key to the etiology of schizophrenia, and suggest that the inability to make accurate distinctions between internal and external mental events can begin following infancy. For instance, studies of infants have demonstrated clear evidence of a sense of self-other differentiation in the first few weeks of life (Stern, 1985), suggesting that self-other constructs are not entirely dependent upon interactional factors during development.

An equally compelling body of evidence that the self-other dissolution in schizo-phrenia could be acquired following years of normal development derives from studies of patients with brain injuries. Patients with various types of brain damage, with no known prior psychiatric disturbance, have been shown to manifest a form of the disso-lution of self that is believed to be a sole consequence of their brain lesions, as dis-cussed in greater detail by Barr (see chapter 7). Patients with hemiplegia—involving paralysis or weakness on one side of the body, usually the left (Cutting, 1978), and visual hemifield neglect—have been observed to deny the weakness of their paralyzed limbs and to develop other abnormal attitudes about their paralysis. This denial of obvi-ous limb weakness is referred to as anosognosia (Babinski, 1914). Some hemiplegic patients experience their weakened or paralyzed limbs as strange or alien, and may believe that they belong to others (Gertsmann, 1942; Cutting, 1978, Critchley, 1974; Levine & Rinn, 1986; Nightingale, 1982; Miller, 1991). Thus, specific brain insult in individuals with no known premorbid psychopathology can lead to severe disturbances in making distinctions between what is part of the self and what is not.

The question to be addressed in this paper is whether patients with schizophrenia who manifest severe disturbances in maintaining the distinction between internally generated mental events and mental events that originate outside of the self have a sim-ilar disturbance to patients with anosognosia. This phenomenon is referred to here as *autonoetic agnosia** in order to distinguish it from similar notions described previously with labels used to suggest or imply an etiology based upon early interpersonal experi-ences, such as boundary disturbances (e.g., Jacobson, 1954; Blatt & Wild, 1976), and to reflect its similarities to other deficits in recognizing specific aspects of perception or cognition that result from brain disorder, such as visual agnosia and anosognosia. It has previously been difficult to determine whether this deficit has specific relationships with other cognitive deficits in schizophrenics, since it has not been rigorously charac-terized or defined with specific criteria that could enhance the reliability and validity of its assessment. The possible cognitive and neuroanatomic correlates associated with autonoetic agnosia will be postulated following a review of studies of normal individu-als, patients with schizophrenia, and patients with brain lesions. One benefit of this approach is that it may contribute to the identification of specific aspects of the phe-nomenology of schizophrenia associated with particular disease processes. Similar approaches have been applied to various aspects of negative (Strauss, Carpenter, & Bartko, 1974) and deficit (Carpenter, Heinrichs, & Wagman, 1988) symptoms to demonstrate the possible neuroanatomic pathways implicated in these symptom clus-ters (Andreasen, 1989; Tamminga et al., 1992). The possible cognitive and neu-roanatomic aspects of delusions and hallucinations have not received as much atten-tion, notwithstanding recent attempts to explore the cognitive processes involved in specific aspects of psychosis in schizophrenia, such as thought echo (David, 1994a) and hallucinations (Gray, Feldon, Rawlins, Hemsley, & Smith, 1991).

---

*This term was developed in consultation with Professor Ralph Rosen of the University of Pennsylvania Department of Classical Studies.

## Determining the Origin of Mental Events: Cognitive Processes and Relevant Neuroanatomy

Before discussing the manner in which autonoetic agnosia and associated symptoms may develop in schizophrenia as a function of cognitive deficits and brain dysfunction known to be present in the disorder, I will review the results of selected studies that point to specific cognitive functions and brain regions underlying the capacity to distinguish between internally and externally generated mental events.

One of the most important functions of the brain is to recognize what is a part of the self and what is not. In terms of basic survival, we need to understand the difference between objects that are part of our bodies and external objects, which may put our health at risk through infectious disease, internal injury, and the like. Yet we place selected nonself objects without ourselves frequently; some obvious examples occur during breathing, eating, sexual activity, medical procedures, and the process of "cleaning the boundaries," such as brushing our teeth and washing our skin. The reduced danger of this entrance depends upon the strength of our immune system, as well as the wisdom of our selections. The importance of these selections is matched by the complexity of the task. Since information about the universe of nonself objects that come into our perception is acquired through the nervous system, this information becomes part of the self in the form of mental representations. One of the primary functions of consciousness is to maintain awareness of internal states, external facts, and the distinction between the two. Thus, the nervous system must devote considerable energy to distinguishing between external objects that are not part of the self and their internal representations, which are. An example of the advantage of this function is that when we are hungry, we recognize that we cannot subsist on the internally generated mental images of the foods we would like to eat!

Recent studies of cortical structure, circuitry, and function suggest that one of the guiding principles of the development of neuronal tissue may be the determination of what is part of the self and what is not (Montague, Gally, & Edelman, 1991). In recent models of neural development, the pattern of neural activity serves as a guide by which terminal axonal arbors are segregated within dendritic fields during the development of neural circuitry. Thus, the structure of neural circuitry may be determined in part by an individual's history of neural activity (Edelman & Cunningham, 1990). Computer-simulation models of human brain functions suggest that this mechanism of neural development can be applied to the development of self-identity in humans (Edelman, 1987). In these computer models, self-identity proves not to be static but, rather, is plastic and dynamic. Even in the adult neuroanatomy, the pattern of neural connectivity that is postulated to be associated with self-identity is in constant flux. Thus, the human brain has the capacity to alter its structure on the basis of its previous function. If the connections between affiliated networks are disturbed, the historical imprint of their relatedness may be disturbed as well. In some cases, this could lead to loss of a previously acquired belief about what is part of the self and what is not.

While these processes are equally important in most living things, unlike most other species, humans have the additional capacity to understand and empathize with the experience of nonself beings. This ability has clear adaptive advantages in such diverse realms as love and war, yet it adds greatly to the complexity of distinguishing which mental events we generate and which have been generated externally. We need not only to make distinctions between externally generated perceptual stimuli and internally generated ideation but also to distinguish our own emotional responses from the emotions of others, and to recognize that our "experience of the other" is internally generated. Before I discuss the cognitive and neuroanatomic dysfunctions in schizophrenia that may make such distinctions difficult, leading to autonoetic agnosia and associated symptoms, I will describe a series of related functions in normal individuals: (1) the process of distinguishing visual images from perceptions; (2) the process of making the distinction between memories of real and imagined events, termed *reality monitoring*; and (3) a proposed internal cognitive system by which thoughts, images, and perceptions are supervised.

## Visual Image Generation and Perception

The relationship between image generation and the perception of stimuli is relevant to the notion of an impairment in schizophrenia, in distinguishing between self-generated and externally generated mental events. Convergent data from psychophysiological, cognitive, and neuroanatomic studies suggest that there are common neural substrates for imagery and perception. In human and nonhuman primate brains, projections from posterior association cortex to frontal areas are inevitably accompanied by projections in the opposite direction (Goldman-Rakic, 1987; Mesulam, 1990). When humans speak, neurons are activated simultaneously in Broca's and Wernicke's areas suggesting reciprocal coupling of these areas (Mesulam 1990). When monkeys see visual illusions in specific aspects of the visual field, neurons in the visual cortex associated with perception of this part of visual space fire despite the absence of actual stimulation. The data from this line of investigation suggest that cognition is not governed by specific brain areas; rather, it is the result of such parallel distributions of neurons acting in concert (Goldman-Rakic, 1987; Mesulam, 1990). The implications of these parallel distributed networks in the visual system, and their relevance to autonoetic agnosia in schizophrenia, will be considered here.

Studies of normal human cognition suggest that there is a spatially organized internal representation of the visual field. When one forms a visual mental image, the specific region of the internally represented visual field where the image is formed undergoes a change of state (Farah, 1989). Brain-damaged individuals show deficits in imagery that parallel their deficits in perception (Farah, 1988; Kossyln & Koenig, 1992) consistent with the notion of parallel pathways for imagining and perceiving visual stimuli. For example, the work of Bisiach (Bisiach & Luzzatti, 1978; Bisiach, Luzzatti, & Perani, 1979) suggests that patients with unilateral visual neglect ignore objects on the same side of space in both perception and mental imagery. In one study (Bisiach et al., 1979), patients with right parietal lobe damage were presented with cloudlike forms moving behind a screen with a vertical slit in the center, such that the shape of the whole forms could be reconstructed from the successive views seen through the slit. The patients were asked to determine whether pairs of forms viewed in this way were the same as or different from each other. Although all stimulus input through the slit was presented to central vision (i.e., providing visual input to both cerebral hemispheres), these patients showed neglect of the left sides of the forms by incorrectly judging forms to be the same when they differed on their left sides. Thus, even though the perception of these forms was not impaired in these patients with hemifield neglect, since the visual stimuli were presented in central vision, there was an impairment in the process by which the forms were constructed in their imagination consistent with their left-side neglect. These data support the notion of a strong relationship between the processes of constructing visual perceptions and visual images.

As described in Kosslyn et al. (1993) and Farah (1988), a variety of evidence suggests that the brain regions involved in vision are also involved in visual mental imagery. Virtually every area involved in vision that has an afferent connection to another area receives an efferent connection from that area, and the forward and backward projections are of comparable size (Van Essen, 1985). The nature of this neuroanatomic structure suggests that the brain maintains the capacity for neural connectivity from areas that mediate the organization of visual inputs to the lower level areas that mediate early aspects of visual stimulus input. The direction of connections reported from area TE (in the anterior inferior temporal lobe) to area 17, the primary visual cortex region in the occipital lobe (Douglas & Rockland, 1992) is consistent with the notion that visual mental images are formed by using stored information to reconstruct spatial patterns received from cortical areas mediating visual stimulus input (Kosslyn et al., 1993).

Further support for the concept of bidirectional neural pathways mediating visual perception and imagery can be found in studies of regional brain activation. Studies using various imaging methods (Farah, Peronnet, Gonon, & Girard, 1988; Goldenberg et al., 1989) have reported that brain regions associated with visual perception are activated when subjects are instructed to generate visual images. Recently, Kosslyn et al. (1993) used PET to distinguish between brain areas activated during visual perception, visual imagery, and a psychomotor control task. The results indicated that a network of regions are activated during visual mental imagery that include primary visual cortex (area 17 in the Talairach and Tournoux, 1988, atlas), superior parietal, inferior parietal and temporal regions, and dorsolateral prefrontal cortex. It is believed that the superior parietal regions are activated in order to disengage attention from one region of visual image to another (Posner & Petersen, 1990), while the inferior parietal areas may be involved in encoding the spatial relations among stimulus parts during the construction of visual images (see Kosslyn et al., 1990). The temporal lobe may be activated during this task in order to recall visual memories that help produce the visual images, while the prefrontal cortex may be involved in helping to construct the visual images, possibly by keeping previously built components of the image on line while the image is being refined and extended (Goldman-Rakic, 1987).

One of the important questions in relating this work to autonoetic agnosia in schizophrenia is the process by which disturbances in processing perceptual input may result in confusion between imagined and perceived stimuli. The finding that imagery affects relatively low-level visual areas raises the possibility that top-down processing may play a greater role in perception than is currently assumed. The results from the PET study of Kosslyn et al. (1993) suggest that visual mental imagery may be used in perception itself when one is faced with fragmentary input. In this study, the processing of degraded visual stimuli resulted in activation of the same brain regions that were activated during a visual imagery task. Thus, when the human brain is faced with fragmentary input from external sources, it appears to call on internal imagery processes in the attempt to make sense of the incomplete data. The possible effect of this process on autonoetic agnosia in schizophrenia will be described below.

## Reality Monitoring

Humans acquire information from a variety of sources, including various sensory organs for perceiving stimuli and internal sources for different types of idea generation. *Reality monitoring* refers to the successful discrimination between internally and externally generated sources of information (Johnson & Raye, 1981). Successful reality monitoring involves a variety of processing components (see Johnson, 1992). Much of the work on reality monitoring has investigated the process of identifying memories to an internal versus an external source. First, memories originating in perception typically have more perceptual information (e.g., color, sound), contextual time and place information, and more meaningful detail, whereas memories originating in imagination typically have more accessible information about cognitive operations—that is, those perceptual and selective processes that took place when the memory was established (Johnson, Foley, Suengas, & Raye, 1988; David, 1993). For example, I know that my fantasies of having beaten Nick Faldo on the final hole of the Ryder Cup Golf Championship are self-generated, since there are so few details about the event available to me: I know nothing about what his reaction was, who else was there with me, what color the sky was, or even how I got to the golf course. A second way in which internally derived imagination and externally derived memories are distinguished is through reasoning. Such processes include retrieving additional information from memory and considering if the target memory could have been perceived or self-generated given these other specific memories or general knowledge. For example, I am further compelled to believe my Ryder Cup memories of victory over Nick Faldo are self-generated, since I have never met Mr. Faldo and I am not a very good golfer.

Empirical studies of normal volunteers suggest that there are a variety of ways in which the process of reality monitoring can fail. First, if there is overlap in the content of memories derived from perception and those generated via imagination, the two may become confused. The more often subjects imagine a picture, the greater the likelihood that they believe they had actually seen it (Johnson, Raye, Wang, & Taylor, 1979). If subjects are asked to imagine hearing a word in another person's voice, they are more likely later to believe they had perceived it from the other person than if they imagined saying it themselves (Johnson, Foley, & Leach, 1988). The increased perceptual similarity between the memory of a perception and the memory of an imagined event can contribute to the confusion. If perceptual qualities of imagined events are unusually vivid, they may be more difficult to discriminate from perceived events. This may occur if reflective processes recruit an overabundance of perceptual processes during imagination. Another possible source of deficit in reality monitoring is that subjects often refer to supporting memories and contextual information to substantiate their perceptions. ("I remember exactly what she wore that day"). Memories derived from perception typically have more contextual information than memories derived from imagination (Johnson, 1988). Supporting memories for events occurring both before and after a target event are used to help specify the origin of a memory. A reduction in the amount of contextual information usually associated with perceived events or an increase in the contextual information associated with imagined events may produce deficits in reality monitoring (Cohen & Servan-Schreiber, 1992). If there is a disruption in the retrieval of contextual memories or the coding of these memories initially, the context of the input of the stimulus is likely to be reduced and the memory may be experienced as more isolated, foreign, and unreal to the individual. A deficit in the ability of an individual to access information during recall of real versus imagined events may similarly disrupt reality monitoring (Johnson, 1988).

### Brain Regions Implicated in Reality Monitoring

No studies to date have investigated the brain regions implicated in the specific task of reality monitoring as described here. However, by inference, the frontal lobes are the most likely brain area to be involved in mediating reality monitoring functions (Johnson, 1991a). Given the importance of the temporal cortex in memory, it is likely to be crucial in recalling whether stimuli were internally or externally generated. Successful reality monitoring is dependent upon the development of contextual associations to memories. Since the establishment of context, particularly with regard to the temporal relationship of events, is mediated by prefrontal regions (Milner, Petrides, & Smith, 1985; Shimamura, Janowsky, & Squire, 1990), dysfunction of the prefrontal cortex may impair reality monitoring by disrupting the process of establishing a context for mental events to be coded, whether externally or internally generated, to be remembered later. This type of disruption could cause internally and externally generated mental events to be recalled similarly, resulting in an individual's inability to distinguish what was perceived from what was imagined.

The anterior cingulate gyrus may also be important in distinguishing internally from externally generated mental events. This proposition is based on the observation that anterior cingulectomy patients often experience spontaneous activation of information with a high degree of perceptual content (Johnson, 1991a). Since one of the functions of the prefrontal cortex, particularly the limbic connections between the orbital prefrontal cortex and the amygdala, is to inhibit inappropriate affective responses (Rolls, 1990; LeDoux, 1992), it is possible that impairments in frontal functions result in inappropriate administration of affective tone to memories of internally derived events. In terms of reality monitoring, this may have the effect of making internally generated mental events appear real to the experiencer.

### The Supervisory Attention System

Access to information about one's own cognitive operations, an important part of executive functions (Stuss and Benson, 1986), is an essential component of identifying oneself as the origin of information (Johnson, 1991b). Sperry (1950) suggested that when a command is sent from higher cortical regions to motor areas to make a motor movement, a parallel message is sent to the perceptual system to be ready for stimulus input. He referred to this mechanism as *reafference* or *corollary discharge*. According to Frith (1987), corollary discharge is part of an internal monitoring system that enables an individual to distinguish between effects due to self-generated actions and events in the external world. Frith suggested that an internal monitor of actions and thoughts not

only makes us aware that an action is about to occur but also communicates information about the source of that action. Frith makes the distinction between stimulus-
driven actions (*stimulus intentions*), self-generated actions (*willed intention*), and
actions currently being initiated. The monitor must be able to compare the information
from these different sources and indicate mismatches, so that current goals, stimulus
meanings, and actions can be modified. Anatomical and behavioral evidence forwarded by Goldberg (1985) and Passingham (1987) substantiate the distinction between
these two pathways to action. In Parkinson's disease, for instance, self-generated acts are
impaired, while stimulus driven acts are unaffected.

Similar to Frith's model, Gray (1982) proposed the function and anatomy of a comparator that continually monitors sensory data from the external world and compares
these with expected perceptions. He locates this monitoring to the septo-hippocampal
system. Frith also argues that the hippocampus plays a significant role in comparing
current sensory information with an internally generated model of the world in which
expected stimuli and suitable responses are specified. However, the dorsolateral prefrontal cortex (DLPFC) is also likely to be involved in this comparative function, as
neurons in area 46 of the *Rhesus* monkey appear to keep recently acquired stimuli
immediately available in working memory (Goldman-Rakic, 1987), and these stimuli
can be compared to stored information. Gray (1982) forwards the notion that relevant
information about responses is passed through the connections between the prefrontal
cortex and the entorhinal area, while projections from the prefrontal cortex to the cingulate cortex are associated with information about anticipated responses. Eventually,
these connections involve the monitoring system of the hippocampus. Frith, Friston,
Liddle, and Frackowiak (1991) propose that information about intended self-generated
acts comes to the monitor from the prefrontal cortex via the entorhinal cortex (hippocampal gyrus), the cingulate cortex, and are realized via the basal ganglia and the
supplementary motor areas. Normal individuals engaged in a task of eye-movement
generation demonstrate maximal activation in the left parahippocampal gyrus (Frith,
Friston, Liddle, & Frackowiak, 1992). While these brain regions are likely to be involved
in the process of differentiating between internally and externally generated mental
events, empirical data do not support the notion of information traveling serially like a
pinball between brain areas, as forwarded in these models. Rather, this complex function is likely to be mediated by neural networks that work in parallel among these different regions (Goldman-Rakic, 1988; Mesulam, 1990). Dysfunctions in these networks may result in the attempt to identify the source of information without adequate
data available. As discussed below, dysfunctions in different brain regions or connections between regions may result in different types of monitoring deficits.

Shallice (1988) suggested that frontal cortical regions subserve a supervisory attentional system that is essential for performance of novel tasks that require self-generated
mental effort, but not for performance of routine tasks in which actions are specified by
the current situation. Evidence for the neuroanatomic distinction between internally
driven and stimulus-driven responses can be derived from studies of lesions in the sup-
plemental motor area (SMA). Such lesions impair internally generated responses, but
not responses elicited by external stimuli (Passingham, Chen, & Thaler, 1989). Recent
PET data suggest that during a willed task (either word generation or finger-movement
generation) compared to a control task (automatic verbal or finger-movement response

to stimuli), significant increases in activation occur specifically in the DLPFC (area 46) and the anterior cingulate gyrus (area 32), while decreases are found in the posterior cingulate gyrus (area 23), superior temporal gyrus (area 22), angular gyrus (area 39), and sensory motor cortex (Frith et al., 1991) In this study, willed word generation was associated with left DLPFC increases only, while willed movement generation was associated with bilateral increases. In a similar word-generation task (subjects gave the use of the word presented—e.g., cake—eat), Petersen, Fox, Posner, Mintun, and Raichle (1988) also found activation of the DLPFC and the anterior cingulate cortex. Deiber et al. (1991) reported that the task of generating random joystick movements into one of four quadrants was associated with bilateral prefrontal activation similar to that in the Frith et al. (1991) study. The results of these activation studies have been interpreted to suggest that the increase in activity of the cingulate cortex is associated with attention to response selection, while the DLPFC is involved in internal response generation (Frith et al., 1991; Petersen et al., 1988). This notion is supported by PET data that the cingulate cortex, but not the DLPFC, is activated by the Stroop Color-Word Task, which demands effortful attention to response selection; but since responses are made to external stimuli, little self-generated activity is required (Pardo, Pardo, Janer, & Raichle, 1990). Conversely, Warkentin, Nilsson, Risberg, & Carlson (1989) reported that a verbal fluency task, which demands self-generated activity, activates the DLPFC but not the anterior cingulate.

In summary, the normal process of making distinctions between internally generated and externally generated mental events involves a supervisory attentional system that continuously assesses the perceptual richness and complexity of information, determines the context of the information, and invokes reasoning processes to determine the origin of the information. Multiple sources of evidence suggest that this important and complex cognitive function may be mediated by a neural network involving the prefrontal cortex. The next section will address how this system may be impaired in schizophrenic patients with symptoms of autonoetic agnosia.

## Cognitive Deficits Associated with the Genesis of Autonoetic Agnosia in Schizophrenia

Since the process of distinguishing between internally and externally generated mental events is extraordinarily complex, it could be impaired by a variety of deficits. Furthermore, severe impairments in determining the origin of information could result from sporadic cognitive deficits that would not always be present in an individual. This is particularly relevant in patients with schizophrenia, since cognitive deficits and psychotic symptoms, present in almost all patients at some phase of their illness, are correlated with one another cross-sectionally in some studies (Green & Walker, 1985) but not others (Goldberg et al. 1993), and the symptoms of psychosis are quite variable in schizophrenia patients over time (Putnam et al., 1993).

Surprisingly little direct empirical data have been collected on the ability of schizophrenic patients to distinguish between information they derived from external sources and information generated internally. In the few studies completed to date, schizophrenic patients have been shown to make more errors than normals in remembering whether words came from a list that they had actually read aloud or from a list that they read silently to themselves and imagined themselves saying (Harvey, 1985; Harvey, Earle-Boyer, & Levinson, 1988; Tanenbaum & Harvey, 1988). While normals also make errors on this task, most of their errors are the result of the belief that they only thought about words that they actually said (Raye & Johnson, 1980). In contrast, schizophrenic patients make errors with an opposite bias: they believe they said words that they only thought about saying (Harvey et al., 1988), suggesting that they mistake internal representations or images for actual events in the external world. Providing a context for memory by asking subjects to generate stories about words with a common theme that they either say aloud or think to themselves reduces the differences between schizophrenic patients and normals, yet schizophrenics still make significantly more errors in discriminating what they said from what they thought they said (Tanenbaum & Harvey, 1988). Patients with hallucinations and Schneiderian delusions may be particularly impaired on tests of reality monitoring. Psychotic patients with hallucinations were found to be more likely than psychotic nonhallucinators to misattribute to the experimenter items they had generated themselves (Benthall, Baker, & Havers, 1991). Among a group of schizophrenic patients, those with Schneiderian experiences of alien control of their thoughts and actions are significantly less likely to make error corrections in the absence of visual feedback, suggesting that these schizophrenics may have particular difficulties monitoring their responses (Frith & Done, 1989). These data suggest that schizophrenic patients manifest deficits in distinguishing between internal and external sources of information. The deficits may be particularly severe in patients with hallucinations and Schneiderian delusions.

One of the important questions about this work is which cognitive deficits are associated with the inability to distinguish between externally and internally generated mental events in schizophrenia. Considerable data have been collected on cognitive deficits in schizophrenia, and will be considered here.

*Reduced Perceptual Input*    The first cognitive deficit to be considered as a possible contributor to autonoetic agnosia and the symptoms that may be produced as a result is an impairment in the normal differences between the phenomenal qualities of perceived and imagined events. Disruptions in the normal flow of perceptual events could result in a relative weakening of the experience of perceptual stimuli compared to internally generated images. This weakening may render the process of making distinctions between internally and externally generated information more difficult. A large literature on the cognitive deficits of patients with schizophrenia suggests that there is severe impairment in the normal attentional processes required to acquire information about the external world of perceptual stimuli (see reviews by Nuechterlein & Dawson, 1984; Holzman, 1987). One of the results of this attentional deficit may be a reduction in the amount and intensity of perceptual stimuli that is received from external sources (Granholm, Asarnow, & Marder, 1991; Serper, 1993), which may make internally generated information seem rich in comparison. Thus, schizophrenic patients with autonoetic agnosia may misinterpret these internally generated stimuli as having the richness of external stimuli. Such a misinterpretation could result in the perception of internally generated thoughts as hallucinations or "new" thoughts that are perceived as novel, and thus are determined to have originated from a noninternal source, as in thought insertion. It is important to note that the reduction of perceptual input does not require a perceptual deficit. However, a sporadic attentional disturbance could result in a reduced amount of perceptual information available for processing.

As suggested by the recent PET work of Kosslyn et al. (1993), the presence of fragmentary perceptual input may result in recruitment of internally generated imagery regulated by top-down neuroanatomic pathways to fill in the gaps in perceptual information. In this manner, these substitute stimuli may be misinterpreted as actual perceptions, resulting in the experience of hallucinations. Thus, if attentional deficits in patients with schizophrenia result in fragmentary perceptual input, imagined input may be used to make perceptions "complete," resulting in confusion between internally and externally generated mental events.

Reduced perceptual input can be a consequence of social isolation, lack of social skills, and deafness—all of which have been associated with the development of delusions (Swann, 1984; Maher & Spitzer, 1984). Not only are these states associated with a reduced capacity or opportunity to test ideas against the social consensus but, in addition, these are conditions in which the number of internally generated mental events increases relative to the number of externally derived mental events. Those people who are restricted from social interaction and external stimulation may engage more frequently in self-generated processes. Thus, if they engage more in imagination than in perception, the imagined processes may gain prominence over those that are based in the real world (Johnson, 1991b). The importance of social isolation in the development of the symptoms of autonoetic agnosia is supported by the documented relationship between premorbid social isolation and later schizophrenic delusions and hallucinations (Lewine, Watt, & Fryer, 1978; Watt, 1978), although a relationship between early attentional disturbance and later schizophrenia has not been established (Cornblatt, Lenzenwegger, Dworkin, & Erlenmeyer-Kimling, 1992; Erlenmeyer-Kimling et al. 1993).

It has been repeatedly suggested that hallucinations may be the result of abnormally vivid mental imagery (Sietz & Malholm, 1947; Horrowitz, 1975) that causes schizophrenic patients to misattribute occasional vivid images to an external source. However, as noted by Neisser (1967), hallucinations are often very difficult to perceive to the patients who suffer from them, yet individuals who do not hallucinate may experience very vivid mental images that they do not regard as real. Thus, the specific cognitive attribution of the experience as having occurred outside the self is critical for autonoetic agnosia and the resultant psychotic symptoms to develop.

*Memory*    Memory deficits, which are well documented in patients with schizophrenia (e.g., Saykin et al. 1991) may lead to autonoetic agnosia in at least two distinct ways. First, the effect of disrupted memory for perceptual events may have the effect of diluting the richness of the original perceptual event, which creates similarities in the phenomenal experiences of memories for actual experiences and self-generated imagined events. Second, memory deficits could result in an individual's inability to retrieve supporting information about the event whose source is under consideration. If the supporting memories of an actual event are not able to be retrieved, the event may appear not to have sufficient context to have taken place in reality. Memories of events that were imagined may thus appear, in contrast, to have equal contextual support as those that were generated by external experience. In general, this impairment may result in confusion between real and imagined events. If this impairment persists over time, false beliefs about the principles on which reality is based could develop. More specifically, the repeated inability to establish an adequate context for memories and other internally generated mental events may result in the interpretation of mental events as coming into and out of awareness as if on their own accord. In the struggle to understand an internal world of contextless memories, thoughts, impulses, and even motor movements, an individual may develop the belief that an external force is in control of the appearance of these mental events, resulting in delusions of thought insertion, thought withdrawal, and delusions of control. As noted by Johnson, Hashtroudi, and Lindsay (1993), delusional individuals often are vigilant about seeking supporting information about their delusions since normal supporting memories are not available. In patients with schizophrenia, delusions have been reported to be richer in perceptual content than real memories and fantasies (David & Howard, 1994). The authors of this study propose that the richness of delusional memories may be attributable to the great amount of attention they receive from the delusional individual, as evidenced by the increased rehearsal and affective tone associated with delusional memories compared with real memories.

*Context*    Autonoetic agnosia could also result from deficits in placing information in the proper context, independent of memory deficits. The deficits of schizophrenic patients on several attention- and language-related tasks have been explained in terms of a disturbance in the internal representation of contextual information (Cohen & Servan-Schreiber, 1992). If memories for internally and externally generated mental events are retrieved adequately, yet they are not placed in the context of the relevant information available about reality, comparisons between internally generated events and external reality may be inaccurate. For example, after having visited his grandmother's grave site, a schizophrenic patient developed the belief that she was sending him thoughts about her painful death. Apparently, he was unable to connect his own memories about her death to the context of visiting her grave. The absence of a proper context for these memories, which was interpreted as having arrived in the patient's head completely out of context, resulted in the experience of thought insertion.

*Reasoning Processes*    Most symptoms that result from the cognitive deficit of autonoetic agnosia suggest a breakdown in the normal reasoning processes. Normal reasoning involves frequent comparisons between ideas and consensually derived reality. While the experiences that may result from autonoetic agnosia, such as the experience of thought withdrawal, are not likely to derive solely from an inability to place one's thoughts in the context of social reality, maintenance of the belief that thoughts are actually regularly withdrawn from one's head by an outside force demands a certain degree of disconnection between internally generated beliefs and general consensus about the powers of the human brain.

The delusions that could result from autonoetic agnosia may initially be borne from an inappropriately lax system for making the judgment whether a particular belief is implausible (Johnson, 1988). The criteria for plausibility are usually set by the context in which a belief is placed. As described by Johnson (1991), people are more lax about detecting peaches in a tree than in detecting enemy planes in the sky. Since schizo-phrenic patients have severe problems with tasks that require establishing a context for internal representations (Cohen & Servan-Schreiber, 1992), they may not be able to determine the plausibility of their beliefs because of chronic deficits in understanding the relationship between a belief and its context.

*Supervisory Attentional System*    The task of keeping the many different components of the self in mind is complex. Any deficit in the supervisory attentional system that com-pares internally and externally generated mental events to one another may result in autonoetic agnosia. As described above, the presence of a specific monitoring system that compares internally and externally generated mental events has been proposed by Gray (1982) and Frith (1987). Gray suggested that an internal comparator continually monitors sensory data from the external world and compares these with expected per-ceptions. Similarly, Frith differentiated between stimulus intentions—responses to envi-ronmental stimuli—and willed intentions—responses to internally generated notions; and suggested that a breakdown of the monitor would lead to confusion about the source of an action or thought, as manifest in the symptoms of schizophrenia.

According to Frith (1987), some of the psychotic symptoms of schizophrenia are experienced when self-generated acts occur but information about willed intentions fails to reach the monitor. The occurrence of mismatches between intentions and actions could be reduced in two ways: the signal to the monitor about willed intentions could be increased, or the signal that initiates self-generated acts could be reduced. The pres-ence of a deficient monitor in schizophrenia and other psychotic disorders is supported by evoked potential studies. Self-generated tones (tones elicited by the subject's button press) in normals results in attenuated evoked potentials compared to randomly occur-ring tones. However, among schizophrenic patients, only 20% attenuate to the self-generated tones, while 40% of nonschizophrenic psychotic patients demonstrate attenuation (Frith & Done, 1988). The model of autonoetic agnosia in schizophrenia presented in this chapter suggests that patients with autonoetic agnosia may be the least likely psychotic patients to demonstrate attentuation to self-generated tones, since self-generated acts are frequently experienced as having been generated externally, and would thus be processed similarly to randomly occurring perceptual phenomena.

The inability to hold information on-line in working memory (Baddeley, 1986) may be a key aspect of a deficit in this system, as any comparison among mental events involves working memory, and an interruption in working memory processes interferes with the ability of the patient to keep a constant self in mind. Working memory, medi-ated by the dorsolateral prefrontal cortex in *Rhesus* monkeys (Goldman-Rakic, 1987), has been shown to be impaired in patients with schizophrenia (Park & Holzman, 1992; Keefe et al., 1995), particularly in schizophrenic patients with severe deficits in their ability to administer self-care (Keefe et al., 1993). Other aspects of a supervisory atten-tional system, such as abstraction and executive functions, have also been demonstrated to be impaired in schizophrenia (Goldberg, Weinberger, Berman, Pliskin, & Podd, 1987).

Deficits in the ability to keep different mental events, such as perceptions and inter-nally generated notions, in mind at the same time may lead to confusion between them. Since perceptions are more stable, and are not under conscious control compared to images, which can be changed at will (Casey, 1976), as loss of control of internally generated images may make them seem more like externally generated events, even perceptual events (Johnson, 1988). A chronic deficit in maintaining the temporal connectedness among different mental events, as evidenced in some patients with schizophrenia, could be experienced as a loss of control of self-generated ideation; consequently, these self-generated ideas could be perceived as having been generated externally.

An impairment in supervisory attentional processes that causes the cognitive deficit of autonoetic agnosia may also lead to impairment of the communication between conscious and unconscious awareness that normally results in insight. An important aspect of insight, as described above, is the capacity of individuals to view themselves (including their mental operations) accurately in the context of the external world and to move without confusion between internal and external perspectives. The structure of cognition suggests that different aspects of cognitive functioning are differentially available to conscious awareness. For example, the brain systems necessary for computing particular visual stimulus properties such as facial identity or object shape are different from those necessary for conscious awareness of these aspects of a stimulus (Farah, 1992). Since the supervisory attentional system is responsible for keeping individuals aware of the information that they hold, and thus maintaining insight, a deficit in this system could result in a discrepancy between mental events and awareness of these events. Insight, in part, thus relies on the ability to be aware of what is part of the self and distinguish it from what is not. Furthermore, in order to see oneself accurately from an external perspective, and thus have insight, one must be able to distinguish between one's internal perspective and one's estimate of an external perspective. If schizophrenic patients with autonoetic agnosia cannot distinguish between internally and externally generated mental events, they may have particular difficulty distinguishing between observer and observed in trying to gain insight about their symptoms, behaviors, and circumstances. A schizophrenic patient with autonoetic agnosia may intend to move his arm, but this intention is not brought into awareness. The resultant experience may be that, since the arm moved, it was moved by an external force. It would be very difficult for a schizophrenic patient with autonoetic agnosia to gain insight into the fact that his belief in the powers of the external force is delusional. In terms of an individual's experience of self, he may be aware that, in general, his identity is different from that of other people, but some of his thoughts, feelings, and actions may not be fully represented in conscious awareness, and may thus result in the insightless belief that they are alien to him. It is thus common for schizophrenic patients with autonoetic agnosia to believe that they are not ill, as they cannot take the perspective of the observer, which is necessary to establish the context—generally a social context—in which their symptoms are placed. For example, a patient with inappropriate affect can thus not recognize its inappropriateness, since that determination requires an understanding of how an individual's behavior is viewed from the perspective of the (social) observer. Since patients with autonoetic agnosia have difficulty distinguishing between internal and external perspectives, they cannot "view" their symptoms as objective observers, and thus lack insight about their pathological nature.

*Motivation*     Amotivation, repeatedly observed in patients with schizophrenia, may contribute to reducing the distinction between internally and externally generated events on many levels. Since the maintenance of this distinction is an effortful process that requires more motivation than the fusion of internally and externally generated events (Johnson, 1992), amotivation could blur the distinction by reducing an individual's ability to gather accurate data about real events, retrieve data about those events, make comparisons between real and imagined events, gather contextual support for real versus imagined memories, and observe one's own cognitive processes with enough vigilance to detect differences between real and imagined events.

### General Considerations

The symptoms manifest as a disturbance of autonoetic agnosia in schizophrenia are likely to develop as a result of persistent deficits. The inability to attain accurate information about the external world owing to attentional deficits, or to retain it owing to memory deficits, is unlikely to result in a direct manifestation of symptoms such as hallucinations or thought insertion. However, over time these deficits, if persistent, may be dealt with in a manner that either does not allow them to receive attention from the patient or that results in the development of a mistrust of internal constructs about how the world operates, as well as about how one's brain functions. The absence of a solid trust in these two realms could lead to attempts to fit the faulty data into constructs that make sense to the individual. In order to compensate for the deficits, patients either isolate themselves (Cornblatt et al., 1992; Erlenmeyer-Kimling et al., 1993) or are forced to try to understand reality on the terms they have been given. These questions are not asked philosophically by the patient, with plenty of time to consider the options; rather, they are asked in a panic to understand the difference between internally and externally generated mental events, and to understand the nature of the world in which the patient must try to survive. The resultant delusions could be particularly unshakable if the deficit is sporadic, as the intrinsic punishment of not perceiving the fit between reality and internal representations would be intermittent, and thus very difficult to extinguish. Support for the notion of a delay between change in cognitive function and change in psychosis comes from data suggesting that the attentional deficits of schizophrenia respond to typical neuroleptic medications early in the course of a successful treatment trial, while the symptoms of psychosis resolve at a later stage (Serper, Davidson, & Harvey, 1994).

It is likely that the symptoms that result from autonoetic agnosia in schizophrenia are the relatively healthy responses of a diseased brain to understand itself and the external world in which it functions. In hemiplegic patients, the manifestation of pure denial of illness appears to precede anosognosic phenomena, such as the belief that a weakened limb is alien, as patients with this type of phenomenon tend to have had their brain injury in the more distant past than patients with complete denial of any deficit (Cutting, 1978). The course of these symptoms in hemiplegic patients suggests that interpretation of the weakened limb as alien is an attempt by patients to resolve their understanding of how the newly acquired deficit fits within the context of who they understand themselves to be. Thus it is possible that symptoms that result from autonoetic agnosia in schizophrenia are an attempt on the part of patients to place their cognitive deficits and disrupted perceptions in the context of what they know about their cognitive operations. For example, in the experience of thought insertion, it is possible that when a patient with schizophrenia has severe attentional disturbances, the disruption in the flow of thought is experienced as so unusual compared to what he expects that he interprets these thoughts as belonging to someone else. While there appears to be an absence of a cross-sectional relationship between anosognosia and anosognostic phenomena, since they rarely occur together (Cutting, 1978), there may be an important developmental relationship between the two. If there is a similar relationship among autonoetic agnosia, lack of insight, and symptoms such as hallucinations or Schneiderian delusions in schizophrenia, it may be detectable only through longitudinal studies, not through typical cross-sectional analyses.

Positing a relationship between autonoetic agnosia and positive symptoms such as hallucinations and Schneiderian symptoms poses potential problems in that the prevalence of these symptoms in patients with schizophrenia varies widely (28–72%) across studies (Mellor, 1982), and the correlations among these symptoms is low (Lewine, Renders, Kirchhofer, Monsour, & Watt, 1982). While Schneider (1959) postulated that his first-rank symptoms were pathognomonic to schizophrenia, empirical studies have suggested that many nonschizophrenic patients manifest first-rank symptoms, including patients with mood disorders (Carpenter & Strauss, 1974; Koehler & Seminario, 1978), temporal lobe epilepsy (Trimble, 1990; Cutting, 1990), and benzodiazepine withdrawal (Roberts & Vass, 1986). However, some studies suggest that Schneiderian symptoms may discriminate schizophrenics and mood psychotics better than any other symptoms (O'Grady, 1990; Junginger, Barker, & Coe, 1992), and cluster analysis of schizophrenic patients suggests that about 25% of patients are characterized specifically by their Schneiderian delusions and severe hallucinations (Shtasel et al., 1992). These data suggest that while these symptoms are not nearly as specific to schizophrenia as Schneider suggested, they are also not completely atypical in schizophrenia.

The assessment of positive symptoms such as delusions and hallucinations can be empirically challenging, since they are based upon the subjective report of the internal state of the patient, and thus the validity of their assessment is never certain (Frith, 1992). It is therefore difficult to determine if the hallucinations and delusions postulated to be associated with autonoetic agnosia may derive from a single underlying pathophysiology. The variable prevalence of these symptoms and the low correlations among them could be attributed to the low validity of assessing symptoms on the basis of patient report. Furthermore, just as some patients with tuberculosis manifest disruptions of normal pulmonary functions while others manifest hepatic dysfunction, both springing from a common etiology, different psychotic symptoms may develop in different patients from a common underlying cognitive deficit. Only empirical studies of the cognitive deficits that may be associated with this cluster of symptoms can address this question.

Although experiences of the dissolution of the boundary between self and nonself are associated with psychosis in schizophrenia, these experiences in nonschizophrenic individuals are not consistently associated with psychopathology. Kohut (1966) argues that fragmentation of the self is common among all people, and that it can be adaptive psychologically in that it creates a need in an individual to determine what characterizes his or her particular self, and what aides in the process of developing a more cohesive concept of self. In an unscreened sample of volunteers from the general population, 39% of respondents reported having experienced feelings of dissolution of self (Wuthnow, 1978). While this dissolution is clearly maladaptive in schizophrenia spectrum disorders, in nonschizophrenic or nonpsychiatric populations it is often associated with feelings of enhanced meaning to one's life and a sense of connectedness to other people, especially in cases of extreme mystical or religious experience (Stace, 1960; Allison, 1968; Deikman, 1982). Thus, the experience of dissolution of the boundary between self and nonself may not be pathognomonic of schizophrenia; rather, it is the specific inability to recognize self-generated ideation as one's own that may be impaired.

## Neuroanatomic Correlates of Autonoetic Agnosia in Schizophrenia

While the specific neuroanatomic involvement in autonoetic agnosia in schizophrenia has not been determined, data from a variety of different sources shed light on the possible regions, and connections between regions, that may be associated with this cognitive deficit and the symptoms of psychosis that may result. Since the cognitive functions involved in distinguishing between internally and externally generated mental events are complex, it is likely that no specific brain region mediates them. Thus, a complex neural network associated with this distinction could fail as a result of several possible regional brain dysfunctions. Evidence for the involvement of the following regions in the symptoms of autonoetic agnosia in schizophrenia will be considered: the temporal lobes, including the hippocampal regions; the anterior cingulate; the dorsolateral prefrontal cortex; and the connections between brain regions, including the stratium.

### Temporal Lobe

A variety of evidence suggests that temporal lobe structures, including the hippocampus, may be involved in the development of autonoetic agnosia in schizophrenia. First, a subgroup of patients with temporal lobe epilepsy manifest some of the symptoms that may result from autonoetic agnosia, including Schneiderian delusions of thought insertion and delusions of control (Perez, Trimble, Murray, & Reider, 1985; Trimble, 1990). In a study of the postsurgical brain tissue of patients with temporal lobe epilepsy, 5% of patients with mesial temporal sclerosis had psychotic symptoms, while 23% of patients with alien tissue (small tumors, hamartomas, and focal dysplasia) had been psychotic (Taylor, 1975). The major difference between these two groups that could account for the increased rate of psychosis was developmental, since mesial temporal sclerosis is a postnatal lesion and a number of the alien tissue disorders are embryonic in origin. Since mesial temporal sclerosis is more damaging to the whole temporal lobe, a nonfunctional lobe may be less likely to produce psychosis than one that is dysfunctional (Taylor, 1975). Thus, among patients with epilepsy, the temporal lobe dysfunction that is most associated with psychosis is that which develops prenatally and which damages less temporal lobe tissue. Cutting (1992) has argued that since Schneiderian first-rank symptoms of schizophrenia were more common along left-side than right-side temporal lobe epileptics (Perez et al., 1985), exaggerated left-side activity in the presence of diminished right-side activity leads to the symptoms of schizophrenia.

The role of temporal lobe structures in memory suggests that they are probably important in distinguishing between internally and externally generated mental events. As described above, since perceptual input is compared to internally generated memories as part of the comparison between internally and externally derived events, the presence of accurate memory is essential for clear-cut distinctions between the two. Both Frith (1987) and Gray (1982) suggest that the hippocampus is important in the comparison of sensory data and expected perceptions based upon an internally generated model of the world derived from stored memories. Dysfunction of the temporal lobes or hippocampal structures, as reported repeatedly in patients with schizophrenia (Lieberman et al., 1992; Weinberger, Berman, Suddath, & Torrey, 1992; Suddath, Christison, Torrey, Casanova, & Weinberger, 1990; Bogerts, Meertz, Schonfledt-Bausch, 1985; Shenton et al., 1992), could contribute to the inability of schizophrenic patients to maintain in memory accurate models of the external world, which disturbs the process of comparing externally and internally generated mental events.

The temporal lobe has also been implicated as a possible site associated with hallucinations. Electrical stimulation of the temporal lobe can produce verbal hallucinations (Penfield & Perot, 1963), and the left temporal lobe is the most common site for epileptic foci associated with auditory hallucinations (Roberts, Done, Bruton, & Crow, 1990). The presence of auditory hallucinations in schizophrenia has been associated with increased perfusion in the left medial temporal lobe, as measured by PET (Liddle, Friston, Frith, & Hirsch, 1992), and in the hippocampus, as measured by SPECT (Musalek et al., 1989); the frequency of auditory hallucinations is negatively correlated with the volume of the left superior temporal gyrus, as measured with MRI (Barta, Pearlson, Powers, Richard, & Tune, 1990).

### Anterior Cingulate Gyrus

The anterior aspect of the cingulate gyrus appears to be involved in maintaining the distinction between imagery and perception, as individuals who have had anterior cingulatomy report spontaneous generation of imagery with perceptual content (Johnson, 1991a). Increased activation of this region during tasks that require responses to external stimuli (Pardo et al., 1990), but not during tasks that require monitoring internal mental events (Frith et al., 1991), suggests that the anterior cingulate may help to amplify externally generated mental events, which, through the cognitive processes involved in reality monitoring, aids in the identification of their origin as external to the self. Frith (1992) proposes that information about intended self-generated acts comes to the monitor from the prefrontal cortex via the entorhinal cortex (hippocampal gyrus) and the cingulate cortex, and are realized via the basal ganglia and the supplementary motor areas. Normal individuals engaged in a task of eye-movement generation demonstrate maximal activation in the left parahippocampal gyrus (Frith et al., 1992). As noted by Liddle (1993), the fact that this region is associated with increased rCBF in schizophrenic patients with delusions and hallucinations (Liddle et al., 1992) suggests that the system of self-monitoring mental events may be impaired in psychotic schizophrenic patients.

This region appears to be abnormal at the cellular level in schizophrenic patients, as decreased neuronal density in the anterior cingulate has been reported (Benes,

Davidson, & Bird, 1986), possibly associated with a developmental disturbance in neuronal migration or differentiation (Benes, 1993). While the presence of such a disturbance is speculative, it may have important implications for the etiology of the symptoms of schizophrenia, since the anterior cingulate is connected to the hippocampal formation via the presubicular region, which shows increased myelination during late adolescence in normal brain (Benes, 1989), and which may be associated with a neurodevelopmental disturbance in schizophrenia (Benes, 1993).

### Prefrontal Cortex and the Striatum

Although the prefrontal cortex has been demonstrated to be dysfunctional in schizophrenia in terms of its structure (Breier et al., 1992), physiology (Andreasen et al., 1992), and cognitive function (Goldberg et al., 1987), the relationship between prefrontal dysfunction and the symptoms of autonoetic agnosia are not known.

The range of functions mediated in part by the human prefrontal cortex is far from completely described. It is generally accepted, however, that this brain region is involved in the guidance of multistep behaviors, including monitoring of ongoing actions, decision making, planning, and creativity, with support from working memory and categorization of knowledge (Benson & Stuss, 1990; Damasio, 1991; Goldberg, 1985; Fuster, 1989; Weinberger, 1993). The supervisory attentional system forwarded by Shallice (1988) is heavily dependent upon prefrontal functions. In addition, the process of placing information in its proper context is mediated by prefrontal regions (Cohen & Servan-Schreiber, 1992). Thus, based upon what is known about the functions of the prefrontal cortex, it plays a critical role in the process of distinguishing between internally and externally generated mental events. Dysfunctions of the prefrontal cortex with associated deficits in working memory, contextual processes, or the supervisory attentional system that monitors the origin of mental events may result in autonoetic agnosia in schizophrenia.

The prefrontal cortex is involved in monitoring mental events in different modalities. As examples, its role in monitoring vision and in monitoring motor behavior will be considered. Visual perceptual processing and visual mental imagery, as described above, appear to activate similar neural networks, with the exception that the neural flow of imagery involves top-down processes while perception involves bottom-up pathways. The network activated during visual perceptual processing includes primary visual cortex, superior parietal, inferior parietal and temporal regions, and dorsolateral prefrontal cortex. Visual imagery activates these same regions, but the direction of the pathway may be reversed; it appears to be generated and monitored by the dorsolateral prefrontal cortex (Kosslyn, Flunn, Amsterdam, & Wang, 1990). Impairments in the prefrontal cortex may result in confusion between visual stimuli that are generated through imagery and visual stimuli that are generated from external perceptions.

Motor behavior is initiated via projections from the prefrontal cortex to the striatum, and then the globus pallidus, which then projects to the anteroventral and ventrolateral nuclei of the thalamus. These thalamic nuclei project to the premotor and supplementary motor areas and the anterior cingulate cortex, and finally to the motor cortex (Frith, 1987). Dysfunction in any of these areas could lead to deficits in self-generated responses, as found in Parkinson's disease and patients with specific prefrontal lesion.

Frith and Done (1988) suggest that the positive symptoms of schizophrenia are related to a failure to monitor actions resulting from a malfunction in the pathways connecting the prefrontal lobes and the striatum. When a motor movement is generated and carried out, yet the region that initiated the process (prefrontal cortex) is disassociated from the movement itself owing to an impairment in the connections between the prefrontal cortex and the motor cortex, the movement may be experienced as having been generated by forces outside the self, as in delusions of control. This model of neural dysfunction in the striatal connections leading to the prefrontal cortex is supported by the development of psychosis in patients with metachromatic leukodystrophy, which is likely to result from impairments in the white-matter connectivity between different cortical regions, particularly in circuitry leading to the frontal cortex (Hyde, Ziegler, & Weinberger, 1992).

This neuroanatomic model of autonoetic agnosia in schizophrenia suggests that this cognitive deficit may be caused by the disconnection of specific brain regions. Computer-generated models of parallel distributed processing in the brain have been used to describe the development of some symptoms that may result from autonoetic agnosia (Hoffman, 1986; Hoffman & McGlashan, 1993) in terms of the intentional stance (Dennet, 1991), in which humans tend to imbue randomly occurring events with intention. For example, people playing chess against a computer tend to perceive the computer as having intentions about the outcome of the match (Dennet, 1971). In computer simulation of Hoffman and McGlashan (1993), when different components of a network are isolated from one another, there are several consequences. First, outputs from the network become bizarre, unrelated to the original inputs. Second, different components become more autonomous from one another. Third, some neural modules begin producing outputs that are independent from information that they receive, and strive relentlessly to reproduce themselves, called parasitic focus (Hoffman & McGlashan, 1993). In applying these results to brain processes, Hoffman and McGlashan suggest that if speech centers were isolated from general motor initiation circuits such as the supplementary motor area through pathology in the neurodevelopmental process of cortical pruning, a form of inner speech may result that would be perceived by the patients to be unintended and independent from other thought processes, and thus independent from the patient's understanding of self, leading to the interpretation of the mental events as hallucinations or thought insertion.

An alternative hypothesis has been forwarded by David (1994b), who proposes that *excessive* activity between brain regions, referred to as *dysmodularity*, is a more accurate explanation of the pattern of cognitive deficits, symptoms, and neuroanatomic findings reported in patients with schizophrenia. As noted by David (1994b), this proposal is supported by the wealth of data suggesting overloaded cognitive systems in schizophrenic patients as well as neuroanatomic data suggesting reduced cerebral asymmetry (Crow, 1990) and lack of gray matter relative to white (which is generally associated with greater connectivity between brain regions) (Jernigan et al., 1991). While the controversy over whether there is reduced or excessive cortical connectivity is far from settled, the presence of some type of abnormality in the connections between brain regions in schizophrenic patients is a promising possibility for future research.

The few relevant imaging studies of the relationship between dysfunctional brain regions or cortical connectivity and schizophrenic symptoms suggesting autonoetic agnosia have yielded conflicting data. Using SPECT, comparisons of relative blood flow in schizophrenic patients while they were experiencing auditory hallucinations and while they were in a nonhallucinating state have suggested significant increases in blood flow in Broca's area associated with hallucinations (McGuire, Shah, & Murray, 1993). These data support the notion that verbal hallucinations are a part of inner speech that is not monitored accurately by other brain systems. However, other studies have yielded findings that do not support this model. If autonoetic agnosia could be attributed to a disconnection between the prefrontal cortex and other brain regions, *diminished* activity in the striatum connecting these regions could be expected. A PET study of resting-state brain metabolism (Cleghorn et al., 1992), however, found that schizophrenic patients who experienced auditory hallucinations, compared to schizophrenic patients without hallucinations, had lower relative metabolism in auditory and Wernicke's regions, and the severity of hallucinations correlated *positively* with relative metabolism in the striatum and anterior cingulate regions. No significant differences in Broca's area were found. A number of speculative explanations of these conflicting data could be generated; it is clear, however, that definitive explanations will require additional studies investigating the relationship between regional brain activation and the hallucinations and delusions associated with autonoetic agnosia.

The notion that a disconnection among brain regions is responsible for autonoetic agnosia has relevance to the loss of insight found in patients with schizophrenia. Since the neurological data discussed above suggest that brain lesions in various regions, including most prominently the right frontal, parietal, and temporal lobes, can result in disturbances in conscious awareness about what is part of the self and what is not, the disconnection between self-generated mental events and the awareness that these mental events were generated by the self is also likely to have correlates in the dysfunction of the neuroanatomy. Since the prefrontal cortex and the striatal connections with other brain regions are the areas most likely to be associated with self-monitoring of mental events (Goldberg, 1985), it is possible that deficits in insight are associated with dysfunctions of these brain regions in schizophrenia. Recent findings of a relationship in schizophrenic patients between poor insight and perseverative errors on the Wisconsin Card Sorting Test support this notion (Young, Davila, & Scher, 1993).

## Conclusions

Several important symptoms of schizophrenia, including poor insight, hallucinations, and Schneiderian delusions, can be understood as a function of autonoetic agnosia—the inability to distinguish between internally and externally generated mental events. This disturbance may be the result of cognitive deficits reported in schizophrenia, including reduced perceptual input, memory deficits, the inability to place information in a relevant context, deficiencies in reasoning processes, and deficits in the ability of a supervisory attentional system to monitor cognitive and perceptual processes. The absence of normal motivation could also account for maintaining the effort required to distinguish internally and externally generated mental events. These deficits could be attributable to general brain dysfunction, as well as to specific regional brain dysfunction in a number of areas. While dysfunction of the prefrontal cortex and the striatal connections to the prefrontal cortex are the most likely to be involved in autonoetic agnosia in schizophrenia, the dysfunction of other regions, such as the temporal cortex and the anterior cingulate, may also have an important role.

While this model of some symptoms of schizophrenia answers few questions about the relationships among symptoms, cognitive deficits, and neuroanatomic dysfunction in schizophrenia, several questions are raised. The specific cognitive deficits that under-lie autonoetic agnosia have not been determined, yet the patterns of cognitive deficit in schizophrenic patients with persistent poor insight, hallucinations, or Schneiderian delusions could be investigated. As discussed above, it is likely that these relationships will not be revealed by cross-sectional data, since cognitive deficits and the symptoms of psychosis in schizophrenia appear to be uncorrelated. Questions about the brain regions or pathways that may be associated with autonoetic agnosia may be less difficult to address, as measures of brain structure and physiologic function tend to be more stable than measures of cognitive performance. However, since the development of the self and the monitoring of self-generated mental events are extraordinarily complex processes involving a multitude of brain regions, it is unlikely that any simple regional brain dysfunction will be associated with autonoetic agnosia.

*Acknowledgments*    This work was supported by a Young Investigator Award from the National Alliance for Research on Schizophrenia and Depression. The author wishes to express gratitude to Drs. William Barr, Philip D. Harvey, Ralph Hoffman, and Marcia K. Johnson for their helpful suggestions on previous versions of this manuscript.

*References*

Allison, J. (1968) Adaptive regression and intense religious experience. *Journal of Nervous and Mental Disease, 145*(6), 452–463.

Amador, X. F., Strauss, D. H., Yale, S. A., & Gorman, J. M. (1991). Awareness of illness in schizophrenia. *Schizophrenia Bulletin, 17,* 113–132.

American Psychiatric Association. (1987). *Diagnostic and statistical manual of mental disorders, 3rd ed.* Washington, DC: Author.

Andreasen, N. C. (1989). Neural mechanisms of negative symptoms. *British Journal of Pyschiatry, 155,* 93–98.

Andreasen, N. C., Rezai, K., Alliger, R., Swayze, V. W., Flaum, M., Kirchner, P., Cohen, G., & O'Leary, D. S. (1992). Hypofrontality in neuroleptic-naive patients and in patients with chronic schizophrenia. *Archives of General Psychiatry, 49,* 943–958.

Babinski, M. J. (1914). Contribution a l'etude des troubles mentaux dans l'hemiplegie organique cerebrale. *Revue Neurologique, 1,* 845–848.

Baddeley, A. (1986). *Working memory.* Oxford: Clarendon Press.

Barta, P. E., Pearlson, G. D., Powers, R. E., Richard, S. S., & Tune, L. E. (1990). Auditory hallucinations and smaller superior temporal gyral volume in schizophrenia. *American Journal of Psychiatry, 147,* 1457–1462.

Benes, F. M. (1989). Myelination of cortical-hippocampal relays during late adolescence. *Schizophrenia Bulletin, 15,* 585–593.

Benes, F. M. (1993). Neurobiological investigations in cingulate cortex of schizophrenic brain. *Schizophrenia Bulletin, 19,* 537–549.

Benes, R. M., Davidson, J., & Bird, E. D. (1986). Quantitative cytoarchitectural studies of Cerebral cortex of schizophrenics. *Archives of General Psychiatry, 43*, 31–35.

Benson, D. F., & Stuss, D. T. (1990). Frontal lobe influences on delusions: A clinical perspective. *Schizophrenia Bulletin, 16*, 403–411.

Bentall, R. P. (1990). The illusion of reality: A review and integration of psychological research on hallucination. *Psychological Bulletin, 107*, 82–95.

Bentall, R. P., Baker, G. A., & Havers, S. (1991). Reality monitoring and psychotic hallucinations. *British Journal of Clinical Psychology, 30*, 213–222.

Bisiach, E., & Luzzatti, C. (1978). Unilateral neglect of representational space. *Cortex, 14*, 129–133.

Bisiach, E., Luzzatti, C., & Perani, D. (1979). Unilateral neglect, representational schema and consciousness. *Brain, 102*, 609–618.

Blatt, S. J., & Wild, C. (1976). *Schizophrenia: A developmental approach.* New York: International University Press.

Bogerts, B., Meertz, E., & Schonfledt-Bausch, R. (1985). Basal ganglia and limbic system pathology in schizophrenia: A morphometric study of brain volume and shrinkage. *Archives of General Pyschiatry, 43*, 36–42.

Breier, A., Buchanan, R. W., Elkashef, A., Munson, R. C., Kirkpatrick, B., & Gellad, F. (1992). Brain morphology and schizophrenia. *Archives of General Psychiatry, 49*, 921–926.

Carpenter, W. T., Heinrichs, D. W., & Wagman, A. M. I. (1988). Deficit and nondeficit forms of schizophrenia: The concept. *American Journal of Psychiatry, 145*, 578–583.

Carpenter, W. T., & Strauss, J. S. (1974). Cross-cultural evaluation of Schneider's first-rank symptoms of schizophrenia: A report from the International Pilot Study of Schizophrenia. *American Journal of Psychiatry, 131*, 682–687.

Casey, E. S. (1976). *Imagining: A phenomenological study.* Bloomington, IN: Indiana University Press.

Cleghorn, J. M., Franco, S., Szechtman, B., Kaplan, R. D., Szechtman, H., Brown, G. M., Nahmias, C., & Garnett, E. S. (1992). Toward a brain map of auditory hallucinations. *American Journal of Psychiatry, 149*, 1062–1069.

Cohen, J. D., & Servan-Schreiber, D. (1992). Context, cortex, and dopamine: A connectionist approach to behavior and biology in schizophrenia. *Psychological Review, 99*, 45–77.

Cornblatt, B. A., Lenzenwegger, M. F., Dworkin, R. H., & Erlenmeyer-Kimling, L. (1992). Childhood attentional dysfunctions predict social deficits in unaffected adults at risk for schizophrenia. *British Journal of Pyschiatry, 161* (suppl. 18), 59–64.

Critchley, M. (1974). Misoplegia, or hatred of hemiplegia. *Mount Sinai Journal of Medicine, 41*, 82–87.

Crow, T. J. (1990). Temporal lobe asymmetries as the key to the etiology of schizophrenia. *Schizophrenia Bulletin, 16*, 433–443.

Cutting, J. (1978). Study of anosognosia. *Journal of Neurology, Neurosurgery, and Psychiatry, 41*, 548–555.

Cutting, J. (1992). The role of right hemisphere dysfunction in psychiatric disorder. *British Journal of Psychiatry, 160*, 583–588.

Cutting, J. (1990). *The right cerebral hemisphere and psychiatric disorders.* New York: Oxford University Press.

Damasio, A. R. (1991). Concluding comments. In H. S. Levin, H. M. Eisenberg, & A. L. Benton (Eds.), *Frontal lobe function and dysfunction* (pp. 401–408). New York: Oxford University Press.

David, A. S. (1993). The neuropsychological origin of auditory hallucinations. In A. David & J. Cutting (Eds.), *Neuropsychology of schizophrenia* (pp. 269–313). Hove, Sussex: Erlbaum.

David, A. S. (1994a). Thought echo reflects the activity of the phonological loop. *British Journal of Clinical Psychology, 33,* 81–83.

David, A. S. (1994b). Dysmodularity: A neurocognitive model for schizophrenia. *Schizophrenia Bulletin, 20,* 249–255.

David, A. S., & Howard, R. (1994). An experimental phenomenological approach to delusional memory in schizophrenia and late paraphrenia. *Psychological Medicine, 24,* 515–524.

Deiber, M. P., Passingham, R. E., Colebatch, J. G., Friston, K. J., Nixon, P. D., & Frackowiak, R. S. J. (1991). Cortical areas and the selection of movement: A study with PET. *Exploratory Brain Research, 84,* 393–402.

Deikman, A. J. (1982). *The observing self: Mysticism and psychotherapy.* Boston, MA: Beacon Press.

DeLisi, L. E., Dauphinais, I. D., Gerson, E. S. (1988). Perinatal complications and reduced size of brain limbic structures in familial schizophrenia. *Schizophrenia Bulletin, 14,* 185–191.

Dennett, D. C. (1971). Intentional systems. *Journal of Philosophy, 48,* 87–106.

Dennett, D. C. (1991). *Consciousness explained.* Boston, MA: Little, Brown.

Douglas, K. L., & Rockland, K. S. (1992). Extensive visual feedback connections from ventral inferotemporal cortex. *Society of Neuroscience Abstracts, 18,* 390.

Edelman, G. M. (1987). *Neural Darwinism: The theory of neuronal group selection.* New York: Basic Books.

Edelman, G. M., & Cunningham, B. A. (1990). Place-dependent cell adhesion, process retraction, and spatial signaling in neural morphogenesis. *Cold Spring Harbor Symposia on Quantitative Biology, 55,* 303–318.

Erlenmeyer-Kimling, L., Cornblatt, B. A., Rock, D., Roberts, S., Bell, M., & West, A. (1993). The New York High-Risk Project: Anhedonia, attentional deviance, and psychopathology. *Schizophrenia Bulletin, 19,* 141–153.

Farah, M. J. (1988). Is visual imagery really visual? Overlooked evidence from Neuropsychology. *Psychological Review, 95,* 307–317.

Farah, M. J. (1989). Mechanisms of imagery-perception interaction. *Journal of Experimental Psychology: Human Perception and Performance, 15,* 203–211.

Farah, M. J. (1992). Agnosia. *Current Opinion in Neurobiology, 2,* 162–164.

Farah, M. J., Peronnet, F., Gonon, M. A., & Girard, M. H. (1988). Electrophysiological evidence for a shared representational medium for visual images and visual percepts. *Journal of Experimental Psychology: General, 117,* 248–257.

Fenichel, O. (1945). *The psychoanalytic theory of neurosis.* New York: Norton.

Freud, S. (1915/1963). The unconscious: In P. Rieff (Ed.), *General Psychological Theory.* New York: Collier.

Freud, S. (1924/1963). Neurosis and Psychosis. In P. Rieff (Ed.) *General Psychological Theory.* New York: Collier.

Frith, C. D. (1987). The positive and negative symptoms of schizophrenia reflect impairments in the perception and initiation of action. *Psychological Medicine, 17,* 631–648.

Frith, C. D. (1992). *The cognitive neuropsychology of schizophrenia.* Hove, England: Erlbaum.

Frith, C. D., & Done, D. J. (1988). Towards a neuropsychology of schizophrenia. *British Journal of Psychiatry, 153,* 437–443.

Frith, C. D., & Done, D. J. (1989). Experiences of alien control in schizophrenia reflect a disorder in the central monitoring of action. *Psychological Medicine, 19,* 359–363.

Frith, C. D., Friston, K., Liddle, P. F., & Frackowiak, R. S. J. (1991). Willed action and the prefrontal cortex in man: A study with PET. *Proceedings of the Royal Society of London, 244,* 241–246.

Frith, C. D., Friston, K., Liddle, P. F., & Frackowiak, R. S. J. (1992). PET imaging and cognition in schizophrenia. *Journal of the Royal Society of Medicine, 85*, 222–224.

Fuster, J. M. (1989). *The prefrontal cortex* (2nd ed.). New York: Raven Press.

Gerstmann, J. (1942). Problem of imperception of disease and of impaired body territories with organic lesions. *Archives of Neurology and Psychiatry, 48*, 890–913.

Goldberg, G. (1985). Supplementary motor area structure and function: Review and hypotheses. *Behavioral and Brain Sciences, 8*, 567–616.

Goldberg, T. E., Gold, J. M., Greenberg, R., Griffin, S., Schulz, S. C., Pickar, D., Kleinman, J. E., & Weinberger, D. R. (1993). Contrasts between patients with affective disorders and patients with schizophrenia on a neuropsychological test battery. *American Journal of Psychiatry, 150*, 1355–1362.

Goldberg, T. E., Weinberger, D. R., Berman, K. F., Pliskin, N. H., & Podd, M. H. (1987). Further evidence for dementia of the prefrontal type in schizophrenia? *Archives of General Psychiatry, 44*, 1008–1014.

Goldenberg, G., Podreka, I., Steiner, M., Willmes, K., Suess, E., & Deecke, L. (1989). Regional cerebral blood flow patterns in visual imagery. *Neuropsychologia, 27*, 641–664.

Goldman-Rakic, P. S. (1987). Circuitry of primate prefrontal cortex and regulation of behavior by representational knowledge. In F. Plum (Vol. Ed.) & V. B. Mountcastle (Sec. Ed.), *Handbook of physiology, Section 1: The nervous system, Volume 5: Higher functions of the brain*. Bethesda, MD: American Physiological Society.

Goldman-Rakic, P. S. (1988). Changing concepts of cortical connectivity: Parallel distributed cortical networks. In P. Rakic & W. Singer (Eds.), *Neurobiology of neocortex*. New York: John Wiley.

Granholm, E., Asarnow, R. F., & Marder, S. R. (1991). Controlled information processing resources and the development of automatic detection responses in Schizophrenia. *Journal of Abnormal Psychology, 100*, 22–30.

Gray, J. A. (1982). *The Neuropsychology of anxiety*. Oxford: Oxford University Press.

Gray, J. A., Feldon, J., Rawlins, J. N. P., Hemsley, D. R., & Smith, A. D. (1991). The neuropsychology of schizophrenia. *Behavioral and Brain Sciences, 14*, 1–84.

Green, M., & Walker, E. (1985). Neuropsychological performance and positive and negative symptoms in schizophrenia. *Journal of Abnormal Psychology, 94*, 460–470.

Harvey, P. D. (1985). Reality monitoring in mania and schizophrenia: The association between thought disorder and performance. *Journal of Nervous and Mental Disease, 173*, 67–73.

Harvey, P. D., Earle-Boyer, E. A., & Levinson, J. C. (1988). Cognitive deficits and thought disorder: A retest study. *Schizophrenia Bulletin, 14*, 57–66.

Heilbrun, A. B. (1980). Impaired recognition of self-expressed thought in patients with auditory hallucinations. *Journal of Abnormal Psychology, 89*, 728–736.

Hoffman, R. E. (1986). Verbal hallucinations and language production processes in schizophrenia. *Behavioral and Brain Sciences, 9*, 503–548.

Hoffman, R. E., & McGlashan, T. H. (1993). Parallel distributed processing and the emergence of schizophrenic symptoms. *Schizophrenia Bulletin, 19*, 119–140.

Holzman, P. S. (1987). Recent studies of physiology in schizophrenia. *Schizophrenia Bulletin, 13*, 48–73.

Horrowitz, M. (1975). Hallucinations: An information processing approach. In R. K. Siegel & L. J. West (Eds.), *Hallucinations: Behavior, experience and theory* (pp. 163–196). New York: John Wiley.

Hyde, T. M., Ziegler, J. C., & Weinberger, D. R. (1992). Psychiatric disturbances in metachromatic leukodystrophy: Insight into the neurobiology of psychosis. *Archives of Neurology, 49*, 401–406.

Jacobson, E. (1954). *The self and the object world*. New York: International University Press.

Jernigan, T. L., Zisook, S., Heaton, R. K., Moranville, J. T., Hesselink, J. R., & Braff, D. L. (1991). Magnetic resonance imaging abnormalities in lenticular nuclei and cerebral cortex in schizophrenia. *Archives of General Psychiatry, 48*, 881–890.

Johnson, M. K. (1988). Discriminating the origin of information. In T. F. Oltmanns & B. A. Maher (Eds.), *Delusional beliefs* (pp. 34–65). New York: John Wiley.

Johnson, M. K. (1991a). Reality monitoring: Evidence from confabulation in organic brain disease patients. In G. P. Prigatano & D. L. Schacter (Eds.), *Awareness of deficit after brain injury: Clinical and theoretical issues* (pp. 176–197). New York: Oxford University Press.

Johnson, M. K. (1991b). Reflection, reality monitoring, and the self. In R. Kunzendorf (Ed.), *Mental imagery* (pp. 3–16). New York: Plenum Press.

Johnson, M. K. (1992). MEM: Mechanisms of recollection. *Journal of Cognitive Neuroscience, 4*, 268–280.

Johnson, M. K., Foley, M. A., & Leach, K. (1988). The consequences for memory of imagining in another person's voice. *Memory and Cognition, 16*, 337–342.

Johnson, M. K., Foley, M. A., Suengas, A. G., & Raye, C. L. (1988). Phenomenal characteristics of memories for perceived and imagined autobiographical events. *Journal of Experimental Psychology: General, 117*, 371–376.

Johnson, M. K., Hashtroudi, S., & Lindsay, D. S. (1993). Source monitoring. *Psychological Bulletin, 114*, 3–28.

Johnson, M. K., & Raye, C. L. (1981). Reality monitoring. *Psychological Review, 88*, 67–85.

Johnson, M. K., Raye, C. L., Wang, A. Y., & Taylor, T. H. (1979). Fact and fantasy: The roles of accuracy and variability in confusing imaginations with perceptual experiences. *Journal of Experimental Psychology: Human Learning and Memory, 5*, 229–240.

Junginger, J., Barker, S., & Coe, D. (1992). Mood theme and bizarreness of delusions in schizophrenia and mood psychosis. *Journal of Abnormal Psychology, 101*, 287–292.

Keefe, R. S. E., Blum, C., Roitman, S. L., Harvey, P. D., Davidson, M., Mohs, R. C., & Davis, K. L. (1993). *Cognitive dysfunction in Kraepelinian schizophrenics*. Presented at the American College of Neuropsychopharmacology Annual Meeting.

Keefe, R. S. E., Roitman, S. L., Harvey, P. D., Blum, C., DuPre, R. L., Prieto, D. M., Davidson, M., Davis, K. L. (1995). A pen-and-paper human-analogue of a monkey prefrontal cortex activation task: Spatial working memory in patients with schizophrenia. *Schizophrenia Research, 17*, 25–33.

Kety, S. S., Rosenthal, D., & Wender, P. H. (1975). Mental illness in the biological and adoptive families of individuals who have become schizophrenic: A preliminary report based on psychiatric interviews. In R. Fieve, D. Rosenthal, & H. Brill (Eds.), *Genetic research in psychiatry* (pp. 147–165). Baltimore, MD: Johns Hopkins University Press.

Koehler, K., & Seminario, I. (1978). 'First-rank' schizophrenia and research diagnosis schizophrenic and affective illness. *Comprehensive Psychiatry, 19*, 401–406.

Kohut, H. (1966). Forms and transformations of narcissism. *Journal of the American Psychoanalytic Association, 14*, 243–272.

Kosslyn, S. M., Alpert, N. M., Thompson, W. L., Maljkovic, V., Weise, S. B., Chabris, C. F., Hamilton, S. E., Rauch, S. L., & Buonanno, F. S. (1993). Visual mental imagery activates topographically organized visual cortex. *Journal of Cognitive Neuroscience, 5*, 263–287.

Kosslyn, S. M., & Koenig, O. (1992). *Wet mind: The new cognitive neuroscience*. New York: Free Press.

Kosslyn, S. M., Flynn, R. A., Amsterdam, J. B., & Wang, G. (1990). Components of high-level vision: A cognitive neuroscience analysis and accounts of neurological syndromes. *Cognition, 34*, 203–277.

LeDoux, J. E. (1992). Emotion and the Amygdala. In J. P. Aggleton (Ed.), *The Amygdala:*

*Neurobiological aspects of emotion, memory, and mental dysfunction* (pp. 339–351). New York: Wiley-Liss.

Levine, D. N., & Rinn, W. E. (1986). Opticosensory ataxia and alien hand syndrome after posterior cerebral artery territory infarction. *Neurology, 36,* 1094–1097.

Lewine, R. R. J., Renders, R., Kirchhofer, M., Monsour, A., Watt, N. (1982). The empirical heterogeneity of first rank symptoms in schizophrenia. *British Journal of Psychiatry, 140,* 498–502.

Lewine, R. R. J., Watt, N. F., & Fryer, J. H. (1978). A study of childhood social competence, adult premorbid competence, and psychiatric outcome in three schizophrenic subtypes. *Journal of Abnormal Psychology, 87,* 294–302.

Liddle, P. F. (1993). The psychomotor disorders: Disorders of the supervisory mental processes. *Behavioural Neurology, 6,* 5–14.

Liddle, P. F., Friston, K. J., Frith, C. D., & Hirsch, S. R. (1992). Patterns of cerebral blood flow in schizophrenia. *British Journal of Psychiatry, 160,* 179–186.

Lieberman, J. A., Alvir, J. M. J., Woerner, M., Degreef, G., Bilder, R. M., Ashtari, M., Bogerts, B., Mayerhoff, D. I., Geisler, S. H., Loebel, A., Levy, D. L., Hinrichsen, G., Szymanski, S., Chakos, M., Koreen, A., Borenstein, M., & Kane, J. M. (1992). Prospective study of psychobiology in first-episode schizophrenia at Hillside Hospital. *Schizophrenia Bulletin, 18,* 351–371.

Maher, B., & Spitzer, M. (1984). Delusions. In H. E. Adams & P. B. Sutker (Eds.), *Comprehensive handbook of psychopathology.* New York: Plenum Press.

McGuire, P. K., Shah, G. M. S., & Murray, R. M. (1993). Increased blood flow in Broca's area during auditory hallucinations in schizophrenia. *Lancet, 342,* 703–706.

Mellor, C. S. (1982). The present status of first rank symptoms. *British Journal of Psychiatry, 140,* 423–424.

Mesulam, M. M., Hersh, L. B., Mash, D. C., & Geula, C. (1992). Differential cholinergic innervation within functional subdivisions of the human cerebral cortex: A choline acetyltransferase study. *Journal of Comparative Neurology, 318,* 316–328.

Mesulam, M. M. (1990). Large-scale neurocognitive networks and distributed processing for attention, language and memory. *Annals of Neurology, 28,* 597–613.

Miller, L. (1991). *Freud's brain: The neuropsychodynamic foundation of psychoanalysis.* New York: Guilford.

Milner, B., Petrides, M., & Smith, M. L. (1985). Frontal lobes and the temporal organization of memory. *Human Neurobiology, 4,* 137–142.

Montague, P. R., Gally, J. A., & Edelman, G. M. (1991). Spatial signaling in the development and function of neural connections. *Cerebral Cortex, 1* (3), 199–220.

Musalek, M., Podreka, I., Walter, H., Suess, E., Passweg, V., Nutzinger, D., Strobl, R., & Lesch, O. M. (1989). Regional brain function in hallucinations: A study of regional cerebral blood flow with 99m-Tc-HMPAO-SPECT in patients with auditory hallucinations, tactile hallucinations and normal controls. *Comparative psychiatry, 30,* 99–108.

Neisser, U. (1967). *Cognitive psychology.* New York: Appleton-Century-Crofts.

Nightingale, S. (1982). Somatoparaphrenia: A case report. *Cortex, 18,* 463–467.

Nuechterlein, K. H., & Dawson, M. E. (1984). Information processing and attentional functioning in the developmental course of schizophrenic disorders. *Schizophrenia Bulletin, 10,* 160–203.

O'Grady, J. C. (1990). The prevalence and diagnosis of Schneiderian first-rank symptoms in a random sample of acute psychiatric in-patients. *British Journal of Psychiatry, 156,* 496–500.

Pardo, J. V., Pardo, P. J., Janer, K. W., & Raichle, M. E. (1990). The anterior cingulate cortex mediates processing selection in the Stroop attentional conflict paradigm. *Proceedings of the National Academy of Science, 87,* 256–259.

Park, S., & Holzman, P. S. (1992). Schizophrenics show spatial working memory deficits. *Archives of General Psychiatry, 49*, 975–982.

Passingham, R. E. (1987). Two cortical systems for directing movement. In *Motor areas of the cerebral cortex: Symposium (CIBA Foundation Symposium 132)* (pp. 151–161). Chichester: Wiley.

Passingham, R. E., Chen, Y. C., & Thaler, D. (1989). Supplementary motor cortex and self-initiated movement. In M. Ito (Ed.), *Neural programming (Taniguchi Symposia on Brain Sciences: No. 12)* (pp. 13–24). Basel: S. Karger.

Penfield, W., & Perot, P. (1963). The brain's record of auditory and visual experience. *Brain, 86*, 595–596.

Perez, M. M., Trimble, M. R., Murray, N. M. F., & Reider, I. (1985). Epileptic psychosis: An evaluation of PSE profiles. *British Journal of Psychiatry, 146*, 155–163.

Petersen, S. E., Fox, P. T., Posner, M. I., Mintun, M., & Raichle, M. E. (1988). Positron emission tomographic studies of the cortical anatomy of single word processing. *Nature, 331*, 585–589.

Posner, M. I., & Peterson, S. E. (1990). The attention system of the human brain. In W. M. Rowan, E. M. Shooter, C. F. Stevens, & R. F. Thompson (Eds.), *Annual review of neuroscience* (pp. 25–42). Palo Alto, CA: Annual Reviews.

Putnam, K. M., Harvey, P. D., Davidson, M., White, L., Parrella, M., & Davis, K. L. (1993). *Symptom stability of geriatric schizophrenics.* Poster presented at the 1993 meeting of the American Psychiatric Association, San Francisco, CA.

Raye, C. L., Johnson, M. K. (1980). Reality monitoring vs. discrimination between external sources. *Bulletin of the Psychonomic Society, 15*, 405–408.

Ricks, D. F., & Berry, J. C. (1970). Family and symptom patterns that precede schizophrenia. In M. Roff & D. F. Ricks (Eds.), *Life history research in schizophrenia.* Minneapolis, MN: University of Minnesota Press.

Roberts, G. W., Done, D. J., Bruton, C., & Crow, T. J. (1990). A 'mock-up' of schizophrenia: Temporal lobe epilepsy and schizophrenia-like psychosis. *Biological Psychiatry, 28*, 127–143.

Roberts, K., and Vass, N. (1986). Schneiderian first-rank symptoms caused by benzodiazepine withdrawal. *British Journal of Psychiatry, 148*, 593–594.

Roland, P. E., & Friberg, L. (1985). Localization of cortical areas activated by thinking. *Journal of Neurophysiology, 53*, 1219–1243.

Rolls, E. T. (1990). A theory of emotion and its application to understanding the neural basis of emotion. *Cognition and Emotion, 4*, 161–190.

Sartorius, N., Shapiro, R., & Jablensky, A. (1974). The international pilot study of schizophrenia. *Schizophrenia Bulletin, 1*, 21–35.

Saykin, A. J., Gur, R. C., Gur, R. E., Mozley, P. D., Mozley, L. H., Resnick, S. M., Kester, D. B. & Stafiniak, P. (1991). Neuropsychological function in schizophrenia. *Archives of General Psychiatry, 48*, 618–624.

Schneider, K. (1959). *Klinische Psychopathologie* (5th ed.). New York: Grune & Stratton.

Serper, M., Davidson, M., & Harvey, P. (1994). Attentional predictors of clinical change during neuroleptic treatment in Schizophrenia. *Schizophrenia Research, 13* (1), 65–71.

Serper, M. (1993). Visual controlled information processing resources and formal thought disorder in schizophrenia and mania. *Schizophrenia Research, 9*, 59–66.

Shallice, T. (1988). *From neuropsychology to mental structure.* New York: Cambridge, University Press.

Shtasel, D. L., Gur, R. E., Gallacher, F., Heimberg, C., Cannon, T., Gur, R. C. (1992). Phenomenology and functioning in first-episode schizophrenia. *Schizophrenia Bulletin, 18*, 449–462.

Shenton, M. E., Kikines, R., Jolesz, F. A., Pollack, S. D., LeMay, M., Wible, C. G., Hokama, H., Martin, J., Metcalf, D., Coleman, M., & McCarley, R. W. (1992). Abnormalities in the left temporal lobe and thought disorder in schizophrenia. *New England Journal of Medicine, 327*, 604–612.

Shimamura, A. P. Janowsky, J. S., & Squire, L. R. (1990). Memory for the temporal order of events in patients with frontal lobe lesions and amnesic patients. *Neuropsychologia, 28*, 803–813.

Sietz, P. F., & Malholm, H. B. (1947). Relation of mental imagery to hallucinations. *Archives of Neurology and Psychiatry, 57*, 469–480.

Sperry, R. W. (1950). Neural basis of the spontaneous optokinetic response produced by visual inversion. *Journal of Comparative and Physiological Psychology, 43*, 482–489.

Spitzer, R. L., Endicott, J., & Robins, E. (1978). *Research Diagnostic Criteria (RDC)*, 3rd ed. New York: New York State Psychiatric Institute.

Stace, W. T. (1960). *Mysticism and philosophy*. Philadelphia: Lippincott.

Stern, D. N. (1985). *The interpersonal world of the infant*. New York: Basic Books.

Strauss, J. S., Carpenter, W. T., & Bartko, J. J. (1974). The diagnosis and understanding of schizophrenia: Part III. Speculations on the processes that underlie schizophrenic symptoms and signs. *Schizophrenia Bulletin, 11*, 61–76.

Stuss, D. T., & Benson, D. F. (1986). *The frontal lobes*. New York: Raven Press.

Suddath, R. L., Christison, G. W., Torrey, E. F., Casanova, M. F., & Weinberger, D. R. (1990). Anatomical abnormalities in the brains of monozygotic twins discordant for schizophrenia. *New England Journal of Medicine, 322*, 789–794.

Swann, W. B., Jr. (1984). Quest for accuracy in person perception: A matter of pragmatics. *Psychological Review, 91*, 457–477.

Talairach, J., & Tournoux, P. (1988). *Coplanar stereotaxic atlas of the human brain*. New York: Thieme.

Tamminga, C. A., Thaker, G. K., Buchanan, R., Kirkpatrick, B., Alphs, L. D., Chase, T. N., & Carpenter, W. T. (1992). Limbic system abnormalities in schizophrenia using PET with fluorodeoxyglucose and neocortical alterations with deficit syndrome. *Archives of General Psychiatry, 49* (7), 522–530.

Tanenbaum, R. R., & Harvey, P. D. (1988). Use of text stimuli normalizes reality monitoring in schizophrenics. *Bulletin of the Psychonomic Society, 26*, 336–338.

Tausk, V. (1919/1948). On the origin of the "influencing machine" in schizophrenia. In R. Fliess (Ed.), *The psychoanalytic reader* (pp. 31–64). New York: International University Press.

Taylor, D. C. (1975). Factors influencing the occurrence of schizophrenia-like psychosis in patients with temporal lobe epilepsy. *Psychological Medicine, 5*, 249–254.

Trimble, M. R. (1990). First-rank symptoms of Schneider: A new perspective? *British Journal of Psychiatry, 156*, 195–200.

Van Essen, D. C. (1985). Functional organization of primate visual cortex. In A. Peters & E. G. Jones (Eds.), *Cerebral cortex*. New York: Plenum Press.

Warkentin, S., Nilsson, A., Risberg, J., & Carlson, S. (1989). Absence of frontal lobe activation in schizophrenia. *Journal of Cerebral Blood Flow Metabolism, 9* (suppl. 1), S354.

Watt, N. F. (1978). Patterns of childhood social development in adult schizophrenics. *Archives of General Psychiatry, 35*, 160–165.

Weinberger, D. R. (1993). A connectionist approach to the prefrontal cortex. *Journal of Neuropsychiatry and Clinical Neurosciences, 5*, 241–253.

Weinberger, D. R., Berman, K. F., Suddath, R., & Torrey, E. F. (1992). Evidence of dysfunction of a prefrontal-limbic network in schizophrenia: A magnetic resonance imaging and regional cerebral blood flow study of discordant monozygotic twins. *American Journal of Psychiatry, 149,* 890–897.

Wuthnow, R. (1978). Peak experiences: some empirical tests. *Journal of Humanistic Psychology, 18,* 61.

Young, D. A., Davila, R., & Sher, H. (1993). Unawareness of illness and neuropsychological performance in chronic schizophrenia. *Schizophrenia Research, 10,* 117–124.

## 9

MARCEL KINSBOURNE

# Representations in Consciousness and the Neuropsychology of Insight

It is now generally agreed that consciousness in some manner arises from the activity of the brain (CIBA Foundation, 1993). Therefore, how one conceptualizes the brain basis of consciousness depends on one's working model of how information flows and is processed and represented in the brain. More specifically, since we are aware of the content of representations that result from processing, and not of the processing itself (Lashley, 1956), the neuropsychology of consciousness deals with representations. It inquires into the nature and distribution of the cell assemblies whose activity contribute that representation of the experience of the moment. In this discussion I shall first consider, in principle, the requirements that any representation has to meet for its content to be reflected in consciousness. Must such representations be in a particular part of the brain, in some special state of activation, and at a particular stage of information processing? Or is any representation eligible to compete for a presence in consciousness? Having reached some provisional conclusions about these matters, I shall apply these conclusions to those representations whose contents include self-awareness, including insight into one's own actions and one's situation in the world.

If the self were embodied in a cell assembly located at a point toward which all input channels converge and from which all output channels originate, then it would be hard to understand how a person can lack insight into his or her activity and situation. If the consciousness module lacked the necessary information because information flow is interrupted, the person should have insight into that fact and might be expected to defer judgment, but not to appear oblivious to or even deny, physical reality. But I shall argue that if the brain is not organized in such a centered fashion, it becomes intelligible that facts about the self might, in certain pathological states, become opaque to the self.

## Does It All Come Together in the Brain?

There is no doubt that information converges on the brain from the body's near and distance receptors in the physical sense of traveling from many organs toward a single one. But functionally, these projections are parallel rather than converging, in that they retain their identities and local sign and do not coalesce all the way to the cerebral cortex. At that point, do they integrate stepwise toward some superordinate locus, according to the functional architecture of the centered brain? This *pontifical cell* assembly, so caricatured by James (1890/1950), would combine an overview of all conscious percepts with one of all intended actions. Alternatively, do they continue throughout as a largely parallel though interactive and differentiated network—a brain organization that is uncentered?

The widely used metaphor that considers consciousness to be something "entered" assumes that, after being represented, information has to be transported to some privileged brain area dedicated to transferring the information into conscious experience. It assumes that for centrally represented information to become conscious, something additional has to be done to it (e.g., Searle, 1992; Nagel, 1993)—that is, consciousness is the product of some presumably exquisitely elaborate transformation (Penrose, 1989). This leads naturally into the gratifying conjecture that perhaps humans alone among species have the neurological wherewithal to accomplish something so sophisticated. A likely consequence for neuropsychology is that there be a particular location in the brain, damage to which can selectively eliminate the hypothesized "consciousness module" or, should the module be distributed rather than focal, disrupt such circuitry. That accomplished, and if consciousness is epiphenomenal, the individual should proceed as before in the moment-to-moment business of living, but bereft of awareness (the zombie scenario). If consciousness has causal efficacy, then, that single lesion should strip all those cognitive processes from the repertoire that rely on consciousness (the automaton scenario). But no such syndrome of selective ablation of conscious experience from continuing information or sweepingly depleted information processing has even been described (although the cerebrum, and consciousness with it, can be switched off by the interruption of ascending activation at specific brain stem loci). Nor have event-related measurements of cerebral functioning revealed a centered cerebral architecture. Metabolic measures have not revealed any awareness area the activity of which is highly correlated with the activity of the areas specifically involved in processing and representing. Subjects studied while performing cognitive tasks typically exhibit the distribution of metabolic activity that would be expected in view of the modality of the input. If there are additional areas of activation, they are prefrontal, should problem solving or an effortful task be involved.

## Parsimony in Representing

There is no evidence that input, including input of which one is aware, is represented in any area other than that which is specialized for its processing. There is nothing to suggest that it is communicated to or entered into any separate place where the attribute of being consciously perceived is grafted on. Any process that transduces activity from one form (domain) into another must in principle be vulnerable to malfunction. The nonexistence of any disorder or any artificial means by which the generation of consciousness from ongoing neural activity can be impaired or abolished implies that consciousness is not, after all, a product derived from neural activity. Instead, it *is* the neural activity, from a particular (subjective) point of view. Being conscious is what it is like to *be* a brain (in certain functional states). Confusion between the mental (i.e., neuronal) activity and its subjective aspect persists to the present day. It is not their "subjective quality" that confers selective advantage on organisms with mental activity, as many have assumed (e.g., Ramachandran, 1993). It is the mental (i.e., neural) activity that confers selective advantage. That activity has a subjective quality from the first-person point of view.

The postulate of the uncentered brain is counterintuitive. The most facile analogy for consciousness in the brain is the person in the world. Nestled in the brain is the consciousness center, for which the rest of the brain is a surrogate world. It has long seemed intuitively obvious that the conscious mind is housed, not in the brain in general, but in some deeply recessed brain center (e.g., Sherrington, 1934), which is specialized to accomplish what must be the highest mental function. Such an organization does conform to people's intuition that they have a unitary self and that their subjectivity is unique, in that it places the subjective (first-person) self at the peak of all processing sequences. We have described this construct as regarding the self as a viewer in a Cartesian theater on the screens of which preprocessed information is displayed (Dennett & Kinsbourne, 1992). This intuition comes easily; it merely projects into the brain the experienced relationship between the individual and the ambient environment. However, as any science matures, it leaves intuition further and further behind. For instance, constructs in contemporary physics, such as the Lorenz contraction, are anything but intuitively obvious but generally accepted nonetheless. In the case of the brain, by now a mass of evidence — anatomical, functional, and clinical — militates against the intuitively pleasing classical (Cartesian)–centered construct of the brain. Neither in the anatomical organization of its pathways nor in the ever more fully specified localizations of its functions can one discern a place in the brain "where it all comes together."

## Design Characteristics of the Brain

The cerebral cortex is a feltwork manifold of neurons with interlocking dendrites and mostly without axons. This neuropil features no boundaries or physical discontinuities between its disparately specialized areas. Nor is it replete with projections that, like private telephone lines, conduct information unidirectionally from center to center, as required by traditional neuropsychological concepts (e.g., Geschwind, 1965). Cortico-cortical connections that sweep out of the gray into the white matter and back again have been well described, but they are bidirectional (Galaburda & Pandya, 1983), with a comparable density of axons sweeping in either direction (Felleman & Van Essen, 1991). Connections are often equally specific in both directions (Mignard & Malpeli, 1991). Topographically specified projections to the cortex from subcortical structures are far more numerous than previously believed, and supply the many receiving areas within each modality with information about different features or properties of a display roughly in parallel. Even within a modality — let alone between modalities — though there are plentiful heterarchical interconnections, there is no overall pattern of hierarchical convergence. The study of cross-modal integration suggests that information does *not* converge on nodal points, as envisaged in serial hierarchical models of information flow.

Dramatically illustrative of the noncenteredness of the brain is the anatomy of the two cerebral hemispheres. From studies of split-brain individuals, each is known to be equipped with enough specialized processors to be able to control behavior, albeit not with equal versatility or efficiency. In the integrated, intact brain, the hemispheres collaborate, but there is no place in either toward which streams information from both sides for, as it were, an overall appraisal. Admittedly, left-hemisphere verbal facilities are more adept at acquainting an audience with the contents of their truncated consciousness in the split-brain state (Gazzaniga, 1993). But that awareness can exist without verbal commentary cannot be doubted, and the disconnected right hemisphere gives signs of having its own consciousness. The hemispheres can even take turns controlling behavior in a multiple personality disorder (Henninger, 1992). But the two hemispheres need not exhaust the disunity of the brain.

Once the centered concept is abandoned, it becomes unclear what theoretical limit might exist for the number of possible coexisting consciousnesses in one brain. If sectors of cortex are disconnected, each might house a "splinter consciousness," meager in content but real nonetheless (Kinsbourne, 1982), down to whatever limiting complexity of the residual neural network underlies its propensity to have consciousness as an attribute. The potentiality of self-consciousness might call for a more extensive network, since it implies a sense of continuity over (past and prospective) time.

## Adapting Concepts to the Uncentered Brain

Against a backdrop of a century and a half of growing understanding of human neuropsychology, the construct of the centered brain long ago outlived its usefulness and even its credibility (Penfield, 1958; Pribram, 1971; Kinsbourne, 1971, 1976). But only quite recently did hierarchical organization disappear, spectacularly, from most informed discourse. This abrupt turnaround, coincident with progress in neurophysiology and the popularity of parallel distributed processing models in artificial intelligence, is more attributable to a change in Zeitgeist than to a better understanding of neuropsychological findings. Its implications for neuropsychology have not been well digested. While most will disavow belief in a central homunculus, theories in which such an assumption is implicit remain prevalent. The challenge of recognizing and revising the many preconceptions that attended belief in the centered brain, in view of the radically different uncentered construct, remains.

The following preconceptions linger from the logic of the Cartesian theater: We become aware of the contents of representations after they are "entered" into some structure (such as a conscious-awareness system or module; e.g., Schacter, McAndrews, & Moscovitch, 1988; deHoan, Bauer, & Grove, 1992), by some mechanism (such as a central executive system; Shallice, 1988), which inscribes the information on some metaphorical scratch pad (Baddeley, 1986), to be viewed by an internal scanning eye (Kosslyn, 1980).

As against these claims, I suggest this alternative: Represented content contributes to awareness by virtue of sustained activation of the pertinent cell assemblies. It does so regardless of their location in the neural network. This activation facilitates the cell assemblies' collective binding into a dominant focus of neural activity. The activation is enhanced by congruence of the contents with current expectation.

What properties render representations eligible for consciousness? The internal representation of a particular external change may contribute to awareness on some occasions but not on others. It follows that its mere existence does not suffice for a represented content to contribute to conscious experience. Input may trigger measurable psychophysiological changes or induce cognitive priming effects, even when the observer disclaims any corresponding percept. What specifications does a representation have to fulfill for its contents to be reflected in consciousness? I propose that any central representation could contribute to the moment's experience if:

1. The cell assembly is (a) sufficiently activated, and (b) sufficiently enduring.
2. It can become integrated into the dominant brain activity that is (subjectively) that moment's conscious experience.
3. The represented contents are (a) congruent with contents in the current focus of attention; or (b) biologically so prepotent as to automatically assume control of that focus, excluding its current contents.

Stipulation 3 is pertinent to insight, in that it refers to the influence of expectancies, which may be distorted in psychosis. According to the integrated cortical field model of consciousness (Kinsbourne, 1988), these conditions are not only necessary but also sufficient. No further transport of information or confluent integration is required for any representation to contribute to consciousness.

A behaviorally sophisticated organism does not rely solely on isolated preprogrammed or overlearned action sequences. The integrated field of consciousness enables actions to be based on, and memories to be referenced to, complex contingencies that occur too rarely to serve as the basis of learning by cumulative growth in habit strength. While response predispositions wax and wane under the influence of cumulative experience, specific exceptions can be related to particular contexts and recovered by episodic memory. The response predisposition can then be overridden as necessary. Consciousness may be the subjective aspect of the integration of modules that enables episodic memory.

## Blindsight

There is no focal cerebral lesion that generally precludes represented information from becoming conscious. But there is a syndrome of unawareness limited to a visual hemifield. Poppel, Held, and Frost (1973) described a patient who was able to localize by pointing to stimuli that he could not see (a syndrome named *blindsight* by Weiskrantz, Warrington, Sanders, & Marshall, 1974). An intensive research effort has dramatically increased the inventory of what blindsight patients can accomplish when put into forced-choice situations—told to respond as best they can although they cannot see what they are responding to and are convinced that they are merely guessing (Weiskrantz, 1990). This startling performance is not altogether unprecedented. Under conditions of speeded response, normal people initiate action before they become conscious of the stimulus (Libet, 1985; Velmans, 1991; Neumann & Klotz, 1994). What blindsight patients can do is what normals do preconsciously. What the blindsight patients do not do betrays the difference that obtains when representations are incorporated into the dominant focus, so that their contents become conscious. Unlike normal subjects who initiate response before becoming aware of the stimulus or, if the stimulus was subliminal, without becoming aware of it, blindsight patients do not initiate response to the unseen display spontaneously. Their responding is a fragmented activity isolated from their mental life. It is not responsive to external change, but to instruction from another person.

Does this mean that consciousness has causal efficacy, in that information has to become conscious to be integrated into context? Not exactly. A more precise statement is that when cell assemblies integrate into a dominant focus, further possibilities for immediate and subsequent processing arise. Being conscious is the subjective aspect of this neural activity. But it is not in itself causal, as distinct from the neural activity of which it is an aspect.

Because the unseen stimulus was correctly processed, it must have been represented. What was missing from this representation that, if supplied, would have brought it into awareness? To shed light on this question, we shall consider another, much more prevalent and familiar, though no less astonishing, syndrome—unawareness and denial-unilateral neglect. Certain details of the symptomatology of neglect are instructive with respect to what it takes to be aware of a body part or a side of space, and the difference between being unaware and merely uninformed. If the analogy is apt, what is missing in blindsight is simply a sufficient level of activation of the affected cell assemblies.

## Unilateral Neglect of Body and of Space

The unilateral neglect syndrome is a selective disorder of awareness that gives rise to extremely disordered behavior. In a severe case, superficially characterized, the patient has lost awareness of the left side of space and/or his body. He neither experiences input from that side nor initiates action toward it. Equally important, the patient is not aware of his or her disuse of left-sided information and of his or her own left limbs, as judged from the lack of any complaint, from what is said in response to questions, and from absence of any compensatory effort. Has a right-hemisphere module for lateral attention been inactivated (Mesulam, 1981)? According to the Cartesian theater, screens that should depict information from the left are blank. But why then does the individual (i.e., the viewer of the screens) not realize that no information is coming in from that side?

Answers to these questions cannot be based on the simplistic idea that a defective attention module underlies neglect. What is observed is not a deficit per se, but the overcontrol of behavior by the residual intact brain—specifically, by an intact and disinhibited left-hemisphere facility that programs orientation to the right. Some explanations follow.

1. *The gradient of attention across the lateral plane.* The patient does not, in fact, ignore all that is to the left of the midline, while faithfully observing all that is to its right. On tests of visual search, such as when canceling targets scattered among distractors on a display, he exhibits a gradient of degree of failure to detect the target,

greatest at the extreme left, but also continuing into the right side of egocentric space. When required to react to targets in a linear array, he reacts faster the more to the right of the display the target happens to be, regardless of its absolute location.

2. *Heightened attention to the right.* The obverse of the failure to attend to the left is an excess of attending to the right of a display (as if magnetically drawn thereto). Overattention to the right is clinically apparent when the patient's gaze swings toward the rightmost visible feature, regardless of instruction. Contrary to the customary Western left-to-right reading habit, the patient scans a letter sequence right-to-left. In speed of reaction to the rightmost of a row of targets, the neglect patient may even outdo the normal control (reviewed by Kinsbourne, 1993).

3. *Overinterpretation of right-sided features.* Not only does the neglect patient orient to the right ends of things, but he draws stronger conclusions about the object as a whole than would normally be considered warranted from right-located features. Shown a sequence of letters that could have been the end of any one of several words, he completes the word backward into one of the set of alternatives (Kinsbourne & Warrington, 1962; Riddoch, 1990). Similarly, he overinterprets fragments that could have been the right sides of forms, reporting that he saw the complete form (Warrington, 1962). He thinks he has completed drawings, the left of which he has not sketched in. This bias in evaluation indicates a higher order defect than would be expected from mere failure to obtain complete information, and it parallels striking aspects of patients' general attitudes to their bodies and the ambient space.

4. *Awareness of deficit.* The patient with neglect shows no sign that he is aware of the degree to which the sensory information available to him is restricted and incomplete. In contrast to the patient with a sensory deficit, who is fully aware of the loss of input, he behaves as if his experience were unchanged from the premorbid state, and also explicitly denies his deficit. He must be accomplishing satisfactory matches between his input and his memory representations, as during health. Given that the percept is restricted to the right end of the object, then to secure a match, his memory representation must also be restricted in this way. It follows that the representational bias in neglect encompasses remembered as well as directly experienced percepts. This is why although the patient draws conclusions that are often grounded in inadequate information, the resulting perceptual experience, veridical or not, seems normal to him.

That memory representations are involved in the neglect syndrome was elegantly demonstrated by Bisiach and Luzzatti (1978). They asked two patients to describe a scene that was well known to them, first from one imagined vantage point and then from the opposite view. In each case, the patient described what he would have seen on his right were he there in person. The landmarks that were omitted from one perspective were included from the other. It follows that the complete scene was potentially available, but only the imagined right side could be brought into awareness.

5. *The effect of lateral ascending activation.* An early empirical finding by Silberpfennig (1949) reveals the nature of the representational insufficiency. He found that caloric stimulation of the ear contralateral to the lesion by lukewarm water, or of the ipsilateral ear by warm water of above body temperature, was, for the duration of its effect in stimulating the vestibular system, capable of correcting the neglect and restoring veridical perception. The irrigation unilaterally increases or decreases the firing of

acceleration sensors in the horizontal semicircular canal. This finding has recently been confirmed both for space (e.g., Rubens, 1985) and for person (e.g., Vallar, Sterzi, Bottini, Cappa, & Rusconi, 1990). Evidently the unilateral vestibular stimulation generated activation of the damaged hemisphere and restored its ability to act as an effective opponent processor in equilibrating representations across the lateral plane. The representations must have been structurally intact: their complete participation in consciousness required the additional activation.

It is equally significant that once the effect of the stimulation has worn off, the patient reverts to his prior state of unilateral neglect and appears to be quite unaware that he only moments earlier had the benefit of a more complete worldview. I suggest that this is because he again cannot represent the spatial domain to which he just had access. One cannot experience a lack of information in a domain that one cannot represent.

By analogy with neglect, the blindsight patient cannot sufficiently activate the cell assemblies that represent visual information to render them competitive in the rivalry for a role in the dominant focus. One reason may be that, although the representations were best expressed in the visual cortex that has become nonfunctional, they are also multiplexed in neighboring cortex. If some external means were to be found to activate this part of the brain, this would bring the represented contents back into awareness.

## Binding into a Dominant Focus

In order to contribute to awareness, representing cell assemblies must be adequately activated. What happens when they are? I have suggested (Kinsbourne, 1988) that at any time in the awake individual there is a *dominant focus* of coordinated patterned neural activity that underlies the phenomenal experience of that moment, the momentarily dominant draft of the multiple drafts that in rapid succession constitute the apparently continuous stream of ever-changing consciousness (Dennett & Kinsbourne, 1992). How are representations assembled into a dominant focus? The answer to this question is not yet clearly established, and there may be more than one answer. However, following observation of excitability cycles in the 30 to 50 Hz range time-locked to the onset of the auditory evoked potential (Galambos, Makeig, & Talamachoff, 1981), much interest has been invested in the possibility that representations integrate (bind) if the cell assemblies in question enter into joint oscillation (von der Malsburg, 1983; Gray & Singer, 1989; Sheer, 1989) or at least spike synchronously (Singer, 1993). The dominant focus may, therefore, consist of synchronously firing cell assemblies. Given the need for multiple simultaneous bindings into individual objects, object clusters traveling together, and panoramic background (to mention vision alone), the cell assemblies presumably oscillate at multiple frequencies. Joint oscillation in the approximately 40 Hz range cannot be a sufficient condition for consciousness, as it is demonstrable in comatose patients (Firsching et al., 1987). But it may be a necessary condition for the neural tissue to be able to fire at such rates. However this may be, the heuristic value of the concept of dominant focus does not depend on being able to identify the mechanism by which it is implemented. When a representation loses activation because attention has shifted, it ceases to be entrained with the dominant focus and consequently slips from awareness. If the representation is underactivated, it will not be incorporated into the dominant focus in the first place. It also will not be incorporated if it is too rapidly superseded by an undated version. In either case, it may nonetheless have an influence on how the brain subsequently represents that or similar inputs—for instance, through priming effects (Farah, O'Reilly, & Vecera, 1993).

## Fluent Multistage Processing and Modularity

Multistage processing is assumed to underlie all the fundamental cognitive processes. For instance, according to Marr (1982), visual input is first represented centrally as a *primal sketch*, then as a 2 ½-D *representation*, and finally as a 3-D *representation*. But we are only aware of the visual array in 2 ½-D, which is 2-D experience imbued with 3-D knowledge. In generating speech, we encode our intended utterance first in terms of its meaning, then its syntax, finally its phonology. We think in words at the level of phonology (Levelt, 1989). We experience our utterances in terms of phonetics (the product of the articulatory gestures). What bars the earlier representations from awareness? Simply that they were too short-lived. It takes appreciable time for a cell assembly's firing to entrain with that of the dominant focus. If representations succeed each other too quickly, as in highly skilled processing sequences such as the ones instanced, then an intermediate representation's entry into consciousness is aborted or too fleeting to be recalled at the time of verbal response (there being no fact of the matter as to whether it was experienced or not; Dennett & Kinsbourne, 1992). Such a fluent processing sequence would have the attribute of impenetrability that, according to Fodor (1983), characterizes a cerebral module.

Jackendoff (1989) has argued that whether a representation is conscious depends on its level. The ones at the highest level (i.e., the ones that arise earliest in output, latest in input processing) are not directly experienced. As a contingent fact, this appears to be so. But perhaps this is not a property of level per se, but of the facility with which levels interact in fluent processing. For instance, when a person speaks, semantics merges too soon into syntax, and syntax into phonology, for the earlier two representations to be experienced other than interpenetrated by phonology.

## Penetrating the Module

The idea that intermediary representations are not experienced on account of their evanescent nature raises an interesting possibility for pathology. If a lesion incapacitates a stage in information processing, then the represented output from the prior stage may persist long enough to be experienced, shattering the module and rendering it penetrable. Not only is the flawed performance that results indicative of the stage at which the processing has been arrested, but the patient experiences what people with intact brains cannot experience. The phenomenology of gradual recovery from cortical blindness may be a case in point (Poppelreuter, 1923). Deviant experiences reported by psychiatric patients could be analyzed from this perspective, including perceptual distortions in schizophrenia and under psychoactive drug influence. The unaccustomed nature of such experiences may make them seem alien, as in the case of thought insertion and hallucinated speech. That does not mean, however, that they are experienced as any less real than the mundane experiences shared by all.

Another possibility is that disease causes the process of entraining into the dominant focus to become sluggish and protracted. A case in point might be the following. Temporal-duration thresholds are generally elevated in patients with posterior cerebral lesions. In some neglect patients, it is possible to demonstrate extinction to double visual simultaneous stimulation by flashing one signal to the intact field and another to the field opposite the lesion. Although each is detected alone, when both are flashed only the one on the intact ipsilesional side is perceived. One can adjust the interstimulus interval so as to have one stimulus lead the other, and so measure the temporal boundary conditions of visual extinction in the particular patient. Kinsbourne and Warrington (1961) found an extreme case in whom the stimulus to the intact side could follow the one to the impaired side by as much as a full second without the patient reporting the stimulus on the affected side. The stimulus representation on the affected side must have been slow to entrain, and therefore been vulnerable to being diverted from doing so by the subsequent ipsilesional stimulus for an unusually long period of time.

Having concluded that what is represented is likely to be experienced if the cell assembly's activity is sufficiently activated and enduring, we now wonder whether this can include representations that are not triggered by bottom-up information flow. If the brain *infers* the occurrence of a movement, or the uninterrupted extension of a contour or pattern, is it then necessary to activated the lower order neurons that would normally have registered such information, had there been a corresponding external change—or is the decision made by *top-down* fiat, after which the brain goes about its further business?

## Unconscious Inference or Filling In

*Unconscious inference*, so named by Helmholtz, resolves ambiguous percepts by inferring a resolution that has the advantage of familiarity or simplicity or both. This type of inference (top-down rather than bottom-up filling in) occurs continually in normal visual perception (Walls, 1954). Initially, contours are extracted and the neuronal activity that responds to the homogeneous surfaces they enclose (the illuminants) is discounted. The presence of the surface is inferred from the nature and disposition of the contours that surround it. Top-down inference also generates such phenomena as apparent movement, in which a single moving stimulus is inferred on the basis of two rapidly successive, appropriately displaced, briefly flashed stimuli. The phenomenal continuity of patterns across the blind spot is an example of filling in discussed by Helmholtz, and its nature is the topic of imaginative demonstrations by Ramachandran (1992). This is bottom-up filling in, with activity detectable in visual neurons that ordinarily respond to stimuli in that location when they are viewed by the other eye (Gattass et al., 1992).

According to a traditional bottom-up converging information flow model of cerebral function, it would be necessary, in generating the appearance of motion, to stimulate in succession the appropriate receptors (or their cortical relay cells) between the points at which the inferred movement begins and ends. This is what one would naturally do, were it one's intention so to inform a centrally located observer or homunculus. But absent displays on the screens of a Cartesian theater, such reenactment is unnecessary.

Instead, once movement is coded (presumably in area MT), the necessary coding is completed (Dennett, 1991). Similarly, if a repetitive pattern is viewed at a focal point, and one of its units is identified—for instance, as a face (perhaps the face of Marilyn Monroe)—then the brain makes the inference that the other elements of the pattern are also exemplars of the same face—something that could be known for sure (as opposed to inferred) only if each were laboriously fixated in serial fashion. This is perceptual filling in, not conceptual filling in (as of information behind one's ears) as claimed by Ramachandran (1993). The individual perceives them all as Marilyns, just as he or she perceives that an object has depth, although the input is a two-dimensional viewer-centered pattern. Once the information is coded, the experience is instantiated. It does not have to be filled-in with bottom-up detail.

Inference tends toward simplification. Demonstrating what he called an artificial blind spot, Ramachandran (1992) presented a shimmering surface spotted by a small gray rectangular area. It appeared to viewers as though the shimmer gradually encroaches upon the rectangle until only an uninterrupted shimmering surface is seen. When the experimenter turns off the shimmer, the rectangular area that objectively was not part of the shimmering surface continues to shimmer for a few seconds before again being seen veridically. My explanation is that the input from the minority source (rectangle) is over time discounted by the perceptual analyzer as deviating from the rest of the signals only on account of noise contamination, and is reinterpreted as just more twinkle. When the twinkling field is turned off, that interpretation is not immediately contradicted, and it is not revised until a little later. Therefore, the rectangular patch of twinkle lingers. In summary, absent information is either filled in bottom up (blind spot) or top down; either results in a complete representation of the content of the experience. It is not necessary for the brain to do both redundantly. When the higher level decision suffices—for example, "something moved from A to B," or "there is a rectangle"—no further sensory activity is called for. If the filling in specifies sensory detail—for example, the detailed sensation of movement; or the specific size, orientation, and location of the rectangle—then feedback from the decision level organizes the local sensory cell assemblies accordingly and both levels are involved in the filling in. That does not, of course, prove that the brain never does *redundant* double filling in. Evolution is not a maximally economical process. But the point of theoretical interest is that, if the brain were organized around a Cartesian theater, it always would.

## Attention Is Needed to Detect the Absence of Information

The above demonstrates that the brain codes its version or draft, and stays with that pending further information. If a draft is in force long enough to integrate with the dominant focus, it is reported in subsequent accounts of subjective experience. As already mentioned, this effect can be grossly exaggerated in pathology. Poppelreuter (1917/1990) first described patients with posterior unilateral cerebral gunshot wounds who, when briefly shown a geometrical figure exposed so as to overlap a hemianopic field, reported seeing the complete figure. This *imaginative completion* is just as readily elicited if there is nothing projected to the blind field (Warrington, 1962) and if incomplete words (e.g., word endings for left hemianopics) rather than incomplete shapes are presented (Kinsbourne & Warrington, 1962), so long as a stimulus interpretable as one end of a shape or a word is projected ipsilesionally. We know from normative research that when an expected part of a familiar figure is missing, an orienting response (to novelty) ensues (Ruchkin, Sutton, Minson, Silver, & McCar, 1981). The patient was not shown the whole figure. Why did he or she not exhibit an orienting response to the place where a piece was missing? I suggest that this is because the patient was incapable of attending to that side of the display (as in neglect). Absent information to the contrary, the brain infers the complete figure, and this is indeed what is perceived. When a percept is based on inference, it is perceived as vividly and convincingly as if it were based on input, bottom up. The individual cannot discriminate the percept that arises from context and expectancy from that which reflects physical change. Obviously, abnormal expectancy in the thought-disordered individual could radically distort what he or she perceives. That percept is experienced as real, whether or not it defies logic.

Similar considerations can be applied to the problem of unawareness of deficit, notably of left hemiplegia in unilateral neglect. The patient fails to attend to the left side of the body. This does not mean that he or she experiences it as missing. It is filled in, top down, as background bodily sensation. In general, the patient with a sensory deficit *from which attention is withdrawn* has a normal perceptual experience, on account of filling in. No contour or demarcation can be experienced between intact and blind visual field if the impaired field offers no positive sensation (white, gray, black), because the presence of a edge depends on there being sensory signals (signaling presence or absence of some visual property) on both sides. If there are not, the visual field dwindles away imperceptibly, just as it does in front of our ears or just below our eyebrows. The brain does not commit itself as to where exactly the visual field comes to an end. By virtue of filling in, there is, as background to the focus of attention, a general sense of the presence of a background (visual, somatosensory, etc.) that is too undifferentiated to reveal any absence of or discontinuity in specific features. Nor is it apparent to the patient with left-somatic neglect that he is not attending to one of his or her body parts, for the reason that this would require that the patient form a mental image of the part in question, which he or she cannot do. The patient is not only unaware of the information in question but, by virtue of filling in, even has the affirmative sense that all is complete and intact. The patient will therefore strenuously resist or steadfastly ignore mere argumentation to the contrary (Kinsbourne, 1995).

## Implications for Lack of Insight

Lack of insight even in brain damage, let alone in psychosis, is usually treated as dynamically motivated explicit or implicit denial (e.g., Weinstein & Kahn, 1955). However, organically based failures of representation may offer a more parsimonious account.

If one cannot activate a representation of a body part either by exposing it to sensory input or by top-down contextual influence, then one has no information about its status and, when one looks at the body part, no sense of ownership. If one cannot form (i.e., represent) the intention to perform a given movement, then one has no way of knowing whether one has lost this movement from one's repertoire. This we know from unilateral neglect. By extrapolation, a schizophrenic patient who cannot represent the intention to think has no sense of ownership of the thought. The thought appears as if externally motivated, while one's own thinking is blocked. If one did not intend to speak, one does not experience the utterance (overt or covert) as one's own. Failure to activate a representation can, as we have seen, result from withdrawal of attention. This might be particularly apt to occur in psychosis, in which the focus and distribution of attention may be deviant. Correspondingly impaired insight would result. When the focus of attention is alternately controlled by different brain territories, multiple consciousnesses may be established, in mutual ignorance, as in multiple personality disorder.

When schizophrenics report that they are experiencing verbal hallucinations, they can be observed to subvocalize (Green & Kinsbourne, 1990). However, it is not convincing to attribute the voices directly to inner speech, because they often are described as sounding like another person or like someone of a different age and gender. Also, not all inner speech is heard as emanating from voices distinct from the patient's own. An additional factor is required. I have suggested (Kinsbourne, 1990) that verbal hallucinations are a consequence of intense expectancies that derive from disordered thought. When one expects to hear something, one forms in one's mind an *anticipatory representation* (Neisser, 1978). If for some reason (its intensity, or a brain-based inhibitory deficit) this representation activates the phonological representations that subserve inner speech, then one hears the very voice, saying the very things that one expected. Because he did not intend to speak, the patient does not attribute the speech to himself but refers it to an external source. The tendency of schizophrenics to speak in strange voices atypical for them may have a similar origin.

There are two complementary parts to any experienced and remembered event. One is the representation of its contents in focal attention, as figure. The other is the representation of the self in relation to that contents as background. I have suggested elsewhere that this representation of the self is in terms of body background sensation (Kinsbourne, in press-b). The concept of the unitary self is abstracted from the sense of ownership of the body. In pathological states, this construct can be dissociated from its foundation in bodily sensation, giving rise to such experiences as depersonalization and autoscopy at the level of perception, and of a monitoring agency at the level of belief. As with neglect, reasoned argument cannot supply what direct experience did not.

Unawareness of verbal deficit in jargon aphasia is a more complex case. The patient accepts his or her own recorded speech as intelligible, but rejects the identical passages when rerecorded and played in another's voice (Kinsbourne & Warrington, 1963). Perhaps the patient fills in meaning by a mechanism that is triggered only when the voice is his or her own. For possible benefits of such self-deception, see Kiersky this volume.

## Insight and Foresight

Lack of insight into disability in neglect results from a failure to represent the affected body part in consciousness. This is a lack of *current* insight. Lack of *prospective* insight (foresight) results from the inability to represent projections into the future.

Prefrontal damage is well known to cause a failure to plan in the absence of dementia or confusion (Fuster, 1989). Planning proceeds by representing the required action step by step, basing each step on the consequences of the previous step. Direct action proceeds similarly, but differs from planned action in that the individual obtains afferent feedback about the changes induced by the previous step. This generates a new and salient here-and-now upon which to base the next action in the sequence. During planning, this influx of supportive information from the exterior is absent. The individual has to update his or her schema of the situation by *reafference*, the internally generated record of the expected consequence of the act. Reafferent information may not be available to the prefrontally injured patient (Teuber, 1964). He can therefore not inform himself of the likely consequences of his actions. Schizophrenics often have poor insight (see Amador, this volume), perhaps on account of prefrontal dysfunction.

The inability to foresee consequences has implications for insight. The patient can appreciate his or her present limitations, but not anticipate how he or she would function under other circumstances. This may lead the patient to entertain aspirations about further activities, employment, or relationships that are unrealistic in view of his or her handicaps. What looks like a motivated denial of a disability may simply be an inability to foresee consequences. Unbuffered by the ability to foresee, the patient is victim to the moment, swinging abruptly between emotional extremes as circumstance change, unqualified by anticipation of what is to come.

Whatever their original cause, failures of insight in psychosis and brain damage may be mediated by a failure to represent or by distortions of representation resulting from neurological dysfunction.

*References*

Baddeley, A. (1986). *Working memory*. Oxford, England: Clarendon Press.
Bisiach, E., & Luzzatti, C. (1978). Unilateral neglect of representational space. *Cortex, 14*, 129–133.
CIBA Foundation Symposium 174 (1993). *Experimental and theoretical studies of consciousness*. Chichester: Wiley.
deHoan, E. H. F., Bauer, R. M., & Grove, K. W. (1992) Behavioral and physiological evidence for covert recognition in a prosopagnosic patient. *Cortex, 23*, 309–316.
Dennett, D. C. (1991). *Consciousness explained*. Boston: Little, Brown.
Dennett, D. C., & Kinsbourne, M. (1992). Time and the observer: The where and when of consciousness in the brain. *Behavioral and Brain Sciences, 15*, 183–247.
Farah, M., O'Reilly, R., & Vecera, S. (1993). Dissociated overt and covert recognition as an emergent property of a lesioned neural network. *Psychological Review, 100*, 571–508.
Felleman, D. J., & Van Essen, D. C. (1991). Distributed hierarchical processing in the primate cerebral cortex. *Cerebral Cortex, 1*, 1–47.
Firsching, R., Luther, J., Eidelberg, E., Brown, W. E., Jr., Story, J. L., & Boop, F. A. (1987). 40 Hz middle latency auditory evoked response in comatose patients. *Electroencephalography and Clinical Neurophysiology, 67*, 213–216.
Fodor, J. A. (1983). *The modularity of mind*. Cambridge, MA: MIT Press.
Fuster, J. M. (1989). *The prefrontal cortex*. New York: Raven Press.
Galaburda, A. M., & Pandya, D. N. (1983). The intrinsic architectonic and connectional organization of the superior temporal region of the Rhesus monkey. *Journal of Comparative Neurology, 221*, 169–184.
Galambos, R., Makeig, S., & Talamachoff, P. (1981). A 40 Hz auditory potential recorded from the human scalp. *Proceedings of the National Academy of Sciences, USA, 78*, 2643–2647.
Gattass, R., Fiorani, M., Rosa, M. G. P., Pirion, M. C. G., Sousa, A. P. B., & Soares, J. G. M.

(1992). Changes in receptive field size in V, in relation to perceptual completion. In R. Lent (Ed.), *Visual system from genesis to maturity*. Boston: Birkhauser.

Gazzaniga, M. A. (1993). Brain mechanisms and conscious experience. In Ciba Foundation Symposium, 174: *Experimental and theoretical studies of consciousness* (pp. 247–257). Chichester: Wiley.

Geschwind, N. (1965). Disconnexion syndromes in animal and man. *Brain, 88,* 237–294.

Gray, C. M., & Singer, W. (1989). Stimulus-specific neuronal oscillations in orientation columns of cat visual cortex. *Proceedings of the National Academy of Sciences, 86,* 1698–1702.

Green, M. F., & Kinsbourne, M. (1990). Subvocal activity and auditory hallucinations: clues for behavioral treatments. *Schizophrenia Bulletin, 16,* 617–626.

Henninger, P. (1992). Conditional handedness: Handedness changes in multiple personality disordered subject reflect shift in hemispheric dominance. *Consciousness and Cognition, 1,* 265–287.

Jackendoff, R. (1989). *Consciousness and the computational mind.* Cambridge, MA: MIT Press.

James, W. (1890/1950). *The principles of psychology.* New York: Dover.

Kinsbourne, M. (1971). Cognitive deficit: Experimental analysis. In J. McGaugh (Ed.), *Psychobiology* (pp. 285–349). New York: Academic Press.

Kinsbourne, M. (1976). The neuropsychological analysis of cognitive deficit. In R. G. Grenell & A. Gabay (Eds.), *Biological foundations of psychiatry* (pp. 527–589). New York: Raven Press.

Kinsbourne, M. (1982). Hemispheric specialization and the growth of human understanding. *American Psychologist, 37,* 411–420.

Kinsbourne, M. (1988). Integrated field theory of consciousness. In A. J. Marcel & E. Bisiach (Eds.), *The concept of consciousness in contemporary science* (pp. 239–256). New York: Oxford University Press.

Kinsbourne, M. (1990). Voiced images, imagined voices. *Biological Psychiatry, 27,* 811–812.

Kinsbourne, M. (1993). Orientational bias model of unilateral neglect: Evidence from attentional gradients within hemispace. In I. H. Robertson & J. C. Marshall (Eds.), *Unilateral neglect, clinical and experimental studies* (pp. 63–86). New York: Erlbaum.

Kinsbourne, M. (1995). Awareness of one's own body: A neuropsychological hypothesis. In J. Bermudez, A. Marcel, & N. Eilan (Eds.), *The body and the self* (pp. 205–224). Cambridge, MA: MIT Press.

Kinsbourne, M., & Warrington, E. K. (1961). A tachistoscopic study of visual inattention. *Journal of Physiology, 156,* 33–34.

Kinsbourne, M., & Warrington, E. K. (1962). A variety of reading disability associated with right hemisphere lesions. *Journal of Neurology, Neurosurgery and Psychiatry, 25,* 339–344.

Kinsbourne, M., & Warrington, E. K. (1963). Jargon aphasia. *Neuropsychologia, 1,* 27–37.

Kosslyn, S. (1980). *Image and mind.* Cambridge, MA: Harvard University Press.

Lashley, K. S. (1956). Integrative functions of the cerebral cortex. *Physiological Review, 13,* 1–42.

Levelt, W. J. M. (1989). *Speaking.* Cambridge, MA: MIT Press.

Libet, B. (1985). Unconscious cerebral initiative and the role of conscious will in voluntary action. *Behavioral and Brain Sciences, 8,* 529–566.

Marr, D. (1982). *Vision.* New York: Freeman.

Mesulam, M. M. (1981). A cortical network for directed attention and unilateral neglect. *Annals of Neurology, 10,* 309–325.

Mignard, M., & Malpeli, J. G. (1991). Paths of information flow through visual cortex. *Science, 251,* 1249–1251.

Nagel, T. (1993). What is the mind-body problem? In Ciba Foundation Symposium, 174: *Experimental and theoretical studies of consciousness* (pp. 1–7). Chichester: Wiley.

Neisser, U. (1978). *Cognition and reality*. San Francisco: Freeman.

Neumann, O., & Klotz, W. (in press). Motor responses to nonreportable, masked stimuli: Where is the limit of direct parameter specification? In C. Umilta & M. Moscovitch (Eds.), *Attention and performance XV: Conscious and nonconscious information processing*. Cambridge, MA: MIT Press.

Penfield, W. (1958). Centrencephalic integrating system. *Brain, 81*, 231–234.

Penrose, K. (1989). *The emperor's new mind: Concerning computers, minds and the laws of physics*. Oxford: Oxford University Press.

Poppel, E., Held, R., & D. Frost (1973). Residual function after brain wounds involving the central visual pathways in man. *Nature* (London) *243*, 295–296.

Poppelreuter, W. (1917/1990). *Disturbances of lower and higher visual capacities caused by occipital damage* (J. Zihl, Trans.). Oxford: Clarendon Press.

Poppelreuter, W. (1923). Zur psychologie und pathologie der optischen wahrnehmung. *Zeitschrift fur die gesamte Neurologie und Psychiatrie, 83*, 26–152.

Pribram, K. H. (1971). *Languages of the brain*. New York: Prentice-Hall.

Ramachandran, V. S. (1992). Blind spots. *Scientific American, 266*, 86–91.

Ramachandran, V. S. (1993). Filling in gaps in logic: Some comments on Dennett. *Consciousness and Cognition, 2*, 165–168.

Riddoch, M. J. (Ed.). (1990). Neglect and the peripheral dyslexias. *Cognitive Neuropsychology, 7*, 369–554.

Rubens, A. B. (1985). Caloric stimulation and unilateral visual neglect. *Neurology, 35*, 1019–1024.

Ruchkin, D. S., Sutton, D. S., Minson, R., Silver, K., & McCar, F. (1981). P300 and feedback provided by the absence of the stimulus. *Psychophysiology, 18*, 271–282.

Schacter, D. L., McAndrews, M. P., & Moscovitch, M. (1988). Access to consciousness: Dissociations between implicit and explicit knowledge in neuropsychological syndromes. In L. Weiskrantz (Ed.), *Thought without language* (pp. 242–278). New York: Oxford University Press.

Searle, J. R. (1992). *The rediscovery of the mind*. Cambridge, MA: MIT Press.

Shallice, T. (1988). Information-processing models of consciousness: Possibilities and problems. In A. J. Marcel & E. Bisiach (Eds.), *Concept of consciousness in contemporary science* (pp. 305–333). London: Oxford University Press.

Sheer, D. E. (1989). Sensory and cognitive 40 Hz event related potentials: Behavioral correlates, brain function and clinical application. In E. Basar & T. H. Bullock (Eds.), *Brain dynamics* (pp. 339–374). Berlin: Springer-Verlag.

Sherrington, C. A. (1934). *The Brain and its mechanism*. Cambridge, England: Cambridge University Press.

Silberpfennig, J. (1949). Contributions to the problem of eye movements. III: Disturbance of ocular movements with pseudo hemianopsia in frontal tumors. *Confinia Neurologica, 4*, 1–13.

Singer, W. (1993). Synchronization of cortical activity and its putative role in information processing and learning. *Annals and Review of Physiology, 55*, 349–374.

Teuber, H. -L. (1964). The riddle of frontal lobe function in man. In J. M. Warren & K. Ackert (Eds.), *The frontal granular cortex and behavior* (pp. 410–477). New York: McGraw-Hill.

Vallar, G., Sterzi, R., Bottini, G., Cappa, S., & Rusconi, M. L. (1990). Temporary remission of the left hemianesthesia after vestibular stimulation: A sensory neglect phenomenon: *Cortex, 26*, 123–131.

Velmans, M. (1991). Is human information processing conscious? *Behavioral and Brain Sciences, 14*, 651–726.

von der Malsburg, C. (1983). How are nervous structures organized? In E. Basar, H. Flohr, H. Haken, & A. J. Mandell (Eds.), *Synergetics of the brain* (pp. 238–249). Berlin: Springer.

Walls, G. L. (1954). The filling-in process. *American Journal of Optometry, 31,* 329–340.

Warrington, E. K. (1962). The completion of visual forms across hemianopia visual field defects. *Journal of Neurology, Neurosurgery and Psychiatry, 25,* 208–217.

Weinstein, E. A., & Kahn, R. L. (1955). *Denial of illness. Symbolic and physiological aspects.* Springfield, IL: Thomas.

Weiskrantz, L. (1990). Outlooks for blindsight: Explicit methodologies for implicit processes. *Proceedings of the Royal Society of London B, 239,* 247–278.

Weiskrantz, L., Warrington, E. K., Sanders, M. D., & Marshall, J. (1974). Visual capacity in the hemianopic field following a restricted occipital ablation. *Brain, 97,* 709–728.

# PART III

## Culture
## and
## Insight

## 10

LAURENCE J. KIRMAYER

ELLEN CORIN

# Inside Knowledge

## Cultural Constructions of Insight in Psychosis

CASE    Martin was a 30-year-old unmarried, unemployed man who presented to the emergency room with the certain knowledge that he was to be admitted to the psychiatric ward to be executed for crimes he did not commit. When asked how he came to this conviction, he reported that he had noticed a license plate on a passing car that read "K2DR" and immediately knew that this was a reference to the "K-2 Diaries," documents that had been forged by the FBI or some other malevolent agency to frame him for murder and, thus, precipitate his incarceration, trial, and execution in a Kafkaesque nightmare.

Despite this terrifying predicament, Martin agreed to voluntary hospitalization on the psychiatric ward, not because he accepted that he was psychotic but because he knew that events were unfolding in an inexorable way and nothing he could do would make any difference to the outcome.

Martin also reported other paranoid delusions, ideas of reference, and uncomfortable abdominal sensations that he believed were due to "subsonic beams" directed at him through the walls from unseen sources. Treated with neuroleptic medication, his ideas of reference, somatic hallucinations, and delusions rapidly abated and he came to accept that he had experienced an exacerbation of his previously diagnosed schizophrenia.

I [LJK] followed Martin as an outpatient in weekly supportive psychotherapy sessions, and because he found it impaired his ability to think clearly, reduced his neuroleptic medication. He continued to have occasional somatic hallucinations and paranoid delusions. He sometimes wore dark blue sunglasses "to block out the laser beams" and continued to complain of "the subsonics." He felt my occasional fidgeting indicated efforts to control him by special gestures. On one occasion, when he described a homeless person he knew as "crazy" because he believed that he had an atomic bomb inside him, I asked Martin how this was different from his own experiences of laser beams and subsonics. He was nonplused and quickly replied, "Dr. K., I'm surprised at you—the laser beams are *real*."

Martin was exceptionally intelligent—he had almost completed an honors degree in philosophy before falling sick in his early twenties—and brought his formidable intellect and extensive reading to bear on understanding his illness. He had been treated in twice-weekly psychoanalytically oriented therapy intermittently for five years, but had left this therapy abruptly, for reasons he never made clear, some months before his emergency room admission.

Martin spoke at length about the knots and quandaries of his family life and offered critiques of R. D. Laing's writing on this theme. He said he planned to write down some of his own thoughts on schizophrenia, to set the record straight, but then added: "You know, my mind is dissolving. Someday I will have no choice but to kill myself." He left this therapy after 18 months, as abruptly as he had left his earlier psychoanalysis, and was lost to follow up. One year later, he jumped from a bridge to his death.

Martin's unusual experiences could be viewed as symptoms of schizophrenia, which itself is a result of disordered neurophysiology. Yet his struggle to understand and make sense of his predicament cannot be reduced to matters of brain chemistry, nor even to individual psychology. In this chapter, we will try to show how Martin's struggle for meaning, and the tradeoffs it entailed, can be understood only in a social and cultural context. The ways in which Martin partitioned unusual experiences into symptoms of affliction and hard-won insights into the human condition reflected his active use of the cultural knowledge available to him to participate in a social world, preserve his self-esteem, and make his often frightening and confusing experience intelligible. Martin's quest for meaning, however, was largely a solitary activity; he received little support or confirmation from others. The psychiatric intepretation of his experience as schizophrenic delusions and hallucinations was of limited use in his efforts to integrate his psychotic experience.

Martin's story illustrates the paradoxes of insight: although he initially claimed not to be ill, he presented himself to the hospital for treatment; although he could recognize another person's delusions as absurd, he steadfastly held to his own; while continuing to experience hallucinations and delusions, he was able to describe his schizophrenic illness in psychologically sophisticated terms and had a clear concept of its prognosis. Clearly, insight is a complex phenomenon, with components that can evolve independently over time.

David (1990) has identified three overlapping dimensions in clinicians' use of the term *insight*: (1) the recognition that one has a mental illness; (2) the ability to relabel unusual mental events as pathological; (3) compliance with treatment. As Martin's case illustrates, these aspects of insight can occur independently and need not follow a fixed sequence or simple hierarchy. Thus, some patients may adhere to treatment, out of trust or coercion, despite disagreement with the clinician over their diagnosis or the meaning of specific symptoms.

Each of these dimensions of insight has many gradations. For example, recognition that one has a mental illness may range from superficial agreement that one is ill to detailed knowledge of the psychiatric model of one's condition. Similarly, the recognition and labeling of unusual mental events may range from interpretations of experience and behavior as "out of the ordinary," as different from that of others or conventional norms, as indicating that something is wrong, and, finally, as symptoms of an ill-ness (which may be recognized and labeled or remain unspecified). Treatment com-pliance may range from passive following of doctors' directions (owing to blind faith in medical authority or acquiescence to the more or less coercive demands of others), to active collaboration in a therapeutic relationship that involves trust in the clinician and creative use of the supportive relationship. This should make it clear that insight is not a fixed attainment but an evolving process of negotiating meanings of experience with clinicians and other significant actors in the patient's world.

The psychiatric concept of insight privileges the professional explanation of events in terms of disorder or disease over the patient's lived experience. But illness admits many possible interpretations that serve different functions for the individual and his or her entourage. The notion that there is a single accurate or correct view of things given by neuroscience or psychology will not suffice when we face the more pressing clinical question of what to do to make chronic illness livable. Martin understood, better than most, the contemporary psychiatric view of his condition: it is no exaggeration to say that he was killed by insight.[1]

As a folk psychological notion, the metaphor of insight implies that self-knowledge is acquired by direct observation of our mental processes and, as a corollary, that lack of insight in psychosis is a function of an impaired ability for self-observation. Social psy-chological studies call into question these connotations of the metaphor and suggest that much self-knowledge is based, not on direct observation of one's own mental functions or even on one's own behavior, but instead on cognitive schemata, collective representa-tions, and ongoing negotiations of meaning. Insight is inside knowledge then, but not in the sense that it involves accurate perception of mental processes: it is a context-sensitive construal of one's own behavior and situation that bears the impress of culture at every turn. We will illustrate the social and cultural construction of insight with an account of the psychotic experiences of the American science fiction writer Philip K. Dick, who left a lengthy record of his struggle to explain his extraordinary experiences.

Much research indicates that the symptomatology, help seeking, and course of schizophrenia, as well as other psychiatric disorders, are strongly influenced by cultural interpretations. If insight itself is such a culturally mediated interpretation, then we might expect that culture acts through insight to shape the "natural history" of these disorders. Indeed, we will argue that this is one possible contributor to the finding that schizophrenia has a better outcome in developing compared to developed countries.

Reflecting changes in the perspectives of cultural psychiatry, our focus in this chap-ter will move from a view of culture as cognitive representations carried by each indi-vidual; to culture as the evolving system of collective representations, social roles, and practices; to culture as local worlds of meaning that are negotiated and contested by patients, families, clinicians, and other actors. Each more sophisticated view of culture suggests new ways of conceiving of insight in research and clinical practice.

## Insight as Metaphor

The metaphor of insight conveys the impression that we possess the ability to look into ourselves and see what is there. Patients who lack insight are simply unable to see what is evident to others: the fact of their own illness. The fact of illness provides a ready explanation for any unusual experiences or deviant behaviors, and mandates specific medical treatment. The insightful patient accepts the doctor's diagnosis, attributes deviant experiences and behaviors to illness, and complies with treatment as prescribed (David, Buchanan, Reed, & Almeida, 1992).

One implication of this notion of insight as direct perception is that, in the normal course of events, insight is unproblematic, and what requires special explanation is *lack* of insight. Marková and Berrios (1992, p. 859) summarize three types of explanation for lack of insight: impaired awareness, self-deception, and misattribution.

*Impaired awareness* implies that some psychotic patients are unable to have insight into their condition because the biological machinery executing the algorithms for self-awareness is disabled by disease. In this view, psychosis arises from disruptions of processes of self-awareness, perception, and cognition that leave people liable to hallucinations and delusions and, at the same time, unable to accurately observe and interpret their experiences in accord with feedback from their actions or information from others.[2] Lack of insight may then be treated as a symptom of an underlying disorder. This view is challenged, however, by the finding that level of insight is not substantially correlated with severity of psychosis (Amador, Strauss, Yale, Flaum, & Gorman, 1993; see David, chapter 17, this volume).

The notion of *self-deception* is central to psychodynamic accounts of the lack of insight as a form of defensive denial. In psychodynamic theory, insight refers to awareness of intrapsychic emotional conflict and of the connections between past events and current feelings, thoughts, and behaviors. In the case of neurotic disorders, insight generally refers to the ability to give a psychological account of one's motivations and actions. Lack of insight then is a motivated response, a form of defensive self-protection against potentially painful or intolerable thoughts and feelings. It results from active efforts to cope with or adapt to distress. Self-deception refers to the defensive avoidance of clarifying and committing oneself to a particular view of reality and self because this is painful or disadvantageous. Of course, to the extent that the necessary faculties are intact, people coping with schizophrenia are likely to use all the same psychological resources marshaled by patients with anxiety, depression, or dissociative disorders, so self-deception is equally relevant to efforts to cope with psychosis.

Finally, lack of insight may be viewed as *misattribution*, a form of cognitive error based on lack of information, systematic biases, or idiosyncratic beliefs. Misattribution implies that there is a correct attribution for symptoms and experiences that is given by common accord or, in doubtful cases, by medical authority. We must consider the possibility, however, that what is called misattribution is really an interpretation of experience that is due neither to a deficit nor to purely defensive functions, but that reflects a genuine alternative construction of reality. While it may not accord with the dominant view of psychiatry, this alternative reality makes sense within the patient's local world of meaning and, hence, confers the benefits of coherence, order, and intelligibility on unusual, chaotic, or disturbing experience.

The transparency of illness experience implied by the metaphor of insight is misleading, in that a wealth of social psychological studies show that, under ordinary circumstances, much self-knowledge is based not on objective self-awareness or direct perception (introspection) but on context-dependent interpretations of one's own behavior and experience based on multiple sources, including observations of others, acquisition of social norms, and active construction of theories about the self (Neisser, 1988; Nisbett & Wilson, 1977; Ross & Nisbett, 1991).[3] These constructions are mediated and constrained by the different situations or social contexts that the individual lives in and through. Far from being a window into the self, insight is a half-silvered mirror held up between the self and others.

Amador and colleagues (1993) suggest that insight involves both awareness and attribution. Awareness and attribution, though, are closely related. Clearly, attribution depends on awareness, since we must notice something to make it the object of explanations. In addition, the way in which we become aware of deviant experience itself carries information relevant to making causal attributions. Attributions or explanatory models also govern the deployment of attention and guide the search for sensations, experiences, or events that fit a niche within the model or schema that may precede awareness. In practice, then, there can be no sharp distinction between awareness and attribution. Indeed, Dennett (1991) has argued against the notion of consciousness as an inner theater of representation implied by the primacy of awareness, and provides compelling evidence that awareness often occurs after the fact as a perceptual, cognitive, or narrative construction in response to specific imperatives—questions, probes, actions.[4] As a corollary, the self is not a homunculus watching the inner theater of representations, but the narrative center of gravity of accounts about the individual's actions and life trajectory. Insight, like other forms of self-knowledge, must then be understood as a process of attribution or, more elaborately, as the construction of narratives about the self.

Insight involves a series of attributions: symptoms are attributed to affliction and the affliction is labeled as a mental disorder with specific causes, course, and outcome. But attributions do not occur in isolation; they are part and parcel of more extended networks of meaning. Such networks influence the perception of what constitutes a symptom or a sign of illness within a given culture (Corin, Bibeau, & Uchôa, 1993; Good & Good, 1980; Kirmayer, 1989).

Accounts of the onset of psychosis reveal a situation of chaos and confusion, where the crucial question for the person and his or her entourage is what interpretations are at hand to organize experience (Bowers, 1974). Sensations that are initially inchoate can be labeled as symptoms of an illness only after an attributional search. In some cases, the psychotic experiences themselves provide their own interpretations, and these are typically religious or supernatural, or in modern society, involve magical applications of technology like lasers and subsonic beams. In other cases, explanations are found after the fact from some sympathetic or authoritative source—but in every case they represent cultural conceptions.

Kleinman (1980) introduced the notion of a patient's explanatory models (EM): information, beliefs, and expectations regarding the cause, symptomatology, course, appropriate treatment, and probable outcome of illness based on a common fund of cultural knowledge, as well as on personal experience. These EMs can be elicited by direct questions to patients in settings where medical authority does not inhibit their willingness to divulge alternate views. These models influence patients' perceptions of diagnosis and treatment, and hence can account for problems in communication and compliance.

However, the EM perspective imputes a greater degree of coherence and rationality to everyday thinking than it actually displays. Often people cannot give ready explanations for their symptoms or problems, and when they do, they may offer multiple, fragmentary, and contradictory accounts. Young (1982) has tried to account for the manifest complexity, incompleteness, and contradictions present in patients' illness narratives by positing at least three different forms of illness representation that coexist and that may conflict: explanatory models, prototypical cases or events, and *chain complexes*—a form of procedural knowledge derived from the sequence of lived experience. Faced with the fragmented and often contradictory character of illness narratives about epilepsy in Turkey, Good and Good (1993) understand them as *subjunctivizing tactics* aimed at preserving the indeterminacy of the future and the openness of the illness to change and cure. In addition, it is important to recognize that the semantic networks that confer meaning on experience are not simply lists of propositions; they include images, practices, and links to external situations that embody collective knowledge (Kirmayer, 1992). This knowledge is used to construct a story or narrative about the meaning of experiences.

Amador and colleagues (1993) found that insight about past and current episodes of psychosis were poorly correlated. Insight about past illness episodes involves the narrative reconstructions of memory; current insight may be more dependent on feedback from control mechanisms (intrapsychic and social feedback loops) that give evidence of dysfunction or lack of match of action with intention. But both forms of insight are highly context-dependent: past reconstruction and current self-perception must be seen as methods of positioning the self vis-à-vis others. Of course, it may be one feature of some forms of illness that individuals' capacity to respond to shifting contexts is impaired, and hence their self-presentation shows greater stereotypy than that of healthy individuals.

The notion of insight as a narrative construction has special significance for psychosis, because there is evidence that the ability to organize discourse at the level of narrative is impaired in schizophrenia (Hoffman, 1986). Narrative is particularly important in the construction of a coherent sense of self against which events are evaluated through the process of self-awareness (Bruner, 1990; Kirby, 1991). If the stability and coherence of this narrative is interfered with, then the capacity for insight may be correspondingly impaired. Further, since the form of narratives varies cross-culturally (Howard, 1991)—including those narratives that are about the self—culture may interact with psychotic impairment of insight at the level of what narratives of the self are available, socially coherent, and credible. Detailed study of the narrative presentation and representation of self in psychotic patients may then offer a way to integrate psychological studies of the cognitive impairments in schizophrenia with the impact of social structure and cultural knowledge.

Deciding that we are sick, labeling particular sensations or behaviors as symptoms, and attributing them to a specific type of illness all depend on cognitively and socially mediated interpretations of experience (Kirmayer, 1989). The matrix of these interpretations of experience is the sum of shared beliefs and practices we call culture. Insight, then, is a culturally constructed version of experience that patients subscribe to, not simply because their cognitive machinery is intact but by virtue of the way it fits with their social world. This cultural constructivist view of insight is at odds with a clinical perspective that measures patients' insight against the clinician's judgment as a gold standard, inasmuch as the clinician's view also is shaped by cultural concepts and values.

## Insight as a Sociocultural Process

If insight is having "a correct attitude toward a morbid change in oneself" (Lewis, 1934, p. 333), then it is a value-laden concept that is likely to change with time and circumstance. "Correct" can be judged only with respect to some goal: cooperation with treatment, good outcome, ratification of professional judgment, or social control. Since outcome is multidimensional, correct with respect to one dimension (e.g., willingness to accept medication) may conflict with correct with respect to other dimensions (e.g., sense of self-sufficiency, hopefulness, coherence of one's life). Further, the notion of correctness raises the question, with respect to who or what authority (e.g., health professional, family, colleagues)? The "correct" attitude toward an illness depends on changing medical concepts of illness as well as social norms for illness behavior, which may also conflict. Insight then is manifested by specific attitudes and attributions that are contingent on changing knowledge and practice.

Yet lack of insight in psychosis seems also to reflect some more general difficulty in maintaining a consensual view of reality. This more general or pervasive difficulty can be characterized by viewing insight as a process distinct from any specific interpretation or attribution. As a process, insight involves acquiring, stabilizing, and deploying consensual explanations for experience. This ability to conform in one's self-understanding and action does not preclude having strange or psychotic experiences. If the person enjoys a sufficient measure of flexibility, irony, playfulness, and self-reflexive awareness, he or she may adopt a complex stance that allows idiosyncratic experiences to coexist with more conventional ones and still preserve a concern for—and ability to succeed in—making his or her experience intelligible to others.

In this regard, it is instructive to look at the response to psychotic experiences of a person without the persistent or recurrent thought disorder of schizophrenia. Consider, for example, the way the American science fiction writer Philip K. Dick generated alternative explanations for his own religious or psychotic experiences. Dick had a history of anxiety problems (probably panic disorder with agoraphobia) from adolescence, and was treated intermittently with amphetamines. However, he had no known episode of psychosis prior to the events to be recounted. He was a prolific and brilliantly inventive writer who gained a wide following, first in Europe and later in the United States. His stories were characterized by a pervasive sense of paranoia—of hidden connections between seemingly unrelated events and the growing intimation that things are not what they appear to be—which was typically confirmed in each story's denouement, when reality fell open to reveal alternate realities, like a series of Chinese boxes, so that the ultimate ground of experience was left in question. In one story, objects in the world dissolve, leaving slips of paper with their names written on them ("Soft-drink stand"); in another, the characters are programs inside a computer, but then the programmers of the computer are themselves revealed to be just programs in a still greater computer. In his stories, Dick made a virtue of paranoia's infinite regress (Kirmayer, 1983).

In 1974, following surgery for an impacted wisdom tooth, Dick answered the door to receive delivery of a prescription for a narcotic analgesic (Darvon):

> There stood this girl with black, black hair and large eyes very lovely and intense; I stood staring at her, amazed, also confused and thinking I'd never seen such a beautiful

girl, and why was she standing there. She handed me the package of medication, and I tried to think what to say to her; I noticed, then, a fascinating gold necklace around her neck and I said, "What is that? It certainly is beautiful," just, you see, to find something to say to hold her there. The girl indicated the major figure in it, which was a fish. "This is a sign used by the early Christians," she said, and then departed. (Sutin, 1989, p. 210)

At the time he felt only a sense of strangeness about this experience; although it felt significant, its meaning was uncertain. Over the next few days, probably intoxicated by the medication, Dick had a series of visions: colorful patterns, abstract painting like compositions, and pink lights. While some appear to have been phosphenes, others were much more complex and constituted a veritable gallery of modern art. While the pink light had first appeared as a sort of prolonged after-image, he now felt it as beams fired into his brain that conveyed vast stores of esoteric information. With this came the increasing conviction that some god or alien intelligence was trying to contact him, that the world as we know it is an illusion, and, finally, that we are all living in the time of the early Christians and that our contemporary oppressors are Romans in disguise. The delivery girl's visit became a portent of this revelation.

Everyday experiences then took on dual significance: they had one meaning in the mundane world of illusion and another, more profound sense in the realm that had been revealed to him. He actively participated in this alternate realm, performing rituals of purification and baptism with his young son. In addition to the new knowledge he seemed to have acquired, he felt that his tastes, habits, and attitudes had abruptly changed. After several weeks the unusual experiences became more sporadic and in a few months they stopped.

Dick spent years generating alternative explanations for these experiences, which he recorded in a lengthy colloquy with himself that he called his "exegesis" (Dick, 1991). In the process, he struggled to give them coherence. He was well aware of how they might appear to a clinician:

> I can see me telling my therapist this. "What's on your mind, Phil?" she'll say when I go in, and I'll say, "Asklepios is my tutor, from out of Pericleian Athens. I'm learning to talk in Attic Greek." She'll say, "Oh really?" and I'll be on my way to the Blissful Groves, but it won't be after death; that'll be in the country where it's quiet and costs $100 a day. And you get all the apple juice you want to drink, along with Thorazine. (Dick, 1991, p. 18)

He considered and rejected dozens of different theories drawn from psychology, religion, and speculative fiction. He considered psychiatric explanations, but found them inadequate to explain the details of his experience:

> There is no known psychological process which could account for such fundamental changes in my character, in my habits, view of the world (I perceive it totally differently, now), my daily tastes, even the way I margin my typed pages. I've been transformed but not in any way I ever heard of. (p. 6)

Note that it was not the hallucinations and delusions that Dick found hard to explain in psychological terms (as a toxic psychosis), but the more enduring changes in personality.[5] What Dick is calling his personality here is more accurately his sense of self and personhood. Changes in sense of self and social personhood are extremely important for the person with chronic schizophrenia and crucial to understanding the process of constructing insight (Davidson & Strauss, 1992).

What sets Dick apart from the patient lacking insight is his ability to generate, entertain, and use multiple explanations, including those of psychiatric disorder.

> I can entertain (hold) two normally contradictory beliefs—explanations—:
> 1. I became totally psychotic & projected & imagined all that religious, supernatural stuff.
> 2. The guide & savior, the figure of the beautiful woman who I met & whose voice I kept hearing, whose existence during my psychosis I imagined, was & is completely real — & I know when the need arises again, I will find her once more, or rather she will find me & again guide me. (p. 38)

This ability to hold contradictory views is not a sign of disordered logic. It is the ordinary condition of us all, save that we usually are not so honest or adept at making our contradictory premises explicit (and when we do we usually try to elide their dissonance). As a common feature in the construction of meaning, it suggests that insight cannot be simply measured as the outcome of agreement with the clinician, but must be viewed as a process of giving due consideration to alternative explanations. Explanations will be adopted if they make sense and work in some region of the person's lifeworld. Psychiatric explanations, along with many of the more outlandish science fiction explanations, were grist for Dick's creative mill. He wrote a trilogy of Gnostic science fiction novels in which a playful alter ego (Horselover Fat) argued with him over the potential meaning of his experiences (Dick, 1990). Considering the psychiatric dimension of his experience did ultimately lead him to seek help for drug dependence, yet he felt strongly that what he had received in his visions were real insights into the human condition and that religion provided the only system to make them coherent in a positive way.

> You see a plan, you see a pattern of events, and if you have no transcendent viewpoint, no mystical view, no religious view, then the pattern must emanate from people. Where else can it come from, if that's all . . . ? And you start sensing a kind of transcendent thing or mystical thing. . . .
> I think . . . paranoia must be pulled inside out. Absolutely inside out. It's not that it should be destroyed. I mean, that the solution to paranoia is to convince the person there is no pattern to the universe, that everything is chaotic, chance, and that people have no intentions. And that he is unimportant. . . . Turn it inside out, rather than just abolish it. That it's benign, and that it transcends our individualities, and so on. The way I feel is that the universe itself is actually alive, and we're in a part of it. And it is like a breathing creature, which explains the concept of Atman, you know, the breath, pneuma, the breath of God. (Williams, 1986, pp. 161–163).

Ultimately, Dick settled on a version of Gnosticism to account for his experiences, drawing heavily on the *Nag Hammadi Library* (Robinson, 1977). It is striking confirmation of the social embeddedness of this most idiosyncratic of visionary experiences that the epilogue to the most recent edition of the *Nag Hammadi Library* (Robinson, 1988) cites Dick as a contemporary rediscoverer of perennial Gnostic truths. This social legitimation might have served to stabilize Dick's own interpretation of his experience, had he survived to appreciate it.[6]

Certainly, Dick's experience was not typical. The flexibility, irony, and humor with which he worked with his hallucinatory revelations—which resemble those of many patients with schizophrenia—were remarkable. No doubt his vocation and social status as a writer, his lifelong creative play with the anxiety of paranoia, and his intelligence served him in good stead in making sense of his experience. He was able to stabilize and defend a particular interpretation of his experience owing to these exceptional personal and social resources. The sense that he made was idiosyncratic in many respects yet deeply embedded in both popular culture and the esoteric tradition of Gnosticism. In religion he found a perspective to valorize and enrich his own sally into madness.

Dick's psychotic episode was prefigured by years of writing stories with a distinctly paranoid cast. His experience suggests that some people form tentative delusions or paranoid hypotheses much of the time as they seek connections between disturbing events. Ordinarily, people reappraise these hypotheses and dismiss them if they do not fit consensual reality, are unpleasant, or interfere with adaptation. If the cognitive machinery of reappraisal is impaired, paranoid delusions may persist and strengthen. The effects of neuroleptic medication may be not so much to block delusion formation as to allow cognitive reappraisal (Hole, Rush, & Beck, 1979). But the appraisal process itself is one of interpreting signs, symptoms, behaviors, and events in terms of tacit social and cultural knowledge.

What distinguishes Dick from the prototypical psychotic patient lacking in insight is his ability to be self-reflexively aware of the process of constructing his own explanations and to adopt, if and when it is necessary, the perspective of the other (whether that other be a doctor, a fellow writer, or a theologian). Dick was insightful, no matter how thoroughly he rejected the pathological origins and nature of his experiences, because he was complexly aware of the nature of his own consciousness and his writing.[7]

In Dick's account, we can see the process of constructing insight. The experience of psychosis—which may be initially inchoate or consist of well-formed, vivid hallucinations that, nevertheless, rend the fabric of consensual reality—is woven into an integrated whole. Dick wove his compelling and evocative psychotic experiences into a life-affirming philosophy. What made this process possible for him was the time away from psychosis when nothing earth-shattering was happening. In this reflective space, Dick was able to construct a complex narrative with links to cultural traditions that legitimated his experience, gave it public anchor points, and supplied him with new metaphors and models to organize his experience. In memory, reconstructed through narrative, madness was made to cohere.

Insight emerges in Dick's exegetical diaries as partial, tentative, always awaiting confirmation and stabilization. In its tentativeness, his experience differs from that of some delusional patients for whom the sense of conviction that they have found the truth is present from the start. Some delusional experiences carry their own interpretations and are self-stabilizing.[8] In Dick's case this stabilization came partly from finding Gnostic religious texts that mirrored, organized, and deepened his own experiences. It also came from his ability to authorize his own constructions, first as the writer's legitimate engagement with an imaginative world and then as published fictions with a playful yet hortatory style.

Although the process of constructing coherent narratives revealed in Dick's diaries is similar to what any person faced with psychotic experiences might engage in, it is distinctive in two important respects. First, Dick did not belong to a society or subculture with a single dominant tradition that offered him ready-made explanations for his experiences. He had to borrow and adapt a range of ideas; concepts drawn from great traditions were melded with themes from science fiction. Second, as we have noted, Dick had unique personal resources and a special social status that allowed him to authorize and stabilize his narrative constructions. This permitted him to experience some degree of satisfying resolution to his search and to use his insights to further his career.

Bateson (1972) called delusions unlabeled metaphors and held that in schizophrenia patients lost sight of the metaphorical status of utterances. Mistaking metaphors for reality, though, is a feature of everyday thinking: we live among unquestioned metaphors taken for natural categories and literal truths (Lakoff & Johnson, 1980). Analogical modes of reasoning and "magical thinking" (e.g., identity by resemblance, contagion by contact, misplaced concreteness) are ubiquitous and often not recognized as irrational (Rozin & Nemeroff, 1990). The crucial difference is whether metaphors are socially sanctioned and pass for literal truths or are idiosyncratic. For idiosyncratic metaphors, if we wish to avoid being labeled odd or crazy, we had better have the rhetorical skills to defend them and the irony and self-reflexive awareness to distance from them. What is characteristic of schizophrenia, then, is difficulty organizing tentative metaphoric constructions at the level of larger narrative structures that take into account the positions of speaker and listener. This overarching narrative structure determines which metaphors are interpreted as literal and which are just loose analogies, "figures of speech," or simply incoherent.

People with schizophrenia engage in the same sort of creative borrowing, adaptation, and play with concepts to explain their experience that Corin (1990) has called *bricolage* (borrowing the term from Lévi-Strauss). In Corin's study of people with schizophrenia in Montreal, she found that some gravitated toward marginal religious systems and ideas that they gleaned from books or from peripheral involvements with religious sects. Ideas borrowed from many places allowed them to develop a patchwork system of explanations that justified their withdrawal from conventional work and relationships; in some cases, informal and idiosyncratic religious practices also provided a degree of structure to both solitude and social contact. Their experience differs from Dick's however, in several ways. The most important difference arises from the persistence and pervasiveness of psychotic experience. Given the tremendous effort over the years that Dick expended on explaining just a few weeks of intense experiences, we can only wonder at the information overload of someone enduring lengthy and repeated psychoses. The need to develop and adopt a system to filter, organize, and make experience cohere is urgent. This may explain the rigidity with which some delusional systems are held—not so much as a primary feature of psychosis but as an effort to stabilize reality in the face of constant intrusions of the strange and ineffable. In many cases, the result is not a richly elaborated system but a sketchy or jury-rigged structure anxiously defended against constant threats to its stability.

Then, too, most schizophrenic patients have neither the personal resources and talents nor the social status, as an accomplished writer, that Dick enjoyed. This means that it is harder for them to construct a coherent explanation, and when they do, still more difficult to have others accept or ratify it. In consequence, they cannot stabilize their interpretation of the world except by withdrawing from others who challenge the picture they have constructed.

Finally, people with psychoses live in societies or subcultures that make different systems of belief available to them. Dick belonged to a liberal subculture in a pluralistic society that tolerates the sort of borrowing and informal adaptation of esoteric religion he attempted. In urban, pluralistic societies, people with chronic psychoses may draw their explanatory concepts from marginal beliefs and practices because these allow greater freedom for idiosyncratic elaboration and are less likely to bring them into direct confrontation with authorities who destabilize or invalidate their tentative constructions (Corin, 1990). People in some traditional societies may engage in constructions of experience that draw from widely accepted beliefs that give religion or the supernatural a more prominent place in everyday life. Hence, authoritative meanings for psychotic experience may be more readily at hand. This may help with personal or collective efforts to make sense of psychotic experience and with the social integration of individuals with chronic psychoses. The greater availability in some cultures of meaning systems that allow people to positively reframe frightening or disturbing experiences should be reflected in an increased likelihood of reintegration following a psychotic episode and a correspondingly better prognosis.

## Schizophrenia in Cross-Cultural Perspective

While schizophrenia can be identified around the world, there are significant cultural and geographical differences in prevalence, symptomatology, and course (Cooper & Sartorius, 1977; Kleinman, 1988; Leff, 1988; Murphy, 1982; Sartorius, et al., 1986). A striking finding of cross-cultural studies of schizophrenia has been the repeated observation of a better long-term prognosis for individuals in some developing countries compared to patients in urban industrialized settings (Leff, Sartorius, Jablensky, Korten, & Ernberg, 1992; Murphy & Raman, 1971; Sartorius, Jablensky, & Shapiro, 1978; WHO, 1979). Early studies, including the International Pilot Study of Schizophrenia (IPSS), have been criticized because they included only patients presenting to westernized psychiatric health care services and used a limited range of outcome measures (Cohen, 1992).[9] More recently, the WHO Determinants of Outcome Study corrected many of the methodological limitations of the IPSS (Jablensky et al., 1992; but see Edgerton & Cohen, 1994). Patients presenting with psychotic symptoms were accrued from many different types of helping agencies, including traditional healers. Again, the two-year follow-up indicated a better course for patients in developing countries compared to their counterparts in developed countries (Sartorius, 1992).

Lin and Kleinman (1988) have reviewed speculations on the underlying mechanisms for better prognosis in developing countries. These hypotheses all have direct implications for the cultural construction of insight because of the reciprocity between patients' self-image and others' views of them.

First, they point to broad differences in the organization of society and the corresponding concepts of self and personhood. The industrialized urban societies of Europe and America foster an individualistic concept of the person and an egocentric sense of self. In this view, the individual is the prime locus of value, choice, and action and enters into relationships voluntarily with others (Bellah et al., 1985). In contrast, the concept of the person in many developing countries is communalistic and sociocentric, emphasizing group membership as the core of identity, so that individuals think of themselves predominately in terms of these larger affiliations, which are valued over and above the individual in many respects.

As Dumont (1986) points out, western individualism is paradoxical in that, at the same time as it claims to respect difference, it is linked to fierce competitiveness and conformity that leave little room for real differences in behavior, values, and life trajectory for individuals. Lin and Kleinman (1988) suggest that this "intensive individualism" of modern Western societies may interfere with recovery for many schizophrenic patients. The emphasis on self-reliance, competition, and individual achievement as sources of self-esteem may contribute to despair in those less able to compete successfully. Schizophrenic individuals who find they cannot compete in conventional terms have no choice but to distance themselves from conventional sources of social status and self-esteem and to accept a position at the margins of society. The rapidity of social change, the frequency of dislocation, and the general sense of alienation undermine basic social solidarity or support and may aggravate the course of illness. Where identity is drawn from group membership, supportive ties may be less likely to rupture with chronic illness, and individuals who are able to conform minimally may still preserve their sense of identity, belonging, and importance.[10]

A second locus of the impact of culture on the prognosis of schizophrenia involves the family milieu. High levels of negative expressed emotion (EE) have been shown repeatedly to predict poor outcome in young male schizophrenics (Leff & Vaughn, 1985). At one-year follow-up, the WHO Determinants of Outcome Study found that high EE could be measured reliably cross-culturally and that it was related to poor outcome (Leff et al., 1987). However, the global index of EE was no longer related to outcome at two-year follow-up (Leff et al., 1990); only initial hostility remained significantly related to subsequent relapse. The actual prevalence of high EE families was found to be lower in some cultures (e.g., Indian). The authors conclude that in India, the tolerant and accepting attitudes of family members may contribute to the good prognosis of schizophrenia. Even more intriguing was the finding that the pattern of emotions associated with EE in India was quite different from that observed in Anglo-American families. This and related findings indicate the need to go beyond the EE construct to explore the nature of emotional relationships in specific cultures (Jenkins & Karno, 1992).

Jenkins's (1988) work with Mexican-Americans suggests that cultural beliefs and practices surrounding mental illness also interact with hostility in the family. In ethnographic research, she found that many schizophrenic patients were given the relatively benign label "*nervios*" (nerves) rather than "*loco*" (crazy) to describe their condition. The culturally appropriate response to an individual with *nervios* is to treat him or her gently and avoid conflict, arguments, and confrontation. The cultural label for psychotic illness, and corresponding attitudes toward illness along with cultural differences in family communication of emotion, thus promote some of the same behaviors advocated in psychoeducational family treatment of schizophrenia. This may lead to a reduced prevalence of high EE families and, hence, a better prognosis in the aggregate (Guarnaccia, Parra, Deschamps, Milstein, & Argiles, 1992; Karno et al., 1987).

The stigma of mental illness may differ across cultures (Fabrega, 1991; Kirmayer, 1989; Lin & Kleinman, 1988; Townsend, 1978). Waxler (1979) offered this as one explanation for the better prognosis for schizophrenia found in Sri Lanka. She argued that the cultural model for psychosis in Sri Lanka was similar to that for other acute illnesses in that it carried expectations for improvement or recovery and little implication that the individual's personhood was permanently damaged or invalidated. Consequently, individuals who do not display overtly bizarre behavior may be more readily re-integrated into the community following an acute episode and may not suffer long-lasting stigmatization.

It is not possible, with current data, to determine which of many covarying factors contribute to the differential prognosis of schizophrenia across cultures (Edgerton & Cohen, 1994; Gupta, 1992). Although speculations have focused on the attitudes and actions of the patient's entourage, sociocultural factors may also exert their influence through the afflicted person's own interpretation of illness experience. In fact, lack of insight was the most frequent symptom of acute schizophrenia identified in the IPSS (WHO, 1973). Insight was assessed with item 104 of the Present State Examination: "Do you think there is anything the matter with you? What do you think it is? Could it be a nervous condition?" Clearly, this sequence of questions measures agreement with a psychiatric opinion rather than the functioning of underlying cognitive-interpretive processes. The high prevalence of lack of insight then may reflect not so much its status as a core symptom of schizophrenia but the diversity of explanations tendered for psychotic experiences around the world.

Cultural concepts of mental disorder are closely related to insight both in terms of what images and explanations the individual has available to explain their symptoms and in terms of their personal and social costs in self-perceived stigma and self-blame. Sociological studies of labeling and stigmatization have dealt extensively with the consequences of attributing deviant behavior to mental illness (Link, 1987; Link, Cullen, Frank, & Wozniak, 1987). These studies suggest that insight has its costs in reduced self-esteem and lower social status for the afflicted individual. Self-labeling also contributes to a sense of impaired efficacy and may maintain vicious circles of emotional distress (Corin & Lauzon, 1994; Thoits, 1985). At the same time, accepting an illness label may lead to treatment adherence and, if treatment is effective, to fewer symptoms and less basis for social stigmatization and rejection (Warner, Taylor, Powers, & Hyman, 1989). These costs and trade-offs must be figured into individuals' willingness and ability to entertain illness attributions for their own deviant experiences or behavior.

The tendency to apply illness labels to deviant behavior and to stigmatize mental illness may also be related to social structure. Raybeck (1988) has discussed how sociological labeling theory that developed in the context of large-scale urban pluralistic societies must be modified to address the realities of small scale societies. In smaller communities, he argues, there is an effort to avoid labeling deviant behavior or eccentricity in a way that would lead to ostracism. We have observed this in our work in small communities in the Arctic and in Africa, as illustrated in the following case:

CASE    A 25-year-old Inuit man living in a remote Arctic settlement became convinced that he had received religious revelations and poured over the Bible, marking it with colored pens and memorizing extensive passages. He carried this Bible in a sling around his waist and responded to most questions about himself with lengthy quotations depicting the coming apocalypse. He began accosting others on the street and in their homes to exhort them to repent because the day of judgment was near. His enthusiasm was tolerated until he began to become visibly angry in his harangues. At the request of the settlement, he was then sent to the city for psychiatric evaluation. There he was found to have religious delusions but was otherwise lucid and appropriate. A provisional diagnosis of schizophreniform disorder was made and he was given neuroleptic medication. On returning to the community he continued to be active in the local church but tempered his attempts to convert others. He stopped taking medication after about a year. At five-year follow-up, he had become less religious and recalled these experiences with some embarrassment but did not think that he had been ill. He held a part-time wage-earning job and participated in group sports and other community activities, although he had no close friends and spent much time by himself. He was perceived by other community members as having been overly intense in his religious convictions but not as having any illness.

In this case, both cultural values and social structure contributed to this man's reintegration into the community following his hospitalization. The tendency to avoid labeling individuals that is so characteristic of small-scale societies, combined with community tolerance of enthusiastic religious expression and a cultural tendency among the Inuit to label behaviors or states rather than personalities, allowed him to escape disabling social stigma and to maintain a view of himself as not afflicted. This view of himself as not sick, in concert with others' acceptance, probably contributed to a relatively good outcome.

## From Individual to Collective Representation

While psychotic behavior is recognized as deviant across cultures (Murphy, 1976), the conceptual category of mental disorder itself is not universal (Kleinman, 1988; Kirmayer, 1993). In many cultures, deviant behavior is viewed first in terms of its interpersonal, social, or moral significance (Kirmayer, 1989). These interpretations may be more salient and credible for both the sufferer and his social circle than accounts that focus on illness. This is so in part because psychotic experience is often uncanny and prompts supernatural explanations. Religious explanations give more complete and satisfactory accounts of experience than illness attributions when the causes and mechanisms of disease remain shrouded from view and poorly worked out. Religious explanation provides a satisfying answer to psychosis not only because it ties up loose ends and gives an appropriate ontology for uncanny (supernatural) experiences, but also because it has esthetic, moral, and rhetorical force.

Very commonly, then, psychotic experiences are viewed as religious, and individuals who are able to function well enough to parlay these experiences into work as a religious healer or ritual expert may continue to be symptomatic while enjoying an enhanced social role. Obeyesekere (1981) provides examples of this history in his accounts of religious healers in Sri Lanka. However, the availability of cultural symbols does not suffice in itself. In a more recent work, Obeyesekere (1991) distinguishes between two ways in which suffering individuals may use cultural symbols: a "progressive" mode that allows them to embed symptoms or conflicts within a larger shared universe of meaning, and a "regressive" mode that traps them in a symbolic realm of archaic fantasies and persistent anxiety. Both psychological and social factors influence the way in which cultural symbols are used.

Even if social functioning is impaired and the sufferer recognizes that something is wrong, the notion that it is an illness does not necessarily follow. Nor, if it is recognized as an illness, need it be a mental illness—i.e., one confined to specific faculties or aspects of the person (Kirmayer, 1988). Many of the great systems of medicine (e.g., traditional Chinese medicine, Ayurveda) do not have detailed theories of mental disorder as distinct from physical illness (Fabrega, 1991). Differences in disease classification are paralleled by ethnopsychological concepts that situate feelings and emotions not within the disembodied psyche of the individual but in the lived body or in social relationships, the environment, or a spirit world (Kirmayer, 1989; Shweder, 1991).

So far we have approached insight as an attainment of the individual that depends on self-perception and self-representation. Culture then impinges on insight through its effect on individual perception and representation. If we wish to characterize a group we can do so through the individual with a sort of "epidemiology" of cognitive representations (Sperber, 1985)—which might be differentially distributed across class, social status, education, occupation, and subcultural lines.

Culture, however, is a matter not only of individual representations but also of collective representations and actions that are embodied or enacted only through interactional processes that involve family, community, and social institutions. Insight, then, is not simply the product and property of the individual—it is a social construction that many actors in the patient's world contribute to and which they, in turn, may use for differing ends.

The interpretation of a particular illness episode is made according to systems of meaning that belong to a culture through a process that involves negotiation among many actors. This is well illustrated by Corin's (1979, 1985) studies of traditional healers in Zaire. When serious health problems occur, particularly when they involve mental or emotional disturbances, a central concern is to assess their underlying nature. This often involves divination rituals that include patients, family members, and healers. Although in divination the healer uses a range of technical methods to give a formal diagnosis, patients and their families are centrally involved in this quest for meaning, both as participants in a long, ritualized dialog with the healer and through other interpretive rituals and performances.

In this collective search for "insight," some rituals directly involve the patient as the key actor. For example, in Zebola, a therapeutic spirit possession cult of central Africa, the patient is possessed by the spirit who speaks through his or her voice and is guided through a dialog with the healer, a dialog in which family members may also participate. The transgression of social norms or the sense of being in a situation of special vulnerability are most often identified as the triggers for a complex etiological process (Corin, 1979).

CASE    A woman began to feel sick and expressed ill-defined complaints a few months after receiving her first wages for a new job in Kinshasa. After visiting several medical clinics, she consulted the Zebola healer who had her undergo a fumigation. While possessed by a spirit, she revealed that she had not sent her first paycheck to her father, who remained in her village of origin. Her father had been angry and went into the forest where he loudly spoke her name. Nature spirits "grasped" her name and entered her body to kill her. A Zebola spirit took pity on her and decide to save her, if she was initiated into the cult through the ritual.

The insight provided by Zebola divination involves two steps: first, under the guidance of the healer, the patient comes to a true understanding of the origin of her symptoms; second, she must acknowledge the action of a Zebola spirit and accept it through ritual initiation. This initiation actually takes months during which she must repeat her acceptance of election by the spirit day after day.

The insight gained through Zebola divination does not simply point to an illness narrowly conceived but is concerned with the predicament of the person in her life-world. The interpretation provided by the divination involves several levels of meaning: (1) the realization by the patient that she is in a situation of special vulnerability to the hostility and "ill words" of others (as expressed on the cultural idiom "They speak too much of her"); (2) the clarification of the interpersonal tensions in which she is caught; and (3) the revelation of specific cultural errors or transgressions that have made her vulnerable to sickness. This process of generating new knowledge is made possible by the fact that it is not the patient herself who is charged to speak, but a possessing spirit who speaks through her. The intervention of the spirit, as a third agent beyond sufferer and healer, allows the afflicted person's social situation to be analyzed with authority. At the same time, the fact that the patient is possessed serves to distance her from those same conflicts by invoking the spirit's protection.

This whole process is supported by traditional cultural practices involving ritualized trance. In the urban milieu, where trance is less a part of ordinary life, a majority of patients prove unable to enter trance and must symbolically "buy" a medium to replace them. However, the cultural importance attached to the patient herself entering trance is indicated by the fact that before the final public dance which manifests her new status as a spirit initiate, the afflicted person must go through a second divination and, finally, enter into trance herself. On this occasion no one else can replace her.

Since it is not always possible to elucidate the patient's problems from the start, the use of a second divination at the end of treatment allows the social and intrapsychic work that follows the first divination to be publically presented and ratified. Between the two divinations, it often happens that the patient has dreams that she discusses with the healer to better understand the many-leveled etiology of her illness and disentangle the complex relational field in which her problems are situated. The ritual context is then used to consolidate the personal insights achieved and to give them social meaning and authority through enactment.

The diagnostic label "Zebola illness" only provides an entree into this process of interpretation and social action, opening the way to a positive reframing of the afflicted person's self-perception and the social negotiation of illness meanings that subserve insight. That this whole ritual process is, in fact, a search for insight is confirmed by the symbolic gesture of the healer who traces a white line around the patient's eyes with chalk (an iconic representation of insight) to signify that she has received a second sight that gives her access to true reality—a reality that includes the world of spirits as well as her personal and family history and relationships. Eliciting the origin of her problem allows the patient and her family to begin to locate a solution. In addition, election by a Zebola spirit sets in motion a series of ritual performances that profoundly and positively transform the identity of the afflicted person.

A feature of the Zebola ritual, which is shared by most types of divination in Zaire, is the requirement that key representatives of the family be present and assent to the procedures by spitting on the patient's head. In many African cultures, spitting is a ritual form of blessing; it can be understood as an iconic representation of the strength of the words pronounced on this occasion. In this case, it signifies the family's willingness to participate in the quest for meaning and to accept the confrontation it may well entail.

It is important to recognize the performative aspect of the divination ritual. In the ritual enactment of divination and possession, cultural symbols are embodied in images, sounds, feelings and practices. The search for meaning cannot be reduced to an individual intellectual or cognitive process; it involves the interplay of personal and collective representations through the pragmatics of performance. In the transactions that take place surrounding the rituals and in the subsequent use of the etiological information, insight becomes pragmatic reality.

## Culture as Contestation

Divination or diagnosis is only one moment in a larger quest for meaning and therapy. As we have seen, in Africa as in most societies, this quest is not an individual matter; it is the responsibility of the family group (what Janzen (1978) calls the *therapy management group*) to decide whom to consult, to evaluate the relevance of the diagnosis, and to monitor the various treatments and their efficacy. Different members of the family may have their own hypotheses regarding the nature of the disease. In the case of serious problems, the consultation of a healer is preceded by discussions and negotiations between the different lineages (father's, mother's, husband's) involved. According to Zempleni (1969), a temporary first consensus on the potential significance of the problem must be achieved in order to decide which healer to consult. This primary consensus is reinforced, complemented, or replaced by a secondary consensus built on the healer's diagnosis.

Even in traditional societies, most belief systems are intrinsically pluralistic, allowing room for choice and confrontation. Different segments of the patient's social network bring to bear different systems of interpretation as a function of their own relationship to traditions. This diversity is intensified during periods of rapid culture change, when members of the same family may rely on different strata of cultural meaning. For example, as described by Ortigues and Ortigues (1966) in Senegal, the generation of grandparents might favor an explanation in terms of *rab* (ancestral spirits) who have concluded an alliance with certain families and who may ask for ceremonial sacrifices. At the same time, parents may focus on malign magic that entails a search for interpersonal conflicts. Young people may appeal to scientific explanations. Often, belief systems within a family are not so clearly demarcated along generational boundaries. Uchôa (1993) shows the multiple and conflicting interpretations employed by different family members in her detailed account of a woman in Mali with repeated psychiatric hospitalizations. Among the factors invoked to explain her difficulties are her status as a twin, raised by a childless stepmother, torn between her Western educational aspirations and her *griot* background, forced to marry against her will a husband who then takes a second wife. Each actor in her drama interprets her behavior from their position within the social and cultural field, thereby reproducing the familial and social contradictions that contribute to her distress.

Acknowledgment of the psychiatric nature of a problem or the decision to seek psychiatric help by an individual or his or her entourage must be situated within such a context of pluralism and negotiation. Conventional Western psychiatric insight corresponds to the acceptance of one possible interpretation. However, in African societies, such insight may be accepted for a variety of reasons, not all of which are salutary. Far from always corresponding to an increased ability to understand the true nature of a disorder, acceptance of a conventional psychiatric diagnosis may be a sign that the family feels helpless to deal with the problem, has exhausted its resources, or cannot reach a consensus. Resort to Western psychiatry may also indicate that the patient has been socially marginalized or excluded from traditional cultural practices. Analogous dynamics can be observed in the context of immigration, where the presence of cultural differences between professional and patient can accentuate the perception that psychiatry is situated outside the patient's lifeworld. It seems clear, then, that if the notion of insight is meant to characterize the patient's position toward the illness, criteria other than mere conformity to the biomedical view must be used.

This is well illustrated in the case from Senegal of a woman, called Animata, who was hospitalized for an acute episode of agitation (Ortigues, Martino, & Collomb, 1967). This episode appeared abruptly, but she had faced many stresses over the previous two years: the deaths of her mother and her 18-month-old daughter, marital conflict, and a fire in her house. The authors described in detail the parallel evolution of her clinical course and her discourse regarding the potential causes of her affliction. An intelligent woman, she expressed herself with clarity, discussing the place of her family's ancestral spirits in her life, the fate of "exceptional" children regarded as reincarnated ancestors, and her expectations of the *marabouts* she consulted. The authors comment: "All has occurred as if she had organized her illness in front of us and this organization has appeared to us as the very moment of her recovery" (p. 121). They conclude that clinicians can benefit from close examination of patients' use of traditional illness beliefs, both to understand the patient herself and also to shed light on diagnosis and prognosis. In his clinical work in Senegal, Henri Collomb (1965) also suggested that the deployment of these traditional interpretive systems allows patients to tame disturbing or frightening experiences and aids in their integration. This is one of the explanations Collomb offered for the apparent fact that in Africa the acute paranoid psychoses (*bouffées délirantes*) are less likely to evolve into chronic psychoses than in Western countries (Stevens, 1987; Okasha, Dawla & Saad, 1993).

In a study done in Montreal with people diagnosed as schizophrenic and their families, Corin observed a parallel quest for meaning (Corin, 1990; Corin & Lauzon, 1992). In this research, the interpretive principles applied to patients' discourse were not based on a grid of symptoms (e.g., simply assessing "is the discourse psychotic?"), but on the type of experiential world that the discourse revealed. This is in line with the distinction made by the European phenomenological psychiatrists Binswanger (1970) and, more recently, Blankenburg (1986), between a view of abnormal behaviors as *symptoms* of a hidden disease and as *phenomena* expressing a basic alteration of the experience of being in the world. In the second perspective, behavior is considered a window on a lifeworld that comprises experience, action, and the presentation of self. In her study, Corin has taken a phenomenological stance and has collected two types of data relevant to the concept of insight. The first, considers the manner in which patients describe their earlier experience and the way in which they seek to rebuild and give it meaning; the second type concerns patients' self-descriptions. In both cases, what emerges is the importance of recognizing individuals' fundamental suffering but, at the same time, its appropriation and "reopening" by the play of symbolic meanings—particularly, the reintroduction of a gap or a multiplicity of potential meanings, in the way in which they characterize themselves. Similarly, the distinction between negative symptoms and the position of *positive withdrawal* associated with a favorable course in Corin's study is to be sought at the level of the afflicted persons' use of specific meaning systems.

In the urban North American context, however, we have been impressed by the fragmented, solitary, and uncertain character of explanations for illness offered by patients and their families. No encompassing framework was available to them through which they could explore and integrate the meaning of the illness. The therapeutic interaction tended to be restricted to a private colloquy between patient and clinician, and the meaning of symptoms was assimilated to the clinician's diagnostic grid rather than reflecting a dialogical understanding of the patient's lifeworld. As the diagnosis did not build on current understanding of patient and family, it was likely to remain external to the person and of little use in organizing the structure and meaning of everyday life. In this Western context, communicating the diagnosis and leading the patient to accept it is a sort of pedagogical enterprise. The patient's task is to accept the authoritative diagnosis and he or she has little freedom or encouragement to rework it in a personal and creative way (Kirmayer, 1994). While the mental illness label is not necessarily disabling in itself (cf. Warner, Taylor, Powers, & Hyman, 1989), it is at least debatable whether the kind of insight that results from this approach is of greater clinical utility and healing efficacy than one supported by the collective symbolic processes found in other societies.

Davidson and Strauss (1992) suggest that the process of rediscovering and reconstructing a valued and functional sense of self is central to recovery from psychosis. The aspects of this process they observed in their longitudinal study of patients include: (1) discovering the possibility of a more active sense of self or agency; (2) taking stock of strengths and weaknesses and of possibilities for change; (3) putting into action some aspects of the self as a reflection of actual capabilities; and (4) using an enhanced sense of self-identity as a refuge from illness and social stigma. They suggest that the self constitutes a fulcrum where both social factors and one's own efforts at self-definition exert comparable force in determining the course of illness.

To the extent that the self is a unitary construct, the multidimensionality of insight pointed out by David (1990) raises issues for dissonance theory; that is, how do people integrate discrepant information about the self? Do they keep it separate from information about the self (as being about symptoms rather than about illness affecting the self) or add premises to their cognitive self-representation to neutralize, reframe, or reinterpret the potentially dissonant information carried by the recognition that they are ill?

In this regard, it is important to note that not all knowledge is directly related to the self and therefore does not demand the same level or type of coherence. Different cultural concepts of the self may allow different experiences and behaviors to be interpreted as either irrelevant to the self or support a view of the self as inherently less coherent and therefore able to tolerate higher degrees of inconsistency. In fact, the whole notion of the self as a unitary construct may be misleading. Information relevant to the self may be acquired and organized in a variety of ways, resulting in a series of selves that are held together by functional relationships and social requirements for coherence. Neisser (1988) distinguishes five types of self with corresponding forms of self-knowledge:

1. The *ecological self*, constructed through feedback from perception and action in the physical environment;
2. The *interpersonal self*, based on the felt-significance of emotional attachments and relationships;
3. The *extended self*, developed through the narratives of autobiographical memory;
4. The *private self*, based on the experience of privileged access to one's own thoughts and feelings;
5. The *conceptual self*, comprising the network of assumptions, models, and metaphors about oneself as a person, encompasing knowledge of social roles, ethnopsychology, and the position of self in a moral universe.

The conceptual self is the inward face of what anthropologists have studied as the cultural concept of the person (Carrithers, Collins, & Lukes, 1985; Markus & Kitayama, 1991; Marsella, DeVos, & Hsu, 1985; Shweder, 1991). Although, these different selves are woven together into a unitary conception of the self through their functional interactions, the process of acquiring knowledge about each of these selves can be quite distinct.

Indeed, it is possible for contradictions to exist between different versions of the self; these discrepancies need not be willful, although it is possible for the person to intentionally maintain scotomata toward certain aspects of self-knowledge. As Markova and Berrios (1992) suggest, such self-deception may be considered a failure to spell out, or to commit oneself to, a version of reality. The term self-deception, however, implies that a cold, clear, accurate vision of one's own status is best, when much work in social psychology suggests that healthy people enjoy many self-serving biases and distortions in their view of self (Greenwald, 1980; Kiersky, this volume; Taylor & Brown, 1988; for a critique of this literature, see Shedler, Mayman, & Manis, 1993). Both intrapsychic and interpersonal factors may lead an individual to adopt a stance of denial, self-deception or positive misconstrual. A social-cultural perspective would emphasize that this stance must be understood as a form of social positioning (or maintaining a fluid position) vis-à-vis others (Davies & Harré, 1990).

## Conclusions

The metaphor of insight implies that self-awareness is based on introspection. Social psychological studies, however, suggest that self-knowledge is largely the product of social processes involving observation of others and acquisition of culture-specific modes of self-description. Insight, then, does not involve a transparent act of self-perception but a cognitive and social construction or construal of the self. As such, it is profoundly shaped by cultural beliefs and practices.

Recognition of the presence of a psychiatric problem is not simply an individual process that depends on the nature or degree of illness. It consists equally of social processes negotiated among patients, families, and experts who may belong to the patient's culture of origin or be situated outside that culture. If we conceptualize insight as defined in the psychiatric literature as a specific form of interpretation contingent on a larger interpretive field, we can appreciate that the link to reality that allows one to gain insight can be through other things than simply the recognition of symptoms. The emphasis on recognition of symptoms reflects the dominant orientation of the current psychiatric system or, more precisely, its naturalistic perspective toward mental illness.

Psychological explanations are based on a culturally distinctive construction of the self that emphasizes privacy, individualism, autonomy, and self-control. While this mode of self-depiction is highly valued in many Western societies, it is only one possible construal of the self. In recent years, much attention has been given to cultures with a more sociocentric notion of the self. This different concept of the self may influence the symptomatology, course, and treatment response of psychotic disorders. Culture influences the psychotic person's insight into his condition in the following ways:

1. Developing habits of self-observation and self-description that allow the person to recognize and communicate alterations in private experience;
2. Drawing attention to certain behaviors or experiences as deviant and hence as signs or symptoms of affliction;
3. Offering specific accounts for deviant behavior and experience that lead the person to categorize his or her own condition as sickness, moral failing, divine visitation, and the like;
4. Providing ways of assimilating psychotic experience into a social identity.

This last is particularly important, since most knowledge—including the sort of self-knowledge that is taken as insight—is not stored as abstract representations but remains implicit in modes of practice or a way of life (Kirmayer, 1992).

Cross-cultural studies of schizophrenia demonstrate the pervasive and profound effects of culture on insight in psychosis. Existing epidemiological studies, while limited by a focus on establishing cross-cultural similarities, have nevertheless indicated substantial variation in the symptomatology, course, and outcome of schizophrenia and other psychoses, with better outcomes reported in some less industrialized countries (Waxler, 1979; Jablensky et al., 1992). Culturally determined modes of insight and explanation may account, in part, for these clinically important differences.

Unfortunately, there is as yet little empirical work on insight in psychosis from a cross-cultural perspective. However, there are studies of social labeling, experience, and social course and treatment of psychosis that have suggestive implications for future work on insight. A sociocultural perspective can do much to clarify issues in this area, in part by insisting that insight be understood as culturally constructed in at least three ways: through culturally informed cognitive schemata, through collective representations and practices that are socially embodied (and hence, not to be found within the individual), and through an understanding of insight as a form of self-presentation or positioning in a local world where meanings and self-ascriptions are negotiated, collaboratively constructed, and often hotly contested. This adds another dimension to efforts to measure insight as some intrinsic property or capacity of the individual, and insists that we attend equally to the social contexts in which insight is being measured and in which it is used.

We began this chapter with the case of Martin to emphasize that culture is not something "out there"—relevant only to exotic peoples in faraway places. All experience is culturally embedded, and the personal and social significance of psychotic symptoms can be understood only with close attention to the history and practices of the sufferer and his milieu.

Ultimately, insight serves not only self-regulatory functions but also social-rhetorical purposes. Consequently, insight and denial must be seen as facets of the afflicted person's stance or position in relationships with health care providers, in the family, and in wider social spheres. The nature and degree of insight is context dependent and must be understood by researchers and clinicians as a response to the cultural meaning of psychotic experience.

*Notes*

1. Nor is this situation exceptional. Suicide among schizophrenics tends to occur within two years of a first episode and to affect mostly better educated subjects; its occurrence cannot be predicted by traditional suicide risk scales nor does it appear to be modified by drug therapy. Becker (1988) describes it as a "syndrome of cognitive despair," which is a consequence of functional impairments, social disabilities, and a loss of realistic hope for recovery.

2. Indeed, the positive symptoms of schizophrenia (e.g., hallucinations and delusions), and the inability to notice that one is sick, could arise from a common underlying mechanism; for example, a disturbance in the feedback loops by which we ascertain the origin of our behavior could lead us to experience our own thoughts or subvocal speech as hallucinatory voices (Green & Kinsbourne, 1990).

3. Ericsson and Simon (1984), however, have argued that under many circumstances we do have knowledge of our own mental processes based on our ability to report the contents of short-term or "working" memory. It is only when processes bypass short-term memory (STM), or when STM decays or is otherwise rendered inaccessible, that we completely lack introspective access to our mental processes. However, many forms of social learning occur without conscious awareness and result in procedural knowledge that, while it can be used, cannot be explicitly described (as can declarative knowledge). Emotionally charged or personally disagreeable information, such as a stigmatized medical diagnosis or a deflating interpretation of exalted psychotic experiences, is likely to be less accessible to conscious recall for all the defensive reasons adduced by psychodynamic theory.

4. Sensory experiences that constitute the *qualia* of consciousness may occur on the basis of perceptual processes prior to narratization (Humphrey, 1992), and awareness of illness simply as pain, dysphoria, or malaise might be based on such preverbal qualia, but the type of awareness referred to as insight is clearly a form of narrative.

5. In fact, Dick generated at least one hypothesis to take in these personality changes: he was the victim of a dissociative process, a shift to a dual personality that had arisen some years earlier at the time of a traumatic amnesia incurred during an automobile accident. He rejected this explanation as it could not account for the specific details of his personality. The current vogue for diagnosing multiple personality disorder in the United States suggests that he was too quick to dismiss this hypothesis.

6. Dick died in 1982, a few months before the film *Blade Runner*, based on his novel *Do Androids Dream of Electric Sheep?*, was released.

7. In his exegesis, commenting on his science fiction writing, Dick noted: "I do seem attracted to trash, as if the clue—*the clue*—lies there. I'm always ferreting out elliptical points, odd angles. What I write doesn't make a whole lot of sense. There is fun & religion & psychotic horror strewn about like a bunch of hats. Also, there is a social or sociological drift—rather than toward the hard sciences. The overall impression is childish but interesting. This is not a sophisticated person writing. Everything is equally real, like junk jewels in the alley. A fertile creative mind seeing constantly shifting sets, the serious made funny, the funny sad, the horrific exactly that: utterly horrific as it is the touchstone of what is real: horror is real because it can injure. . . . I certainly see the randomness in my work, & I also see how this fast shuffling of possibility after

possibility might eventually, given enough time, juxtapose & disclose something important & automatically overlooked in more orderly thinking" (Sutin, 1989, pp. 154–55).

8. This sense of conviction that accompanies delusions and some hallucinations may arise from several mechanisms: (1) the sensory-affective qualities of delusional thought and experience may be so vivid and compelling that they admit no doubt as to their significance (David & Howard, 1994); (2) cognitive appraisal mechanisms may be malfunctioning so that alternative explanations cannot be generated or tested; or (3) ordinary doubt itself may become emotionally threatening and aversive.

9. Acute psychoses with rapid resolution (brief reactive psychoses) appear to be more common in non-Western countries as well and may contribute to the better prognostic picture in studies that do not use a duration criterion for the diagnosis of schizophrenia (Guinness, 1992; Okasha, Dawla, & Saad, 1993; Stevens, 1987). These psychoses may be more closely related to affective and dissociative disorders than to schizophrenia.

10. One should, however, not to fall into a stereotyped opposition between purely sociocentric selves in developing countries and purely egocentric selves in Western societies. Individual and social aspects of the person are important in all societies. It is more a matter of differential emphasis on one of the two broad orientations based on the availability of collective symbols and rituals for valuing and working out each dimension of the person (Corin, 1980, 1985). The sense of self varies along many other dimensions across cultures and also shows enormous intracultural variation.

*References*

Amador, X. F., Strauss, D. H., Yale, S. A., Flaum, M. H., & Gorman, J. M. (1993). Assessment of insight in psychosis. *American Journal of Psychiatry, 150*, 873–879.

Bateson, G. (1972). *Steps to an ecology of mind*. New York: Ballantine Books.

Becker, R. E. (1988). Depression in schizophrenia. *Hospital and Community Psychiatry, 39*(12), 1269–1275.

Bellah, R. N., Madsen, R., Sullivan, W. M., Swidler, A., & Tipton, S. M. (1985). *Habits of the heart: Individualism and commitment in American life*. Berkeley: University of California Press.

Bowers, M. B., Jr. (1974). *Retreat from sanity: The structure of emerging psychosis*. Baltimore: Penguin Books.

Bruner, J. (1990). *Acts of meaning*. Cambridge, MA: Harvard University Press.

Carrithers, M., Collins, S., & Lukes, S. (Eds.). (1985). *The category of the person*. Cambridge: Cambridge University Press.

Cohen, A. (1992). Prognosis for schizophrenia in the third world: A reevaluation of cross-cultural research. *Culture, Medicine, and Psychiatry, 16*(1), 53–77.

Collomb, H. (1965). Bouffées délirantes en psychiatrie africaine. *Psychopathologie Africaine, 27*, 167–239.

Cooper, J., & Sartorius, N. (1977). Cultural and temporal variations in schizophrenia: A speculation on the importance of industrialization. *British Journal of Psychiatry, 130*, 50–55.

Corin, E. (1979). A possession psychotherapy in an urban setting: Zebola in Kinshasa. *Social Science and Medicine, 13B*, 327–338.

Corin, E. (1980). Vers une réappropriation de la dimension individuelle en psychologie africaine. *Revue canadienne des études africaines, 14*(1), 135–156.

Corin, E. (1985). La question du sujet dans les thérapies de possession. *Psychoanalyse, 3*, 53–66.

Corin, E. (1990). Facts and meaning in psychiatry: An anthropological approach to the lifeworld of schizophrenics. *Culture, Medicine and Psychiatry, 14*, 153–188.

Corin, E., Bibeau, G., & Uchôa, E. 91993). Eléments d'une sémiologie anthropologique des troubles psychiques chez les Bambara, Soninké et Bwa du Mali. *Anthropologie et sociétés, 17*(1-2), 125–156.

Corin, E., & Lauzon, G. (1992). Positive withdrawal and the quest for meaning: The reconstruction of experience among schizophrenics. *Psychiatry, 55,* 266–278.

Corin, E., & Lauzon, G. (1994). From symptoms to phenomena: The articulation of experience in schizophrenia. *Journal of Phenomenological Psychology, 25*(1), 3–50.

David, A. S. (1990). Insight and psychosis. *British Journal of Psychiatry, 156,* 798–808.

David, A., Buchanan, A., Reed, A., & Almeida, O. (1992). The assessment of insight in psychosis. *British Journal of Psychiatry, 161,* 599–602.

David, A. S., & Howard, R. (1994). An experimental phenomenological approach to delusional memory in schizophrenia and the late paraphrenia. *Psychological Medicine, 24,* 515–524.

Davidson, L., & Strauss, J. S. (1992). Sense of self in recovery from severe mental illness. *British Journal of Medical Psychology, 65,* 131–145.

Davies, B., & Harré, R. (1990). Positioning: The discursive production of selves. *Journal for the Theory of Social Behavior, 20*(1), 43–64.

Dennett, D. C. (1991). *Consciousness Explained*. Boston: Little, Brown.

Dick, P. K. (1990). *The VALIS trilogy*. New York: Book-of-the-Month Club.

Dick, P. K. (1991). *In pursuit of Valis: Selections from the exegesis*. Novato, CA: Underwood-Miller.

Dumont, L. (1986). *Essays on individualism: Modern ideology in anthropological perspective*. Chicago: University of Chicago Press.

Edgerton, R. B., & Cohen, A. (1994). Culture and schizophrenia: The DOSMD challenge. *British Journal of Psychiatry, 164,* 222–231.

Ericsson, K. A., & Simon, H. A. (1984). *Protocol analysis*. Cambridge, MA: MIT Press.

Fabrega, H., Jr. (1991). Psychiatric stigma in non-western societies. *Comprehensive Psychiatry, 32*(6), 534–551.

Good, B., & Good, M. J. D. (1980). The meaning of symptoms: A cultural hermeneutic model for clinical practice. In L. Eisenberg & A. Kleinman (Eds.), *The relevance of social science for medicine* (pp. 165–196). Dordrecht: D. Reidel.

Good, B. J., & Good, M.-J. D. (1993). Au mode subjonctif. La construction narrative des crises d'épilepsie en Turquie. *Anthropologie et sociétés, 17*(1-2), 31–42.

Green, M. F., & Kinsbourne, M. (1990). Subvocal activity and auditory hallucinations: Clues for behavioral treatments? *Schizophrenia Bulletin, 16*(4), 617–625.

Greenwald, A. (1980). The totalitarian ego: fabrication and revision of personal history. *American Psychologist, 35,* 603–618.

Guarnaccia, P. J., Parra, P., Deschamps, A., Milstein, G., & Argiles, N. (1992). Si Dios quiere: Hispanic families' experiences of caring for a seriously mentally ill family member. *Culture, Medicine and Psychiatry, 16,* 187–216.

Guinness, E. A. (1992). Brief reactive psychosis and the major functional psychoses: descriptive case studies in Africa. *British Journal of Psychiatry, 160(Suppl. 16),* 24–41.

Gupta, S. (1992). Cross-national differences in the frequency and outcome of schizophrenia: A comparison of five hypotheses. *Social Psychiatry and Psychiatric Epidemiology, 27,* 249–252.

Hoffman, R. E. (1986). Verbal hallucinations and language production processes in schizophrenia. *Behavioral and Brain Sciences, 9*(3), 503–548.

Hole, R. W., Rush, A. J., & Beck, A. T. (1979). A cognitive investigation of schizophrenic delusions. *Psychiatry, 42,* 312–319.

Howard, G. S. (1991). Culture tales: A narrative approach to thinking, cross-cultural psychology, and psychotherapy. *American Psychologist, 46*(3), 187–197.

Humphrey, N. (1992). *A history of the mind: Evolution and the birth of consciousness*. New York: Simon & Schuster.

Jablensky, A., Sartorius, N., Ernberg, G., Anker, M., Korten, A., Cooper, J. E., Day, R., & Bertelsen, A. (1992). Schizophrenia: Manifestations, incidence and course in different cultures: A World Health Organization Ten-Country Study. *Psychological Medicine* (monograph suppl. 20).

Janzen, J. M. (1978). *The quest for therapy in Lower Zaire*. Berkeley: University of California.

Jenkins, J. H. (1988). Ethnopsychiatric interpretations of schizophrenic illness: The problem of nervios in Mexican-American families. *Culture, Medicine and Psychiatry, 12*, 303–331.

Jenkins, J. H., & Karno, M. (1992). The meaning of expressed emotion: Theoretical issues raised by cross-cultural research. *American Journal of Psychiatry, 149*(1), 9–21.

Karno, M., Jenkins, J. H., de al Selva, A., Santana, F., Telles, C., Lopez, S., & Mintz, J. (1987). Expressed emotion and schizophrenic outcome among Mexican-American families. *Journal of Nervous and Mental Disease, 175*(3), 143–151.

Kirby, A. P. (1991). *Narrative and the self*. Bloomington: Indiana University Press.

Kirmayer, L. J. (1983). Paranoia and pronoia: The visionary and the banal. *Social Problems, 31*(2), 170–179.

Kirmayer, L. J. (1988). Mind and body as metaphors: Hidden values in biomedicine. In M. Lock & D. Gordon (Eds.), *Biomedicine examined* (pp. 57–92). Dordrecht: Kluwer.

Kirmayer, L. J. (1989). Cultural variations in the response to psychiatric disorders and emotional distress. *Social Science and Medicine, 29*(3), 327–339.

Kirmayer, L. J. (1991). The place of culture in psychiatric nosology: Taijin kyofusho and DSM-III-R. *Journal of Nervous and Mental Disease, 179*(1), 19–28.

Kirmayer, L. J. (1992). The body's insistence on meaning: Metaphor as presentation and representation in illness experience. *Medical Anthropology Quarterly, 6*(4), 323–346.

Kirmayer, L. J. (1993). Is the concept of mental disorder culturally relative? In S. A. Kirk & S. Einbinder (Eds.), *Controversial issues in mental health*. Boston: Appleton-Century-Croft.

Kirmayer, L. J. (1994). Improvisation and authority in illness meaning. *Culture, Medicine and Psychiatry, 18*(1), 183–214.

Kleinman, A. M. (1980). *Patients and healers in the context of culture*. Berkeley: University of California Press.

Kleinman, A. (1986). *Social origins of distress and disease*. New Haven: Yale University Press.

Kleinman, A. (1988). *Rethinking psychiatry*. New York: Free Press.

Lakoff, G., & Johnson, M. (1980). *Metaphors we live by*. Chicago: University of Chicago Press.

Leff, J. (1988). *Psychiatry around the globe: A transcultural view*. London: Gaskell.

Leff, J., Sartorius, N., Jablensky, A., Korten, A., & Ernberg, G. (1992). The International Pilot Study of Schizophrenia: Five-year follow-up findings. *Psychological Medicine, 22*, 131–145.

Leff, J., & Vaughn, C. (1985). *Expressed emotion in families*. New York: Guilford Press.

Leff, J., Wig, N. N., Bedi, H., Menon, D. K., Kuipers, L., Korten, A., Ernberg, G., Day, R., Sartorius, N., & Jablensky, A. (1990). Relatives' expressed emotion and the course of schizophrenia in Chandigarh: A two-year follow-up of a first contact sample. *British Journal of Psychiatry, 156*, 351–356.

Leff, J., Wig, N. N., Ghosh, A., Bedi, H., Menon, D. K., Kuipers, L., Korten, A., Ernberg, G., Day, R., Sartorius, N., & Jablensky, A. (1987). III. Influence of relatives' expression emotion on the course of schizophrenia in Chandigarh. *British Journal of Psychiatry, 151*, 166–173.

Lemert, E. M. (1962). Paranoia and the dynamics of exclusion. *Sociometry, 25*, 2–20.

Lewis, A. (1934). The pyschopathology of insight. *British Journal of Medical Psychology, 13*, 332–348.

Lin, K-M., & Kleinman, A. (1988). Psychopathology and clinical course of schizophrenia: A cross-cultural perspective. *Schizophrenia Bulletin, 14*(4) 555–567.

Link, B. G. (1987). Understanding labeling effects in the area of mental disorders: An assessment of the effects of expectations of rejection. *American Sociological Review, 52,* 96–112.

Link, B., Cullen, F. T., Frank, J., & Wozniak, J. F. (1987). The social rejection of former mental patients: Understanding why labels matter. *American Journal of Sociology, 92*(6), 1461–1500.

Marková, I. S., & Berrios, G. E. (1992). The meaning of insight in clinical psychiatry. *British Journal of Psychiatry, 160,* 850–860.

Markus, H. R., & Kitayama, S. (1991). Culture and the self: Implications for cognition, emotion, and motivation. *Psychological Review, 98*(2), 224–253.

Marsella, A. J., DeVos, G., & Hsu, F. L. K. (Eds.). (1985). *Culture and self: Asian and Western perspectives.* New York: Tavistock.

Melges, F. T., & Freeman, A. M., III (1975). Persecutory delusions: A cybernetic model. *American Journal of Psychiatry, 132*(10), 1038–1044.

Murphy, H. B. M. (1982). *Comparative psychiatry: The international and intercultural distribution of mental illness.* New York: Springer-Verlag.

Murphy, H. B. M., & Raman, A. C. (1971). The chronicity of schizophrenia in indigenous tropical people. Results of a twelve-year follow-up survey in Mauritius. *British Journal of Psychiatry, 118,* 489–497.

Murphy, J. M. (1976). Psychiatric labeling in cross-cultural perspective. *Science, 191,* 1019–1028.

Neisser, U. (1988). Five kinds of self-knowledge. *Philosophical Psychology, 1,* 35–59.

Nisbett, R. E., & Wilson, T. D. (1977). Telling more than we can know: verbal reports on mental processes. *Psychological Review, 84*(3), 231–259.

Obeyesekere, G. (1981). *Medusa's hair: An essay on personal symbols and religious experience.* Chicago: University of Chicago Press.

Obeyesekere, G. (1991). *The work of culture: Symbolic transformation in psychoanalysis and anthropology.* Chicago: University of Chicago Press.

Okasha, A., El Dawla, S., & Saad, A. (1993). Presentation of acute psychosis in an Egyptian sample: a transcultural comparison. *Comprehensive Psychiatry, 34,* 4–9.

Ortigues, M.-C., Martino, P., & Collomb, H. (1967). L'utilization des données culturelles dans un cas de bouffée délirante. *Psychopathologie Africaine, 121–147.*

Ortigues, M. C., & Ortigues, E. (1966). *Oedipe africain.* Paris: Plan.

Raybeck, D. (1988). Anthropology and labeling theory: A constructive critique. *Ethos, 16,* 371–397.

Robinson, J. M. (Ed.). (1977). *The Nag Hammadi library.* New York: Harper & Row.

Robinson, J. M. (Ed.). (1988). *The Nag Hammadi library in English,* 3rd rev. ed. Leiden: E.J. Brill.

Ross, L., & Nisbett, R. E. (1991). *The person and the situation: Perspectives of social psychology.* Philadelphia: Temple University Press.

Rozin, P., & Nemeroff, C. (1990). The laws of sympathetic magic: A psychological analysis of similarity and contagion. In J. W. Stigler, R. A. Shweder, & G. Herdt (Eds.), *Cultural psychology* (pp. 205–232). Cambridge: Cambridge University Press.

Sartorius, N. (1992). Commentary on Prognosis for Schizophrenia in the third world by Alex Cohen. *Culture, Medicine, and Psychiatry, 16*(1), 81–84.

Sartorius, N., Jablensky, A., Korten, A., Ernberg, G., Anker, M., Cooper, J. E., & Day, R. (1986). Early manifestations and first contact incidence of schizophrenia in different cultures. *Psychological Medicine, 16,* 909–928.

Sartorius, N., Jablensky, A., & Shapiro, R. (1978). Cross-cultural differences in the short-term prognosis of schizophrenic psychoses. *Schizophrenia Bulletin, 4*(1), 102–113.

Shedler, J., Mayman, and Manis, M. (1993). The *illusion* of mental health. *American Psychologist, 48*, 1117–1131.

Shweder, R. A. (1991). *Thinking through culture: Expeditions in cultural psychology.* Cambridge, MA: Harvard University Press.

Sperber, D. (1985). Anthropology and psychology: Towards an epidemiology of representations. *Man, 20*(1), 73–89.

Stevens, J. (1987). Brief psychoses: Do they contribute to the good prognosis and equal prevalence of schizophrenia in developing countries? *British Journal of Psychiatry, 151*, 393–396.

Sutin, L. (1989). *Divine invasions: A life of Philip K. Dick.* New York: Harmony Books.

Taylor, S. E., & Brown, J. (1988). Illusion and well-being: a social psychological perspective on mental health. *Journal of Personality and Social Psychology, 48*, 285–290.

Thoits, P. A. (1985). Self-labeling processes in mental illness: The role of emotional deviance. *American Journal of Sociology, 91*(2), 221–247.

Townsend, J. M. (1978). *Cultural conceptions and mental illness.* Chicago: University of Chicago Press.

Uchôa, E. (1993). Espace dévolu, espace désiré, espace revendiqué. Indifférenciation et folie d'Ajaratou. *Anthropologie et sociétés, 17*(1-2). 157–172.

Warner, R., Taylor, D., Powers, M., & Hyman, J. (1989). Acceptance of the mental illness label by psychotic patients: Effects on functioning. *American Journal of orthopsychiatry, 59*(3), 398–409.

Waxler, N. E. (1979). Is outcome for schizophrenia better in nonindustrial societies? The case of Sri Lanka. *Journal of Nervous and Mental Disease, 167*(3), 144–158.

Williams, P. (1986). *Only apparently real: The world of Philip K. Dick.* New York: Arbor House.

World Health Organization. (1973). *The International Pilot Study of Schizophrenia*, Vol. 1. Geneva: Author.

World Health Organization. (1979). *Schizophrenia: An international follow-up study*, New York: John Wiley.

Yamashita, I. (1993). *Taijin-Kyofu or delusional social phobia.* Sapporo: Hokkaido University Press.

Young, A. (1982). Rational men and the explanatory model approach. *Culture, Medicine and Psychiatry, 6*, 57–71.

Zempleni, A. (1969) La thérapid traditionelle des trouble mentaux chez les Wolof et les Lebou (Sénégal): Principes. *Social Science and Medicine, 3*, 191–205.

# 11

YOSHIHARU KIM

# Japanese Attitudes Toward Insight in Schizophrenia

The aim of this chapter is to give an overview of how insight in schizophrenia has been understood and discussed in Japanese psychiatry. The chapter is divided into four sections. In the first, I will briefly review the significance of this issue in the development of modern Japanese psychiatry, for the benefit of readers who are not familiar with the history of psychiatry in Japan. The second and third sections deal with selected theoretical debates and clinical practices concerning this issue. The last section outlines some evidence-based Japanese studies and representative attitudes of Japanese psychiatrists toward this matter.

## Historical Background

The development of modern Japanese psychiatry was inaugurated after the Meiji Reformation in 1867. Pre-Meiji Japan had few asylums or hospitals to segregate the mentally ill as existed in Europe, and had only certain temples that offered through water bathing treatment. Through Japan's long history, officials had taken a fairly generous attitude toward the mentally ill: records show few incidents of political persecution against them, and in 701, it was already determined that the mentally ill should be treated medically. During the Edo era (1604–1867), the criminal law admitted insanity as a mitigating circumstance. Unlike the situation in Europe, where stigmatization of the mentally ill aroused moral protest by Philippe Pinel and Jean-Etienne-Dominique Esquirol, there had been only a weak social and political tendency to alienate them in Japan. Moreover, the modern scientific urge to classify natural phenomena promoted in Europe by Carl Linnaeus and Charles Darwin had no basis in traditional Japanese

221

culture, which consequently experienced little systematic discussion of how to define and classify mental illness. Scant interest was paid to the subject of insight in the mentally disordered, a feature whose lack was regarded in late 19th-century Europe as a kind of agnosia that was sometimes claimed to be the definition of mental illness (Pick 1882; Dagonet 1881).

During the late Edo period, with the development of industry, incidents of discrimination against the mentally disordered, including deportation from their villages and confinement to private prisons, increased. After the Meiji Reformation, a number of psychiatric asylums were founded in the naïve belief that it was more humane to treat the mentally disordered in hospitals than to leave them in their homes or villages. Since that time, Japanese psychiatric practice has been largely based upon such inpatient treatment, borrowing its methodology mainly from German, and to a lesser degree French and English, psychiatry. The school of psychopathology that was methodologically founded by Jaspers (1913), especially his assertion of the incomprehensibility of psychoses and the lack of insight in schizophrenia, became so influential in Japan as to determine the view of the majority of psychiatrists.

After World War II, an influence of American psychiatry reached this country in the form of a more flexible view of possible recovery from schizophrenia. Klerman (1991) stated that this American optimism was originally derived from experience with soldiers who suffered from reactive psychosis during wartime and who had recovered afterwards. Despite the fact that reactive psychosis was not always included in a narrower definition of schizophrenia used in Japan at that time, this new attitude stimulated the interest in the social rehabilitation of schizophrenics of a number of Japanese psychiatrists. Especially after introduction of antipsychotic drugs in 1955, Japanese psychiatric treatment started to move toward outpatient management, social rehabilitation, and day-care treatment. In 1958, Utena and his colleagues at Gunma University instituted the *Seikatsu-rinshou*, a long-term program for the social rehabilitation of schizophrenics that still continues today.

Under these circumstances in 1963, a symposium on insight in schizophrenia was held by the Japanese Conference of Psychopathology, with the aim of reevaluating the definition of insight promoted by Jaspers. This definition had divided sense of illness from insight, regarding the former as a vague feeling of sickness without precise awareness of its nature and extent, and viewed the latter as an exact consciousness of the illness, including its type, severity, and symptoms. The criticism made by Japanese psychiatrists at that time was brought about because ongoing changes in clinical practice of schizophrenia came to require more positive and flexible views of schizophrenics' attitudes toward their illness.

Unfortunately, in 1964, the then-U.S. Ambassador to Japan, Edward Reischauer, was attacked and nearly assassinated by a young Japanese schizophrenic. Because the Japanese government wanted to avoid diplomatic conflict with the United States, it decided to revise the Mental Hygiene Law toward the seclusion and confinement of psychiatric patients in order to demonstrate that Japan was determined not to let such an incident happen again. Construction of psychiatric hospitals was accelerated, with the result that the number of psychiatric inpatients increased from 100,000 in 1960 to 300,000 in 1970. Regrettably, these additional inpatients were sometimes managed by an insufficient number of staff and even by doctors who lacked psychiatric training and knowledge. In this climate, Jaspers's notion of lack of insight was superficially popular-ized and sometimes used as an excuse for involuntary admission, a situation that was subsequently deplored by a number of psychiatrists, including Kumakura (1987). In those days, some untrained psychiatrists actually said that there was no use persuading schizophrenics to accept inpatient treatment because they were by definition incom-prehensible and lacked insight. One of the most unfortunate consequences of such a distorted view of insight in schizophrenia was the Utsunomiya Hospital Case, where a number of involuntarily admitted psychiatric patients suffered from humiliating, some-times even violent treatment. In 1984 the hospital was finally inspected by a commit-tee of the International Congress of Jurists (ICJ). The case resulted in considerable social interest in the inhumane treatment conducted by several Japanese psychiatric hospitals and led to the 1987 legislation including the current mental health acts ori-ented toward legal assurance of patients' rights.

The antipsychiatric movement of the 1960s, joining forces with the student move-ment, became so influential in Japan as to temporarily occupy the Japanese Society of Psychiatry and Neurology. Psychopathological study was also criticized as practically useless, as stigmatizing the mentally disordered, so that at times it was difficult even to hold open meetings for psychopathological discussions. During this period, efforts to challenge the pessimistic view of schizophrenia as characterized by poor insight were rarely introduced by psychopathologists, but rather were made by the clinicians men-tioned below, who were interested in psychotherapeutic approaches. As the latter were not strongly bound by the methodology of German academic psychiatry, they felt rela-tively free from Jaspers's narrow concept of insight.

In the 1980s, the movement toward open-door psychiatric treatment was accelerated. In 1987, with enactment of a new, socially oriented mental health law, a Japanese foren-sic psychiatrist came out strongly against the notion of lack of insight, on the grounds that it had come to be used as an excuse for involuntary admission of schizophrenics into hospitals. In a symposium held in 1988, several outstanding Japanese psycho-pathologists argued this issue, not only criticizing the traditional concept but also propos-ing their own alternatives. (See section on "Debates in the 1980s" following.)

Today, as discussed below, many Japanese psychiatrists believe clinical interventions can improve various aspects of insight in schizophrenia. In the coming decade, it is expected that this problem will be discussed more concretely, using empirical data; to this end, several Japanese investigations have already been initiated.

## Insight as a Psychopathological Issue

Japanese psychopathological discussion of insight in schizophrenia has struggled to overcome the strict definition made by Jaspers that virtually dominated Japanese psy-chopathology. It will be shown in this section how Jaspers's notion of insight was first accepted, then criticized and challenged by Japanese psychopathologists.

### Classical Views

For several decades after the Meiji Reformation, Japanese psychiatrists generally fol-lowed the European notion of insight in mental illness and the discussions of its absence in schizophrenia or dementia praecox. In late 19th-century Europe, according to Nakatani (1989), insight was often discussed in terms of a general self-monitoring ability of one's mental state. Pick (1882) and Dagonet (1881) mentioned the relations between the various forms of insight and mental disorders, while other researchers regarded its lack as a defining principle of mental illness. Although it had been gradually noticed that some of the mentally disordered maintained insight into their illnesses, a number of celebrated European psychiatrists took a relatively pessimistic view of this issue, especially in the case of schizophrenia. Bleuler (1911), for example, asserted that schizophrenics rarely had sufficient insight into their illness, even in remission. The strict definition of insight proposed by Heilbronner (1904) and Jaspers (1913) hardly challenged such a pessimistic view, which was prevalent in Japanese academic psychiatry for several more decades. *Insight*, in its strict definition by Jaspers, would be difficult to achieve even for patients with somatic diseases. It is no wonder that Jaspers's definition, together with his definition of psychosis by incomprehensibility, contributed to the generally pessimistic and segregated view of schizophrenia in Japan, as well as in some European countries. As a result, lack of insight has been regarded in Japan as a quasi-definition of schizophrenia, even by several contemporary psychiatrists.

*Debates in the 1960s*

It was not until 1963 that some Japanese psychopathologists began to criticize Jaspers's restricted notion of insight in schizophrenia. Nishizono (1963) compared Jaspers's notion of insight with insight into illness derived from psychoanalysis, claiming that the latter concerns not only an intellectual but also a profound emotional understanding of the illness, associated with a deep change of psychodynamics. Thus, he held, schizophrenics could sometimes learn about their illness but lacked this psychological insight. Doi (1961) interpreted this phenomenon as a kind of resistance to confronting the psychotic experience. In Japan, this resistance is based particularly on the sentiment inherent in Japanese culture called *ama'e*—reliance and dependence—whose most typical example can be observed in the relationship between infant and mother. In Japan, *ama'e* is not something that grown-ups should strictly overcome or avoid; it constitutes the backbone of basic human trust among healthy individuals. But Japanese schizophrenics who are not willing to confront their psychotic experience sometimes assume this attitude of *ama'e* in front of psychiatrists, and may seem as if they are babies at their mothers' breasts, not caring to think about the bothers of real life. Contrary to Freud, Nishizono contended that this defense mechanism is related to the intact self of schizophrenics, and could be a focus of psychotherapy to increase patients' insight into their psychotic experience.

Ohashi (1963) discussed the denial of illness as seen in anosognosia, defined by Babinski, and maintained that this denial concerned not only focal neurological symptoms such as paralysis but also the total mental state of the patient and thus could not be regarded as a disturbance of any single sensorial pathway. Kajitani (1963) argued that insight is not a solid attribute of the disease, and that the information obtained from schizophrenics about insight in Jaspers's sense would be dependent on the relationship between doctor and patient. An admission of psychosis would necessarily evoke a deep sense of *haji*—harassment and shame—which must be strictly avoided according to Japanese ethical code.

Shimazaki & Abe (1963) followed the argument of Meyer-Gross (1920), maintaining that although schizophrenics were incapable of insight in the narrow sense defined by Jaspers, they were able to have a *Stellungsnahme*—an attitude toward their illness. Shimazaki examined 35 first-episode schizophrenics in complete or incomplete remission, and classified them into six groups according to their attitudes toward their illness. The first group remembered the psychotic episode as something like a natural disaster, which is transitory and leaves no pathological wake. Patients in this group were ready to admit that they had been ill, but would not reconsider the details of their illness. The second group considered their illness to be a precious experience in terms of their mental maturation, although these explanations were delusional in some cases. The third group was in some despair. They could not find any explanation for their psychosis, which they perceived as something vague and horrible. In the fourth group, the memory of the psychosis was still so vivid that the patients were at a loss as to how to express their feelings or opinions about it. In the fifth group, the patients had a rather childish and optimistic attitude, stating that they were quite relieved and relaxed after their illness. They did not seem to have any conflicts or any desire for a productive future. The sixth group consisted of patients who seemed to be totally indifferent to their disastrous experience.

Shimazaki suggested that these different attitudes toward the psychotic experience should be included in the clinical definition of insight. As a consequence, insight would not be something that ranges linearly from null to full, but would be composed of several dimensions of different qualities. He criticized those clinicians who would consider only the patients' direct statements and tended to discuss the presence or absence of insight in schizophrenics, emphasizing instead the importance of a clinical knowledge of how schizophrenics tried to incorporate their illness into their lives.

Ishikawa (1963) pointed out that insight in Shimazaki's sense was already preferred in clinical practice, and that he would evaluate not the lack of, but rather the presence of, insight in schizophrenics. This would be in terms of a positive attitude toward the future, notwithstanding its being a delusional explanation of the psychotic experience.

## Debates in the 1980s

In the mid 1980s, debates concerning insight in schizophrenia were resurrected in response to social criticism of the involuntary admission of schizophrenics and a new movement toward outpatient management and social rehabilitation.

Kondoh et al. (1985) surveyed 60 schizophrenic inpatients, asking the following: "Why are you coming to (staying in) the hospital?" "What is worrying you the most?" "In what sense do you think you are ill?" "Is something wrong with your body?" "What is mental illness?" "Do you have some hope for your treatment with your doctor?" Kondoh concluded that all the subjects possessed an awareness to some extent that they had something wrong with them. Interestingly, only 4 of the patients were judged by their clinicians to have insight into the illness, 42 to have a sense of illness (incomplete insight), and 14 to have no insight at all. Although the definition of insight used in this study was not clear, it seemed that 22 years after the work of Shimazaki, the doctors involved with this study were still influenced by a narrow definition of insight and tended to dismiss various aspects of the patients' attitudes toward schizophrenia.

The debates were especially stimulated by Kumakura (1987), a forensic psychiatrist who tried to reconsider the notion of lack of insight in schizophrenia in the light of the medical paternalism characteristic of Japanese psychiatry. His work must be considered against a background of the 1960s, when the increasing number of psychiatric beds were occupied by patients who were, in the name of paternalism, involuntarily admitted and insufficiently informed of their treatments and rights. In part, this rough paternalism was the inevitable consequence of a hastened increase in psychiatric beds, a development whose main aim was more the protection of society than the treatment of patients. Psychiatrists, especially those engaged in the antipsychiatric movement, made this situation a target of protest in the 1970s. Kumakura argued that the conflict between paternalism and antipaternalism is inherent to psychiatric practice, and that in Japan the former had been sustained with the naive assumption that psychiatric patients are incapable of judgment, with lack of insight used as an excuse. This is evidently too broad an interpretation of Jaspers's definition, which applied the concept of insight only to an awareness of psychotic experience.

Several psychopathologists contributed to Kumakura's contention, emphasizing the distinction between insight as a subjective experience and insight as an objective recognition. They claimed the former to be particularly important, for schizophrenics do have a certain understanding of their psychotic experience—a fact which had been partly demonstrated earlier by Shimazaki. They further maintained that there was no use in discussing whether this insight was true or false, because it constituted a perceived reality for the patients. An attempt to criticize this subjective view of insight in light of objective medical knowledge would be, in this way of thinking, akin to old Marxists blaming ordinary citizens for not having a knowledge of dialectical materialism. Even since the 1960s, many psychiatrists had paid little attention to their patients' cognitive efforts to incorporate their catastrophic experience into their intact, healthy selves. Jaspers's narrow notion of insight was not aimed at describing this integrative aspect of subjective insight; its central purpose was to define the lack of objective insight that was presumed to be an essential feature of psychoses like schizophrenia. Jaspers himself admitted that psychopathology, as a branch of science, could not touch the subjective aspect of insight, which he regarded as an existential matter. Matsumoto (1988) criticized this attitude as too rigid, and asserted that there was room in clinical practice for the clinician to deal with patients' subjective perceptions of their illness. Nakayasu (1988) pointed out that the Jasperian notion of lack of insight in schizophrenia could not be regarded as a symptom experienced by patients, but as a sign measured by an observer through a certain method or a frame of reference — which in this case is standard medical knowledge of mental illness. He also noted that the symptoms used to define the notion of schizophrenia, such as delusion and hallucination, are mainly observed phenomena, and would be better regarded as signs than as symptoms. A similar view was expressed later in Europe by Bitter, Jaeger, Agdeppa, and Volavka (1989), who stated that delusions and hallucinations should be regarded as objective rather than as subjective symptoms. Nakayasu (1988) regarded lack of insight as one of those objective signs that define schizophrenia from the viewpoint of medical science.

Yasunaga (1988) describes the *awareness of deportment* that reflects insight as a subjective perception. By this term he implied the sense of self that is projected onto one's perception of the position and movement of one's body and mind. This sense is different from any static knowledge, and concerns integrated physical as well as mental activities. It is a sense of the whole activity itself, and does not necessarily concern a precise knowledge of every part of an action. To understand this explanation, think of a golf swing. Good golfers are aware of their swing and may explain it as if throwing their club away to the green. This type of awareness does not need to coincide with an observation of actual body movement. It is often wise to advise to swing as if throwing the club away rather than telling the golfer to keep the left elbow three inches above eye level. According to Yasunaga, we all have this type of awareness of physical and mental activity—the awareness of deportment—but it becomes altered in schizophrenia and other mental disorders.

The core of Yasunaga's discussion is that psychiatrists should synchronize their minds with the patients' and use their own awareness of deportment to understand the patients' experiences so that they can give them appropriate advice. To that purpose, doctors should try to incorporate the patients' physical and mental activities into their own selves and maintain an awareness of the whole therapeutic situation. To illustrate the latter, Yasunaga cites a saying of Ze'ami, a famous 15th-century Japanese Nohu actor, that a performer should be aware of the whole stage, even that part that is behind him. A similar view was expressed by Kandabashi, a Japanese psychotherapist, making us wonder whether such a metaphorical explanation is characteristic of Japanese culture. However, a similar experience of intermingled self boundaries between the doctor and the patient is also described in the theory of empathy put forth by Kohut (1959), in the works of Sullivan (1953), and by Schwing (1940). A certain number of Japanese psychiatrists seem to balance a meditative way of understanding patients with a modern scientific knowledge of mental disorders.

## Insight as a Clinical Breakthrough

Apart from the above-mentioned psychopathological debates, a number of clinical psychiatrists have tried to improve various aspects of insight in schizophrenia. Although most of these efforts were reported individually, two outstanding groups of clinicians seem to have succeeded in integrating theory and practice. Shinkai and his colleagues (1986, 1988) demonstrated a unique technique called *soyegi*, or splint, therapy, a name derived from the basic therapeutic attitude of standing beside a person with schizophrenia to serve as a splint to sustain their deep sorrow. The group *Seikatsu-rinshou*, or the Clinic for Social Life, whose main purpose is to improve schizophrenics' social lives and promote their social insight, has also made an important contribution in this area.

### Soyegi *Therapy*

This therapy is based upon observation of the rapid alteration of transient micropsychotic experiences and recovery from them in the acute and chronic phases of schizophrenia. The occurrence of micropsychotic experiences is regarded as activated by certain verbal and interpersonal stimulus, called *sainen-fukatsu*, or activation-resurgence, said to occur in every interpersonal situation, including therapeutic interviews. When a schizophrenic is interviewed by a psychiatrist, for example, the patient not only recalls the past psychotic experience but can also become recaptivated by micropsychosis newly provoked by the inquiries. As a consequence, the patient may demonstrate delusion or hallucination, or become thought disordered, making it difficult to continue the interview. The term *psychotic* is used in this school to refer, not only to the emergence of positive symptoms such as hallucinations, delusions, or thought disorder, but also to the patient's involvement in those experiences. When a schizophrenic recalls and tends to believe in the reality of the past psychotic experiences rather than in the logical intervention given by a doctor, the patient is considered to be recaptured by psychosis. *Soyegi* therapy tries to profit as much as possible from these *sainen-fukatsu* phenomena in order to promote insight in the following three ways: (1) awareness of the abnormality of psychotic experiences; (2) awareness of the causal relationships of verbal stimulus to the resurgence of psychosis, and (3) awareness of the patient's own resistance to admitting that he or she had been ill.

For clinical convenience, three phases are postulated during recovery from psychosis. The first phase is characterized by the presence of active psychotic symptoms, the second by the feelings of deep sorrow and desperation, and the third by chronic fatigue and exhaustion. These three phases do not always occur in order and can coexist. The first two phases, described below, are considered to be particularly important and require deliberate interventions.

In the first phase, even in the midst of severe psychotic symptoms, there is a waxing and waning in intensity, and schizophrenics may even experience some instances when they regain their *shohki*, or sanity. The main therapeutic task of this phase is to call for the sanity of the patients using a deeply empathetic attitude. Shinkai (1986, 1988) maintains that *shohki* can be gained or recked by prudential or rough words spoken by doctors and staff.

The second important task is to help the patient recognize that he or she is experiencing an alternating movement of falling into psychosis and emancipating from it through a certain stimulus. In this phase it is not insight as a judgment or knowledge that is important, but insight for therapeutic possibility, which is totally dependent upon the therapeutic relationship. The sorrow components of the second phase slip into the first phase, making it difficult for schizophrenics to confront the psychosis, and can deprive them of any hope to manage the illness on their own. Schizophrenics' healthy desire to regain their sanity does not necessarily encourage them to confront their past psychotic experiences, but rather often leads them to a superficial denial of their illness and refusal to treatment. To support schizophrenics in this phase requires considerable patience and maturation on the part of doctors who are expected to serve as a *soyegi*, or splint. Concerning this phase, Shinkai (1986, 1988) seems to be cautious about presenting a rapid formulation, and only a few case reports and preliminary reports are available that demonstrate heated discussion and training within the school.

### Seikatsu-rinshou: *The Clinic for Social Life*

This therapy was started in 1958, with the aim of improving the quality of life for schizophrenics by means of all possible interventions, including rehabilitation and occupational therapy, as well as individual psychotherapy. According to Utena (1965), one of the founders of this method, *Seikatsu-rinshou* uses pragmatic knowledge founded upon empirical methodology. Its aim is to prevent rupture of the patient's actual life by reducing adverse events, and to accumulate experiences of overcoming difficulties in social adaptation. It is hoped that this method will bring about healing and maturation of the patient's personality. Instead of using traditional psychopathological terminology, this school has generated original terms to describe various aspects of the social coping and adaptation of schizophrenics. As for insight, awareness of dysfunction is looked upon as crucially important.

Schizophrenics' attitudes toward social adaptation are divided into active and passive types. It should be noted that this classification is derived from actual case management and not from any hypothetical background. The description of these attitudes comes from schizophrenic patients who struggled for social adaptation in Gunma, a rural city of Japan, during the 1960s, when the country was possessed by a fever for economic growth.

The patients of the *active* group are characterized by a strong desire to become independent and a tendency to complain continually about their social situation. Because they cannot leave their tasks to other people, their excessive efforts to manage by themselves sometimes cause conflicts in occupational settings. They are usually sensitive to criticism and cling to minor achievements that they can be proud of, such as promotions, licenses, or college diplomas.

The reason for this attitude is that they feel ashamed of the psychotic experience associated with their stay at the psychiatric hospital. According to Katoh et al. (1996), their desire for honor and prestige can be understood as a kind of compensation, although their goals may appear trivial in the eyes of ordinary people. Or else it may be a healthy wish of their intact selves to overcome the handicap caused by the illness. However, their coping style is so stereotyped and lacking in flexibility that they are often irritated by obstacles they may encounter. Because they cannot tolerate or conceal this irritation, it works against them. Combined with the rigid coping style itself, it causes their social adaptation to fail. Usually they become quite at a loss in those critical situations when they have to make a decision about how to behave in order to reduce social stress.

In contrast, the *passive* group is composed of patients who are socially withdrawn. Because they do not seem to be willing to seek social activities, they rarely experience disastrous interpersonal conflicts. Katoh et al. (1966), who examined the social life of 140 schizophrenics discharged from Gunma University Hospital from 1958 to 1962, reported that 71 of the 103 who could be traced belonged to the active type, 30 to the passive, and 2 to both. His study maintained that the main focus of intervention should be on the active group to prevent a collapse of the patients' social lives and a relapse of psychosis.

The main part of the clinical intervention consists of providing practical advice when patients cannot tolerate complaints deriving from basic inferiority feelings or when they either try to make inadequate decisions or cannot make any decision at all. It may be useful, for example, to help them understand how to cope with actual difficulties in their workplace or make sound decisions. Although promoting insight is not a direct aim of this method, the patients are encouraged to have insight into their social adaptation and its associated stresses. It is obviously regarded as desirable that schizo-phrenics become able to correct maladaptive aspects of their behaviors and make suit-able decisions by themselves, so that they can avoid social conflicts and reduce stress rather than merely obeying the advice prescribed by doctors. Yuasa (1972) writes that the aim of this method is to help people with schizophrenia cultivate their own wisdom in order to arrange or reform their actual living settings.

*Seikatsu-rinshou* is usually referred to as a branch of social psychiatry. However, this method should also be evaluated as an important and almost a unique Japanese con-tribution to the notion of social insight in schizophrenia—that is, the awareness of dys-function in social adaptation. This contribution is particularly valuable because it has been developed through clinical trials rather than through theoretical arguments of psychopathology. It has the advantage of using colloquial expressions to describe vari-ous aspects of schizophrenics' social coping styles, making it easier to communicate with patients. Until the present, a considerable part of the literature of this practice has been devoted to presenting clinical activities rather than examining clinical hypothe-ses. This task will be an important research theme for the coming generation.

## Insight in Clinical Settings

In this section three contemporary, empirically based studies on insight in schizophre-nia conducted in clinical settings are reviewed. All of them are ongoing and detailed results will be published elsewhere.

### *How Is Insight Viewed?*

We have seen that the topic of insight in schizophrenia has been eagerly discussed by a number of psychopathologists and clinicians. At the same time, it has been criticized for being superficially misused to imply the total incapacity of schizophrenics to make any reasonable judgment. Such a discrepancy in the clinical usage of the term leads us naturally to one question: what kind of attitudes do contemporary Japanese psychia-trists have toward this issue?

To survey this, the author has sent a questionnaire to 120 randomly selected psychi-atric sections of the 488 national and public hospitals in Japan and has received 55 responses at present. The items of the questionnaire are shown in table 11.1. Each item is answered on a 6-point scale, ranging from Definitely to Never. Insight is defined here by 5 dimensions: awareness of the need for treatment, being mentally ill, the abnor-mality of past psychotic experiences, subjective sufferings, and social difficulties. The first three items correspond to David's insight scale (David, 1990); the fourth derives from another study being conducted by the same author (see below), and the last from the work done by the *Seikatsu-rinshou* group. The definition of schizophrenia was not operationally determined, for the purpose of this survey was to examine the image of schizophrenia and insight held by Japanese clinicians in their actual clinical settings. The responders were asked to answer according to patients they had actually seen and were still treating.

All the responders were chiefs of the psychiatric sections of their respective hospitals. Their psychiatric careers varied from 3 to 42 years (mean 18.9). Their preferred diag-

TABLE 11.1 Items of the Questionnaire on Japanese Views of Insight in Schizophrenia

---

Answer the following with regard to the actual schizophrenics you are in the course of treating; use your most preferred definition of schizophrenia.

1. (POOR INSIGHT)   Does the concept of schizophrenia you use include lack of insight in the following five dimensions? (Only when one of the answers is definite should you skip the other questions that concern the same dimension.)

   a. Need for treatment
   b. Being mentally ill
   c. Abnormality of psychotic experiences
   d. Subjective suffering
   e. Social difficulties

2. (OPTIMISM)   Will schizophrenics gain insight in each of those five dimensions when appropriately treated?

3. (TREATMENT PRIORITY)   Is intervention promoting insight in each of those five dimensions important among all possible treatments for schizophrenics? Consider in the case of:

   a. Acute inpatient
   b. Acute outpatient
   c. Partial remission, inpatient
   d. Partial remission, outpatient
   e. Full remission, inpatient (long-stay patients)
   f. Full remission, outpatient

4. (INFLUENCE)   Is insight in those five dimensions influenced by any of the following factors?

   a. Pharmacotherapy
   b. Psychotherapy
   c. Social rehabilitation, day care
   d. Medical education of patient and family
   e. The quality of the initial interview of the treatment
   f. Inpatient's attitude of hospital staff

5. (Several questions about the responder's career, specialty in psychiatry, preferred definition of schizophrenia, etc.)

---

nostic concepts of schizophrenia were Schneider's first-rank symptoms (80%); Bleuler's basic symptoms (53%); negative symptoms (53%); Praecox Gefühl (bizarre social contact; described by Rümke, 1941) (42%); *DSM-III, DSM-III-R* (33%); and *ICD-9, ICD-10* (31%). One third specialized in psychopathology or psychotherapy.

The responders' views of insight in schizophrenia are shown in figure 11.1. Many psychiatrists estimated that schizophrenics show a considerable lack of insight in each of the five dimensions. Although the views in these five dimensions had a significant positive correlation ($p = .05$) to one another, their distribution patterns are not the same. The first three dimensions and the last two seem to form separate distribution groups, the peak of the former being nearer to the lack of insight pole than that of the latter. Despite such a relatively negative view of the presence of insight, the responses also showed a fairly optimistic view of the therapeutic possibility for improvement, a

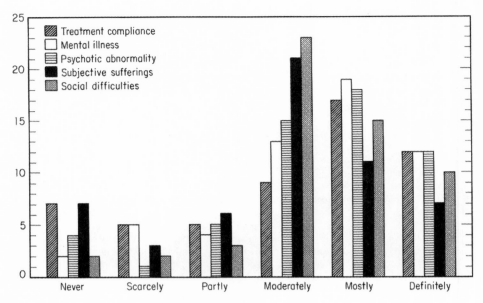

FIGURE 11.1  Insight in Schizophrenia Viewed by Japanese Psychiatrists (N = 55)

high priority placed on treatment toward that aim, and high expectations of influenc-ing insight through various factors. Interestingly, the poor insight scores in general had a significantly *positive* correlation with the scores for optimism, priority, and expecta-tion of influence.

These data may reveal that although Japanese psychiatrists on average have a rather strict view of the presence of insight in schizophrenia, or they underestimate the degree of the patients' insight as stated by Kondoh and colleagues (1985), they nevertheless believe in the possibility of improving it through various clinical inter-ventions, to which they give high priority in the clinical setting. This relatively nega-tive view of the presence of insight might be inherited from the classical psy-chopathology that still serves as the basic framework of Japanese psychiatry, or it may be a reflection of the fact that a majority of schizophrenics do show a lack of insight in a variety of ways (Carpenter, Strauss, & Bariko, 1974; Wilson, Ban, & Guy, 1986; Ama-dor, Strauss, Yale, & Gorman, 1991). However, lack of insight no longer seems to be regarded by the majority of Japanese psychiatrists as an inevitable attribute of schizo-phrenia leading to clinical pessimism. Despite the fact that we do not have any previ-ous data to compare, we can say that the long debates regarding this issue must have been rewarding if they have resulted in these positive attitudes toward clinical man-agement of insight in schizophrenia.

## How Is Insight Determined?

In the usual clinical setting patients feel they might be ill and seek treatment because they have become aware of certain painful or abnormal symptoms. Does the same apply to schizophrenic patients? Is there some correlation between awareness of symptoms and that of need for treatment and of being ill?

Two Japanese studies are currently being undertaken to examine the nature and determinants of insight in schizophrenia. Miyaoka et al. (1993) examined 40 DSM-III-R schizophrenics who had been so diagnosed for more than five years from first onset, and whose age varied from 40 to 60 years. Half were outpatients who had not been hospitalized for more than one year, while the others were inpatients who had been treated in closed psychiatric wards for more than one successive year. Psychopathology was measured by the Positive and Negative Symptom Scale (PANSS), while insight was evaluated by the researchers' own scale invented for clinical use in Japan. This scale aimed to measure the awareness of being mentally ill and the recognition of symptoms including not only psychotic but also neurotic, somatic, and drug-related side effects. This recognition was assessed according to whether the patients regarded it as a symptom of illness and whether they believed that it required counselling or pharmacotherapy.

The total score from the insight scale varied significantly between inpatient and outpatient groups, the former being the poorer. The item scores for recognition of illness and the need for pharmacotherapy were also poorer in the former, while those of the appropriate understanding of the illness and the need for counselling did not differ. A sound awareness of delusion and hallucination was maintained more often in the outpatient group, which, however, did not always correlate with an awareness of the need for treatment.

Kim et al. (1994) are conducting research on the correlation between subjective experience and insight in schizophrenia. To examine the subjective symptoms, an original scale was invented because the ordinary symptom-lists for schizophrenia do not give sufficient emphasis to subjective symptoms. As Strauss (1989a, 1989b) has pointed out, the symptoms that concern the subjective experience of schizophrenia, such as delusion and hallucination, are based upon the judgment of the observers and thus cannot be regarded as pure descriptions of subjective symptoms.

The preliminary subjects were 22 ICD-10 schizophrenics, 10 males and 12 females, 9 of whom were outpatients while the remaining 13 were inpatients. Three dimensions of insight were measured by David's scale: the need for treatment, awareness of illness, and awareness of the psychotic features of experienced delusion. Other psychopathology was measured by the Brief Psychiatric Rating Scale (BPRS), the Scale of the Assessment of Negative Symptoms (SANS), and the Hamilton Depression Scale (HDS; through a structured interview devised by Williams, 1990, with permission).

The data revealed no significant positive correlation between any dimension of insight and any item or the total score of the subjective experience scale, BPRS, SANS, or HDS. A weak negative correlation was detected between the total insight score and the overall BPRS and HDS. Significant negative correlations were found between insight and the HDS items of suicidal ideation, depersonalization, and paranoia—probably because these depressive symptoms deprive the patients of a sound self-monitoring ability and the motivation for treatment. Although the data are preliminary, it seems unlikely that insight in David's sense has a significantly positive correlation to subjective experience—in other words, the awareness of subjective suffering.

The two studies discussed above suggest one common finding: insight in schizophrenia, in the sense of an awareness of the need for treatment, does not always correlate with an awareness of the presence of psychotic, neurotic, or subjective symptoms. The latter can be included in the definition of insight: insight of symptoms. What, then, determines insight of the need for treatment and makes people with schizophrenia come to outpatient clinics? Also, what will insight into symptoms bring about if not insight for the need of treatment? A single answer cannot be expected for these questions, which may include some cultural aspects, whose Japanese components will perhaps be clarified through more detailed investigations in the future.

## Conclusions

Like other fields of science, modern Japanese psychiatry was founded upon knowledge imported from Europe that reached this country during the late 19th century. Later, considerable efforts were made to understand the new perspective brought by European psychiatry and to incorporate it into Japanese culture. The issue of insight came to be known to Japanese psychiatrists as Jaspers's assertion that schizophrenics lacked insight into their illness. Insight was very strictly defined by Jaspers to include a precise and reasonable understanding of the disease. Gradually some Japanese psychiatrists started to criticize this view, using their clinical experience, such that a strict definition of insight missed various important attitudes that schizophrenics assumed toward their illness. A number of Japanese psychiatrists promoted other aspects of insight in schizophrenia, challenging the old, pessimistic view of this illness.

It is a regrettable fact that the rapid construction of psychiatric hospitals urged by the government in the 1960s resulted in a superficial popularization of the notion of lack of insight, used by some psychiatrists as a quasi-definition of schizophrenia or as an excuse for involuntary admission. In response to severe criticism, the current mental health act enforced more open and socially oriented treatment of psychiatric patients, as well as establishing a supervisory system to guarantee patients their basic human rights. In this stream of change, the issue of insight has attracted broad attention from contemporary psychopathologists and clinicians. Thus, insight in schizophrenia, which is dependent upon the relationship between patient and doctor as Kajitani (1983) stated, also reflects the extent to which psychiatrists are concerned about community treatment and the basic human rights of schizophrenics.

Different aspects of insight have been pointed out by several Japanese psychiatrists, especially those engaged in clinical psychotherapy of schizophrenia using a particular sensitivity to other people's feelings that is inherent in Japanese culture. Yasunaga's (1988) argument about the sense of deportment derives from the 15th-century Japanese literature of Noh theater. This sense signifies the insight into loss of balance in one's mental and physical activities as a whole, and may include awareness of the total therapeutic situation, which can be promoted through metaphorical rather than analytical suggestions. Shinkai (1986, 1988) focuses upon a subtle micropsychotic change during clinical interviews, helping schizophrenics become aware of that change so they can develop insight into their past psychotic experiences. Utena (1965) distracted several social codes, such as shame, self-esteem, or competency, which are closely related to the social conflicts Japanese schizophrenics experience in the recovery process. This argument concerns a kind of awareness of the dysfunction in social adaptation, with improvement expected through practical advice for resolving actual social conflicts.

Although most of these practices have been conducted separately, not under a single rubric of insight, they seem to share the characteristic of not viewing schizophrenia as an endogenous disease process but rather as a mixture of social and interpersonal transactions. These practitioners do not deny a biological hypothesis of schizophrenia and they use antipsychotic medications. Nor do they hesitate to regard schizophrenia as a disease. However, the plausible assumption that there is some biological basis for schizophrenia does not mean that clinical manifestations of this illness are a result of neural disease in the same way that paralysis is caused by cerebral lesion. There may exist modifiers between basic biological findings and the manifestation of schizophrenia as troubled human transaction. It is possible that, in some cases, several modifiers have even stronger determinative power for the clinical appearance of schizophrenia than do a biological disturbance postulated to initiate the disease process. To this author's eyes, such a view is held by a number of, if not a majority of, Japanese psychiatrists. These doctors conduct their treatment of schizophrenics not only by counting symptoms and selecting drugs but also by focusing on the *patients'* motivation for treatment and awareness of illness, interpersonal conflicts, and social handicaps. Insight, or self-monitoring and -regulatory function of self, could be one of those strong modifiers, although some schizophrenics seem to lack it, not because of a kind of agnosia caused by the illness but because of some psychological defenses. Why, then, do they hesitate to use this precious mental function? Is it because of the psychological trauma during psychosis, the social handicap and stigma due to the illness, or the overwhelming power and authority of medical staff? The answer should be closely related to the cultural codes of each patient and, in most cases in Japan, to the preference of the clinicians of what kind of method to use and goal to set.

Such an ambiguity highlights the importance of clinical studies of insight in Japan, where the promotion of insight will play a significant role in therapeutic settings in favor of more open treatment for schizophrenia. Some preliminary studies in this country indicate that insight in schizophrenia is composed of several *independent* dimensions, such as the motivation for treatment, the awareness of delusion and hallucination, and the awareness of subjective suffering. Some of the confusion in past Japanese discussions of insight can be explained as a result of confounding these different dimensions. For example, the absence of a differentiation between awareness of psychosis and that of treatment need has resulted in superficial use of Jaspers's notion of lack of insight as the excuse for involuntary admission of schizophrenics. It is hoped that, through further clarification of robust components of insight in schizophrenia, we will be able to evaluate the phenomena of insight more precisely and integrate various clinical attempts for its promotion. The diversity of views about insight that have been aggregated in this book should encourage us toward greater investigation of effective interventions for schizophrenia.

*Acknowledgments*   I wish to thank Dr. Shinkai and Dr. Kobayashi for their detailed advice in translating some basic concepts of *soyegi* therapy. To our pleasure, a more detailed English review of *soyegi* therapy will come out in the near future. I also thank Dr. Miyaoka and his colleagues for permitting me to look into their valuable ongoing study. I learned a lot from comparing their study with our own, the results of which were most helpful in writing this chapter.

*References*

Amador, X. F., Strauss, D. H., Yale, S. A. (1991). Awareness of illness in schizophrenia. *Schizophrenia Bulletin, 17*, 113–132.
Bitter, I., Jaeger, J., Agdeppa, J. (1989). Subjective symptoms: Part of the negative syndrome of schizophrenia? *Psychopharmacology Bulletin, 25*, 180–184.
Bleuler, E. (1911). Dementia Praecox oder Gruppe der schizophrenien. Leipzig: Franz Deuticke.
Carpenter, W. T., Strauss, J. S., & Bartko, J. J. (1974). The diagnosis and understanding of schizophrenia. Part 1: Use of signs and symptoms for the identification of schizophrenic patients. *Schizophrenia Bulletin, 1*, 37–49.
Dagonet, H. (1881). Conscience et aliénation mentale. *Annales Medico Psychologiques, 39*, 368–397.
David, A. S. (1990). Insight and psychosis. British Journal of Psychiatry, *156*, 798–808.
Doi, (1961). The insight into illness. *Psychiat. Neurol. Jap., 63*, 4–11.
Heilbronner, K. (1904). Über Krankheitseinsicht. *Allg. Zeitschr. Psychiat., 58*, 608–631.
Ishikawa, K. (1963). Über Krankheitseinsicht der Schizophrenien und neurose. *Seishin-igaku, 6*, 105–110.
Jaspers, K. (1913). *Allgemeine psychopathologie*. Berling: Springer-Verlag.
Kajitani, T. (1963). Zum Wesen und Erfassen der Krankheitseinsicht. *Seishin-igaku, 5*, 131–140.
Katoh, T., Tajima, A., Yuasa, S. (1966). Characteristics of the social life of discharged schizophrenic patients. *Psychiat. Neurol. Jap., 68*, 1076–1088.
Kim, Y., Sakamoto, K., Kamo, T., Sakamura, Y., & Miyaoka, H. (1997). Insight and clinical correlates in schizophrenia. *Comprehensive Psychiatry*, in press.
Klerman, G. (1991). An American perspective on the conceptual approaches to psychopathology. In: H. McCleiland, & A. Kerr (Eds.), *Concepts of mental disorder* (pp. 74–83). London: Gaskell.
Kohut, H. (1959). Introspection, empathy, and psychoanalysis. *Journal of the American Psychoanalytic Association, 7*, 459–483.
Kondoh, H., Iwakata, T., Onizawa, T., Musha, M., & Ohira, T. (1985). Byoushiki-ronno shuhen [On insight in schizophrenia]. *Psychiat. Neurol. Jap., 87*, 114.
Kumakura, N. (1987). Some considerations on "paternalism" and "self-determination" in psychosis. *Psychiat. Neurol. Jap., 89*, 593–614.
Matsumoto, M. (1988). Eine Kritische Überlegung zum Begriff der Krankheitseinsicht. *Seishinka-chiryogaku, 3*, 25–31.
Meyer-Gross, W. (1920). Über die Stellungnahme zur abgelaufenen akuten Psychose. *Zeitschr ges. Neurol. Psychiat., 60*, 160–212.
Miyaoka, H., Sakai, T., Tatsumi, M., Nozaki, S., Yoshimura, Y., Ota, A., Tadokoro, C., Idei, T., & Kamijima, K. (1993). The assessment of insight of schizophrenic patients. *Proceedings of the Japanese Society for Psychiatric Diagnosis 13*, 718–719.
Nakatani, Y. (1989). Schizophrenia and "insight into disease": Some problems of the terminology. *Jap. J. Clin. Psychiat., 18*, 11–16.
Nakayasu, N. (1988). "Loss of insight into disease" as a method of descriptive phenomenology. *Seishinka-chiryogaku, 3*, 33–42.
Nishizono, M. (1963). Psychodynamics of "Krankheitseinsicht." *Seishin-igaku, 5*, 111–119.
Ohashi, H. (1963). Anosognosia: denial of illness. *Seishin-igaku, 5*, 123–130.

Pick, A. (1882). Uber Krankheitsbewusstsein in psychischen Krankheiten: Eine historisch-klinische Studie. *Arch. Psychiat. Nervenkr.*, *13*, 518–581.

Rümke, H. (1941). *Ned Tijdschr Gneeskd 81*, 4516–4521.

Schwing, (1940). *Ein Weg zur Seele des Geisteskranken*. Zurich: Rascher-Verlag.

Shimazaki, T., & Abe, T. (1963). Ein Aspekt der "Krankheitseinsicht" in der Schizophrenie. *Seishin-igaku, 5*, 97–103.

Shinkai, Y. (1986). Psychotherapy for schizophrenia, its retrospect and status quo. *Seishinka-chiryogaku, 1*, 595–604.

Shinkai, Y. (1988). About the attitude of schizophrenics to their illness from the viewpoint of Soyegi. *3*, 51–60.

Strauss, J. S. (1989a). Subjective experiences of schizophrenia: Toward a new dynamic psychiatry II. *Schizophrenia Bulletin, 15*, 179–187.

Strauss, J. S. (1989b). Mediating processes in schizophrenia: Towards a new dynamic psychiatry. *British Journal of Psychiatry* (suppl. 22–8).

Sullivan, H. S. (1953). *The interpersonal theory of psychiatry*. New York: W.W. Norton.

Utena, (1965). Tenkanki ni tatsu bunretsubyo no chiryou [New perspective of the treatment of schizophrenia]. *Kitakanto-igaku, 15*, 327–331.

Williams, J. B. (1990). Structured interview guide for the Hamilton rating scales. In P. Bech, A. Coppen (Eds.), *The Hamilton rating scales*. Berlin: Springer-Verlag.

Wilson, W. H., Ban, T. A., & Guy, W. (1986). Flexible system criteria in chronic schizophrenia. *Comprehensive Psychiatry, 27*, 259–265.

Yasunaga, H. (1988). From "self-judgement of illness" to "awareness of deportment." *Seishinka-chiryogaku, 3*, 43–50.

Yuasa, S. (1972). Seikatsu-rinshou kara mita bunretsubyou kanja [Schizophrenics viewed from the clinic for social life]. In T. Doi (Ed.), *Bunretsubyou no seishinbyouri* [Psychopathology of schizophrenia], vol. 1 (pp. 19–31). Tokyo: University Press.

# PART IV

*Insight
and
Behavior*

# 12

ALEC BUCHANAN
SIMON WESSELY

# Delusions, Action, and Insight

Do psychotic patients act on their delusions? Not in the opinion of Bleuler (1924):

> They really do nothing to attain their goal; the emperor and the pope help to manure the fields; the queen of heaven irons the patients' shirts or besmears herself and the table with saliva. (p. 392)

Bleuler's contemporaries shared his view (Kant, 1927; Jaspers, 1963). Since then, those writers who have not ignored the issue have argued that delusional action is rare (Anderson & Trethowan, 1973; Fish, 1974; Merskey, 1980; Slater & Roth, 1969). We are unaware of any major text or paper suggesting that acting on delusions is a common occurrence.

There are few data to support this conclusion, however, and some suggestions that it may not be correct. In a study of pretrial prisoners, Taylor (1985) noted associations between delusions and violent offending and between violent behavior and the presence of passivity experiences. In Gibbens' (1958) review of 115 cases of homicide admitted to New Jersey State Hospital, one third of insane murderers had well-structured delusional motives for their crimes. And Lanzkron (1963) reported that 40% of insane homicide occurred "as offspring of a delusional system."

These studies have concerned prisoners, in many ways an atypical group. We have recently been part of a team[1] that undertook a study of acting on delusions in a general psychiatric population. The study investigated the prevalence and phenomenological correlates of acting on delusional beliefs and has been described in detail elsewhere (Buchanan et al., 1993; Wessely et al., 1993; Taylor et al., 1994). The purpose of this chapter is to discuss some theoretical aspects of acting on delusions, to review the results of the study, and to discuss the relationship between delusional action and insight.

What form might this relationship take? One possibility is that the level of delusional action falls as the degree of insight increases. If I have a suspicion that my persecutory ideas are the result of illness, I may be less likely to defend myself. On the other hand, it may be that some delusional actions have the effect of challenging the veracity of the delusion itself, as when a jealous man rifles through his wife's handbag and finds nothing incriminating. In such cases delusional action might be expected to be associated with increased levels of insight. Our group's research sheds some light on these issues, which will be discussed later in the chapter. First, however, an attempt will be made to outline some theoretical aspects of the relationships among abnormal beliefs, action, and insight.

## Theoretical Considerations

This section will first discuss the role of normal beliefs in determining behavior. While essential to the discussion that follows, this is not an area that has been extensively examined by psychiatric researchers; debate has focused principally on information drawn from the fields of psychology and philosophy. The second part of the section will review the various types of delusional belief that have been implicated in action. Among the many factors that may affect the likelihood of a psychotic patient's acting on a delusional belief—factors such as personality and previous experience—will be elements of the psychosis distinct from the belief itself. One of these is insight, while perceptual changes, motor symptoms, and cognitive functioning are others. These elements will be reviewed in the third part of the section.

Mention must also be made of what will not be discussed in this review of the theoretical aspects of delusional action. A considerable literature now exists pertaining to the nature of delusions, much of which is discussed elsewhere in this volume. Principal-components analyses by workers such as Kendler, Glazer, and Morgenstern (1983) and Garety and Hemsley (1987) have identified dimensions such as conviction and preoccupation. These dimensions bear some similarity to the criteria for delusional beliefs described by reviewers such as Kraupl Taylor (1983). It might be expected that each of these dimensions would affect substantially the likelihood of a belief being acted upon, but to the authors' knowledge, little research was conducted in this area prior to that described in the next section. For the purposes of this paper, the definition of delusion will follow the criteria suggested by reviewers such as Kraupl Taylor and Mullen (1979)—namely, that they are false beliefs, held with conviction and regarded by the subject as self-evident, which are not amenable to reason and inherently unlikely in content.

### Beliefs and Behavior

A review of the link between abnormal belief and behavior demands some discussion of the role of normal beliefs in the genesis of action. In the 1940s and 1950s, early behaviorists (e.g., Hull, 1943; Guthrie, 1952) opposed the then widespread notion that action must be explained in terms of purpose. They argued that human behavior could be better explained in terms of receptor impulses and movements. The elucidation of these primary principles would in turn allow a rigorous definition of terms such as *purpose* and *intention*. In the words of Hull,

> The present approach does not deny the motor reality of purposive acts (as opposed to movements), of intelligence, of insight, of goals, of intents, of stirrings or of value; on the contrary, we insist upon the genuineness of these forms of behaviour. We hope ultimately to show the logical right to the use of such concepts by deducting them as secondary principles from more elementary objective primary principles. (Hull, 1943, pp. 25–26)

While beliefs are clearly important if behavior is to be explained in terms of purpose, their role is less apparent when this behavior is explained in terms of primary principles. Hull was clear that purposive behavior could be derived from postulates involving only stimulus and movement.

The role of goal-directed thought was similarly dismissed by Guthrie (1952), who suggested that thinking, like action, was a product of conditioning and tended to occur when action was blocked. These authors aspired to a science that was more rigorous and quantitative. As Hull wrote in 1951,

> The continuous quantitative use of relevant postulates and corollaries will hasten the elimination of errors and the day when mammalian behaviour will take its place among the recognised quantitative systematic sciences. (p. 2)

But it was not the advocacy of a rigorous scientific method that concerned other authors; rather, it was the theory that lay behind the writings of Guthrie and Hull. Keith Campbell (1970) noted that behaviorists had placed the mind not behind an action but in the behavior itself and hence, worryingly for a philosopher, omitted the casual element in mental concepts. In the second half of the 20th century, philosophers' arguments have followed two related themes, both of which allow a pivotal role for belief in the explanation of action.

The first has been expanded by Papineau (1978), who argues that the reasons behind an action involve, first, a desire and, second, a belief that the action will contribute to the satisfaction of that desire. He acknowledges that everyday explanations of action commonly invoke only a desire or a belief, but he argues that both are in fact required; we mention only that part of the cause that is most surprising, least generally known, or most morally significant. The second theme has been described by Charles Taylor. Taylor (1964) explains behavior in terms of Aristotelian teleology; that is, he argues that our present use of the terms *action* and *behavior* do not allow them to be broken down into units of stimulus and response, but require an explanation of behavior in terms of its purpose. Thus, he differs from Papineau in regarding behavior as "pulled" into existence by its purpose, as opposed to "pushed" into existence by the belief and desire of its agent. Taylor's teleological explanation of human behavior clearly implies certain knowledge or beliefs on the part of the subject as well as a desire to act. The author refers to the Canute view of those who reject purposive explanations of action and is graphic in his description of the logical consequences of behaviorist theory,

> The area in which we can attribute responsibility, deal out praise or blame, or mete out reward or punishment, will steadily diminish until in the limiting case, nothing will be

left; the courts will be closed or become institutes of human engineering, moral discourse will be relegated to the lumber-room of history. (pp. 42–43)

The emotive quality of Taylor's plea is not a new feature of the debate. In the 16th century, the use of teleological arguments to demonstrate the existence of a deity led Francis Bacon to compare teleological explanations to vestal virgins: "They are dedicated to God, and are barren" (quoted by Papineau, 1990).

Even as they were written, the views of Hull and Guthrie were not universally held. William Hunter (1930) referred to the importance of symbolic processes in influencing people's instinctive behavior, invoking a model more cognitive than that allowed by some behaviorists. In 1932, Krechevsky published his claim to have found empirical evidence that rats running mazes formed hypotheses to assist them in solving problems. In the second half of the 20th century, writers in medicine and psychology have been more prepared to entertain a cognitive view of behavior where a subject's knowledge and beliefs assume a greater role. Austin (1956–7) described some of the elements in his "machinery of action" as consciousness, voluntariness, self-control, knowledge, and foresight. Fulford (1989) developed this theme in *Moral Theory and Medical Practice*, writing "in the case of raising my arm, what has to be specified, in addition to the state of motion of my arm, is my purpose in raising it" (p. 112). Psychologists such as Spence (1956) and Mowrer (1960) still draw heavily on a view of learning based on Pavlovian conditioning, but Mowrer's references to subjects' learning to be afraid and learning what to do make it clear that he gives greater weight to the cognitive processes of his subjects than did his predecessors. McGinn (1979), developing the work of Davidson (1971), divides bodily movements into active and passive. Action is based on reasons and reasons for actions are based on a combination of desires and beliefs; in McGinn's words, "desire without belief is blind, belief without desire is purposeless" (p. 25). He adds several qualifications to this description of action. First, he argues that desires and beliefs exist in a dynamic state in the conscious mind, and that interaction occurs between them: "Beliefs must then be reckoned in the light of the pattern of desires" (p. 39). Second, he argues that no general law of action can be derived from this framework; "what was sufficient to make me cross the road on a certain occasion will almost certainly not be repeated" (p. 39). Finally, he considers that belief and desire are not in themselves sufficient to produce the will to act and that this will is dependent on what he calls *noticings*, internal or external cues that precipitate action.

In the second half of the 20th century, the influence of purely behaviorist explanations of human action has diminished. Recent medical and psychological writing has focused more on the influence of belief on human action, and this reflects the tenor of philosophical writing on the subject. The role of beliefs in behaviorist theory is vague, and this may go some way to explaining the lack of research in the psychological literature into actions based on delusions.

### Delusions Implicated in Action

The literature pertaining to the behavioral consequences of delusional beliefs will now be reviewed. Ideally, such a review would be informed by epidemiological data providing information as to the likelihood of a particular type of delusion being acted upon. Unfortunately, most reports in this area are anecdotal and allow no such estimate of risk. In the absence of such data, reference will be made, where the original literature allows, to descriptions of phenomenology to illuminate the link between abnormal belief and behavior.

*Delusions of Persecution*    Reports of actions based on delusional beliefs most frequently concern persecutory delusions; often these reports focus on violence inflicted on others. On January 20, 1843, Daniel M'Naghten, apparently under the impression that he was attacking the prime minister, Sir Robert Peel, fired at and mortally wounded Edward Drummond, who was Sir Robert's private secretary. At his trial it emerged that M'Naghten believed he was the victim of a conspiracy and that he was being followed by spies sent by Catholic priests with the aid of the Tories, of whom Peel was the leader. At his trial he stated,

> The Tories in my native city have compelled me to do this. . . . They have accused me of crimes of which I am not guilty; they do everything in their power to harass and persecute me; in fact, they wish to murder me. (Rollin, 1977, p. 92)

M'Naghten was found not guilty and the M'Naghten Rules, which govern the use of an insanity defense in British courts, were the direct outcome of his case. In this century many authors have recorded persecutory delusions in mentally ill offenders, but often make only vague reference to the motive for the crime. Bach-y-rita (1974) and Bach-y-rita and Veno (1974), examining 62 violent prisoners, found 13 who demonstrated "subtle delusional systems" and who "warranted a diagnosis of paranoid schizophrenia." Green (1981), looking at 58 male homicidal patients in Broadmoor Hospital, reported that in 27 cases the act of killing "appeared to be a response" to the patients' persecutory beliefs. Shore, Filson, and Johnson (1988) and Shore et al. (1989) examined the subsequent criminal records of mentally ill people arrested near the White House, in many cases trying to see the president. They found that among those with no record of violent behavior, persecutory delusions were significantly associated with future violence. They gave no further details as to the nature of the delusions.

Other authors give fuller descriptions. Maas, Prakash, Hollender, and Regan (1984) describe the case of a man who killed both parents, claiming that they had tried to kill his children by drowning them in battery acid. Reviewing the records of 10 men charged with patricide, Cravens, Campion, Rotholc, Covan, and Cravens (1985) found 4 cases where the father was considered by the patient to pose threats of "physical of psychological annihilation." Mawson (1985) found 14 patients with delusions of poisoning in a case note study at Broadmoor Hospital and "in all but one the symptom seemed an important antecedent factor to serious violence." In a study of 15 matricidal men, Campion et al. (1985) refer to a schizophrenic patient who killed his mother because he was convinced that she was a sadist who tortured him. Other authors have reported actions based on persecutory beliefs in association with Capgras delusions (Crane, 1976; Weinstock, 1976; Christodoulou, 1978; Romanik & Snow, 1984; Tomison & Donovan, 1988); De Pauw and Szulecka (1988) report that a patient attacked her mother, believing that every time her mother put on her glasses she changed into a local woman whom she disliked intensely. Hafner and Boker (1973) found that 8% of their sample of 263 violent schizophrenics exhibited "paranoid feelings of malaise" and felt that these patients were especially likely to act on their delusions when they perceived an immediate threat to their lives or when persecutory beliefs were accompanied by bodily hallucinations or delusions of bodily harm.

Persecutory delusions have also been described in cases of self-harm, but here again the degree to which the delusional belief motivates the act is often unclear. In some cases, such as that described by Mintz (1964), where a cook on board ship cooked and ate his index finger in an attempt to "rise above his persecutors in the way that Christ had," it is difficult to see any logical link. In other cases, such as those of ocular self-mutilation described by Shore, Anderson, and Cutler (1978); Shore (1979); and Yang, Brown, and Magargal (1981) or of auto-castration described by Mendez, Keily, and Morrow (1972), the link between persecutory belief and action seems vague. Blacker and Wong (1963) are more specific, describing the case of a man who castrated himself believing that evil spirits were using his body to perform unnatural acts. Standage, Moore, and Cole (1974) describe a case of genital self-mutilation in a female schizophrenic who believed that the men in her community were going to sexually molest her. Fire setting, eating, and hospital attendance have also been claimed to be influenced by persecutory delusions. Virkkunen (1974) found that 3 out of 30 cases of arson committed by schizophrenics represented an attempt to escape persecutors. In 1911, Bleuler had described the case of woman refusing to drink milk because she believed it was poisoned, and Lyketsos, Paterakis, Beis, and Lyketsos (1985) have described cases where the eating habits of chronic schizophrenics have been influenced by similar fears. Hutchesson and Volans (1989) have described patients whose persecutory delusions led them to attend hospitals with unsubstantiated complaints of being poisoned.

*Delusions of Jealousy and Grandiose Delusions*    The propensity of jealous delusions to be acted upon in a manner dangerous to others has been described by Shepherd (1961) and Mowat (1966). Gillies (1965) described the case of a schizophrenic who murdered his wife, telling his psychiatrist, "a mysterious power told me she was being unfaithful." More recently, Hafner and Boker (1973) noted delusions of love and jealousy in 11.2% of their sample of violent schizophrenics as against 1.4% of nonviolent schizophrenic controls. Of the 14 patients at Broadmoor with delusions of poisoning described by Mawson (1985), 6 also had delusions of jealousy.

Actions based upon grandiose delusions were described in 1823 by John Haslam. Shortly after the New Bethlem Hospital was built in St George's Fields in London, Haslam described the case of Thomas Lloyd, whose confidence in his madrigal and linguistic abilities led him to dance and sing in public and address foreign visitors in miserable French. In the presence of a hypomanic affect, however, it becomes debatable whether such phenomena should be attributed to the mood state or to the delusional belief. Kraines (1957) wrote that

> the manic patient who says that he is the son of God is not expressing a delusion of symbolic significance as would be true in schizophrenic thinking, but has merely left unsaid the feelings that he is superior, that he is capable of undertaking any enterprise, that he is superior enough to be as powerful as the poetic concept of "Son of God." (pp. 280–281)

Should such a patient attempt to walk on water, it is not clear whether this would occur as a consequence of his belief or his mood. This point will be returned to in the discussion of drive, motivation, and affect.

*Delusions of Passivity, Ill Health, or Bodily Change*    The influence of delusions of passivity on behavior was alluded to by Tomison and Donovan (1988) in their description of a 23-year-old man who attacked two others with a Stanley knife, but no details were given. Two studies of matricidal men (Campion et al., 1985; Green, 1981) have also mentioned passivity, but in association with command hallucinations. Planansky and Johnston (1977) are more explicit. Looking at 59 male schizophrenics who had attacked others or made verbal threats to kill, they identified 9 cases where the subject "had to attack against their will, as if directed by others or by an impersonal force." Delusions of passivity have also been described in cases of self-mutilation (Rosen & Hoffman, 1972; Sweeney & Zamecnik, 1981); Shore et al. (1978) describe the case of a man who enucleated both of his eyes, believing that a force had overpowered him and had taken control of his actions.

Delusions of ill health or bodily change have been described by Green (1981) in matricidal men and by D'Orban and O'Connor (1989) in women who kill their parents. Jones (1965) studied 13 chronic schizophrenic patients with stereotypies. One of his cases touched his ear repeatedly, explaining that it controlled the pumping of his blood. Hafner and Boker (1973) considered that delusions of bodily harm, when linked with persecutory delusions, were associated with violence in schizophrenics. Delusions of bodily change leading to self-harm were described in 1928 by Lewis, while Beilin (1953) reported the case of a Polish laborer who amputated his penis, claiming that there had been a change in his body contour and that he was assuming the form of a woman. Sweeney and Zamecnik (1981), reviewing predictors of self-mutilation in patients with schizophrenia, described instances of patients acting on beliefs that their blood needed to be cleansed or that a limb required surgical investigation.

*De Clerambault's Syndrome and Capgras; Delusions of Guilt*    De Clerambault (1942), in his original description of the eponymous syndrome, quoted by Goldstein (1987), included a description of a man who repeatedly struck his ex-wife in public. Goldstein reviewed 7 cases of erotomania and found that all had acted on their delusions, several to the extent of making physical assaults. Enoch, Trethowan, and Barker (1967) and Taylor, Mahendra, and Gunn (1983) both emphasized the possibility of physical assaults consequent upon the imagined infatuation, but a recent review referring to the "spectre of dangerousness" in de Clerambault's syndrome has concluded that "the evidence that it usually represents anything more than an apparition remains unconvincing" (Bowden, 1990). Capgras syndrome has been linked with violent behavior in several case reports (Weinstock, 1976; Crane, 1976; Szulecka, 1988; Tomison & Donovan, 1988; Silva, Leong, Weinstock, & Boyer, 1989); Romanik and Snow (1984) described the case of a 57-year-old woman who pointed a loaded gun at two meter readers, believing that one of them was a homosexual who had been impersonating her by wearing a mask since he was 8; he had acted like a prostitute and sullied her reputation. Fishbain (1987) attempted to quantify the frequency of Capgras delusions, but his paper highlights the methodological problem that Capgras delusions are usually reported only when attention is drawn to them by violent behavior.

Reports of delusions of guilt associated with behavior usually involve self-harm. Numerous examples exist in the literature of such an association in depression (e.g., Albert, Burns, & Scheie, 1965) and even mania (Hartmann, 1925), and in depression the frequency of suicide attempts has been shown to correlate with delusional ideation (Miller & Chabrier, 1988). In schizophrenia, MacLean and Robertson (1976) described the case of a man who enucleated his own eye when preoccupied with his "sins." Numerous reports exist of self-inflicted eye injuries (Westmeyer & Serpass, 1972; Shore et al., 1978; Crowder, Gross, Heiser, & Crowder, 1979) and genital self-mutilation (Beilin & Gruenberg, 1948; Greilsheimer & Groves, 1979; Waugh, 1986) in the presence of delusions of guilt that do not appear to be mood congruent.

*Religious and Sexual Delusions*    Delusions with religious or sexual themes are common in psychiatry and similar themes are evident among those delusions that are acted upon. Witherspoon, Feist, Morris, and Feist (1989), reviewing the literature on self-inflicted eye injuries, found that 34 out of 85 patients gave religious reasons for their action. Often these were associated with delusions of guilt. Waugh (1986) describes a schizophrenic man who severed his testicles with a razor blade, stating that he felt evil and that self-castration was the only way to gain forgiveness. In other cases, religious beliefs in themselves seem to have motivated an act of self-harm. Kushner (1967) quotes a schizophrenic who was "sure that he had castrated himself in search of purification and not because of feelings of guilt." In many cases, the religious motivation is described in very general terms (Gorin, 1964; Anaclerio & Wicker, 1970; Tapper, Bland, & Danyluk, 1979; Crowder et al., 1979; Sweeney & Zamecnik, 1981); Tenzer and Orozco (1970) describe the case of a woman who removed her own tongue after receiving a message from God that "duty demanded it." In other cases, the motivation seems more specific. Shore (1979) describes a patient who was found with a pencil lodged in his right eye, who quoted Matthew (5:29, "And if they right eye offend thee, pluck it out, and cast it from thee, for it is profitable for thee that one of thy members should perish, and not that thy whole body should be cast into hell." Greilsheimer and Groves (1979) describes a case of genital self-mutilation invoking a similar passage of Matthew 18:7–9. Waugh (1986) describes a man who castrated himself in response to a later passage in Matthew 19:12, "There are eunuches made so by men and there are eunuches who have made themselves that way for the sake of the Kingdom of Heaven." A religious component is frequently present in delusionally based acts that harm others (Maas et al., 1984); Campion et al. (1985) report the case of a 23-year-old man who killed his mother, believing she was the devil. Sexual ideation was present in the motivation of 21 out of 85 cases of ocular self-mutilation reviewed by Witherspoon et al. (1989). Frequently associated with guilt in such cases (e.g., MacLean & Robertson, 1976; Crowder et al., 1979), such ideation may also be implicated when the harm is directed at others. Cravens et al. (1985) described homosexual delusions focused on the father in 3 out of their 10 cases of patricide.

## Other Psychotic Phenomena Affecting Action

In the cases described, a delusional belief is an important contributor to the psychotic individual's course of action. In many cases, however, the belief in question was held for a considerable period before being acted upon. And many patients hold similar beliefs without doing anything about them. As mentioned in the discussion of theoretical considerations, McGinn (1979) has argued that, in addition to a belief itself, *desire* and *noticings* are required to explain an action. It is possible to find equivalents for these terms in psychiatric phenomenology and hence use McGinn's model as a framework to investigate delusional action? This section will consider those elements of psychosis that affect the likelihood of a belief influencing a patient's behavior.

*Insight*    As discussed in the beginning of this chapter, insight might be expected to influence the likelihood of a patient's acting on his or her delusions. A persecuted man might be less likely to take defensive measures if he had a suspicion that his persecutory beliefs were part of a psychiatric illness. Little research has been conducted in this area. Roback and Abramowitz (1979) studied the behavior of schizophrenics in hospitals and found that patients with a greater level of insight were rated as better adjusted behaviorally on 9 out of 12 measures. Van Putten, Crumpton, and Yale (1976), Lin, Spiga, and Fortsch (1979), and Bartko, Herczeg, and Zador (1988) all found that compliance with treatment was improved in patients who were rated as exhibiting more insight. The principal methodological problem with all four studies is that decreased insight and behavioral disturbance could both be indicators of the severity of a patient's illness. The patients of Roback and Abramowitz who were insightful and behaviorally adjusted may have been less ill, and the subjects in the other three studies may have possessed insight and complied with medication for the same reason. In any case, influencing behavior in general is not the same as influencing actions based on delusions.

*Perceptual Changes*    Foremost among these elements may be the perceptual changes associated with schizophrenia. These will be examined with regard to two areas—namely, the perception of form and the perception of emotion. Cutting (1985) considers that although basic visual processes are probably normal in schizophrenia, a deficit exists in the appreciation of visual form. He quotes Levin and Benton (1977), who demonstrated that chronic schizophrenics were worse than neurotics in their ability to recognize faces. Auditory perception may also be affected and, reviewing other modes of perception, Cutting concludes that there is evidence of disorder of body image perception in some patients (Weckowicz & Sommer, 1960; Cleveland, Fisher, Reitman, & Rothaus, 1962). Examples given by the authors make clear the threatening nature of these perceptual changes: Weckowicz and Sommer quote the case of a man who's eyes were being pulled out so that in the mirror they appeared to be completely out of their sockets. Several workers have commented on the propensity of perceived threat to lead to violent action in psychosis (e.g., Mullen, 1988).

Perception of emotion has been found by several authors to be abnormal in schizophrenia. Dougherty, Bartlett, and Izard (1974) showed photographs of facial expressions to schizophrenic and control subjects, and found that schizophrenics were significantly worse at identifying the emotion shown. Iscoe and Veldman (1963) found that schizophrenics did worse than controls when asked to arrange nine drawings in order from happy to sad, and argued that they had difficulty in perceiving "subtle emotional graduations." Spiegel, Gerard, Grayson, and Gengerelli (1962) found schizophrenics "normally sensitive to the nuances of facial expression" but found that, while they were able to arrange facial expressions in order from angry to happy, they were unable to derive the criteria they were using. Similar findings have been described with reference to emotion in speech. Turner (1964) tested the ability of 60 schizophrenics and 30 controls to identify the emotional flavor of a taped nonsense sentence, and found that the performance of schizophrenics was impaired. Studying 24 acute schizophrenics, Jonsson and Sjostedt (1973) found that they did worse than controls when asked to identify the emotional intonation of spoken single words. Perceptual changes such as these may correspond to the "noticings" described by McGinn (1979) as triggers for action based on belief. The abnormal sensitivity of schizophrenics to certain emotional themes (Brodsky, 1963; Cutting, 1985) may also affect the likelihood of their acting on their delusions. Finally it is possible that the decreased empathic ability of schizophrenics described by Milgram (1960) allows them to act in ways that cause harm to others.

The importance of these perceptual changes has been alluded to by several authors. MacLean and Robertson (1976) considered that a perception that an alarming change was occurring in one's body contributed to self-mutilation in psychotic patients. Mowat (1966) found that many of his sample of morbidly jealous murderers described, as grounds for their delusional beliefs and subsequent action, a change in their wives' emotional attitudes. In their review of homicidal aggression in schizophrenic men, Planansky and Johnston (1977) conclude that "transient misperception of danger to life, very frightening and potentially ominous, was distinctly revealed by some men." Of relevance here may be the work of Bemporad (1967) and Reich and Cutting (1982), showing that schizophrenics faced with visual problems were more likely to approach them by concentrating on details rather than on any overall view. In the words of Shakow (950), "If there is any creature who can be accused of not seeing the forest for the trees, it is the schizophrenic." It may be that schizophrenia renders sufferers prone to concentrate on one or two threatening aspects of a situation that would be innocuous if viewed in overall perspective.

*Motor Changes*    In depression, psychomotor retardation inhibits all types of action, and the increased risk of suicide attendant on the lifting of this retardation with treatment has long been recognized. In schizophrenia, the catatonic symptoms have been reviewed by Abrams and Taylor (1976). Of these, the possibility of explaining stereotypies in delusional terms has already been mentioned (Jones, 1965). As pointed out by Mayer-Gross, Slater, and Roth (1960), however, this is very different from establishing a psychological cause; in any case, the behaviors described by Jones are invariably of little consequence. Other catatonic symptoms, such as negativism and stupor, will influence actions based on delusions in the same nonspecific and inhibitory way in which they influence all behavior.

*Drive, Motivation, and Affect*    Perhaps more important influences on motor behavior in psychosis are such factors as drive, inclination, and motivation. These concepts are very close to that of *desire* as described by McGinn (1979), who considered it a prerequisite for action based on belief. They also bear comparison with the concept of *affectivity* described by Bleuler in 1924:

> Action is for the most part influenced by affectivity, if one at least agrees with us when we designate the force and direction of the impulses, or of the "will" as partial manifestations of the affects. He who is happy, sad or furious will react accordingly. (p. 143)

In normal subjects, the drive and inclination to act are closely linked to the affective and emotional aspects of a belief. It seems possible that the likelihood of a delusional belief being acted upon will be influenced by similar factors. In depression, the link between a delusional belief and its affective component is so close that it becomes impossible to distinguish the two; the fact that psychiatrists use the term *mood congruent* to describe certain delusions reflects the fact that these delusions are regarded as having an emotional quality that is inseparable from the belief itself. Any discussion of whether a psychotically depressed patient kills himself because of what he believes or because of what he feels rapidly becomes one of semantics. Similarly, in mania it is difficult to differentiate between grandiose delusions and hypomanic affect as the cause of a patient's extravagant behavior.

In chronic schizophrenia, a reduction in the capacity to experience pleasure has been described by several authors (Harrow, Grinker, Holzman, & Kayton, 1977; Watson, Jacobs, & Kucala, 1979; Cook & Simukonda, 1981). It is unclear whether a similar reduction occurs in the capacity to experience other emotions, although work previously mentioned describing schizophrenics' difficulties in perceiving such emotions as anger (Spiegel et al., 1962) provides some circumstantial evidence that this is the case. If this is so, it might be expected that the delusional beliefs of schizophrenics — charged with less emotion than those of others — should be acted upon less often. Other workers, however, have reached different conclusions. Feffer (1961) presented neutral and emotionally charged words to schizophrenic subjects and normal controls, and found that schizophrenics avoided words with an affective connotation. Garety and Hemsley (1987) found that a high proportion of deluded subjects found their delusions distressing. The work of Vaughn and Leff (1976), showing that schizophrenics living with high expressed emotion (EE) relatives were more prone to relapse, and later work (Leff, Kuipers, Berkowitz, Everlein-Vries, & Sturgeon, 1982), showing that relapse rates fell when EE was reduced, would suggest that in some cases schizophrenics are oversensitive to emotion. It seems likely that the emotional responsiveness of schizophrenics is not simply reduced but is altered in quality. It may be that schizophrenics may attach emotion inappropriately to certain beliefs, including delusional ones, and are then more likely to act upon them.

*Cognitive Factors*    In this connection, mention must be made of cognitive factors that may influence delusional behavior. With regard to depression, the effect of psychomotor retardation has already been discussed. With regard to schizophrenia, several mechanisms have been proposed while little confirmatory evidence has emerged. An impaired ability to make probabilistic judgments has been described (Huq, Garety, & Hemsley, 1988). Frith (1987) described a model for first-rank symptoms and negative signs in schizophrenia. First-rank symptoms, he argued, are consequent upon defective monitoring of action, while negative signs result from an imbalance between willed intentions and stimulus-based intentions. A later paper (Frith & Done, 1989) provided some experimental evidence for the first of these proposals, but not for the second relating to negative symptoms and the implications for delusional behavior are unclear. Robertson and Taylor (1985) tested a group of men held in prison or maximum security hospital on criminal charges, and found that their deluded group showed a deficit of "immediate memory." It is possible that such memory deficits are the result of impaired use of mnemonic strategies. Bauman (1971) showed that schizophrenics' memory for three-letter sequences failed to improve even when it was pointed out to them that the sequences began with consecutive letters of the alphabet. Robertson and Taylor argued that, as a consequence of their memory deficits, deluded patients were likely to misinterpret external stimuli. Other specific cognitive deficits have been invoked with regard to perception and have already been discussed. In more general terms, it has been argued that the relatively intact cognitive function of chronic paranoid patients is associated with a greater propensity for planned violence than is the impaired cognitive function of patients with an acute psychosis (Krakowski, Volavka, & Brizer, 1986; Wessely, 1993). It is not clear that this association represents a causative link, however, or what form such a link might take.

Although a distinct thread has yet to emerge from the investigation of cognitive function in schizophrenia, this area of research does offer some correspondence with theoretical writing on the subject. The views of Fulford (1989) with regard to the importance of belief in the genesis of action have already been mentioned. The work of the same author offers the tantalizing suggestion that the link between a delusional belief and an ensuing action may be impaired in a way that is inseparable from the genesis of the belief itself. Fulford rejects the conventional definitions of delusion, pointing out, *inter alia*, that many delusions are not beliefs at all but value judgments. He suggests that delusions could better be described as defective reasons for action. Could these defective reasons be the products of defective reasoning of a type not previously described? Fulford argues that the nature of the deficit is unclear, and that considerable clinical and philosophical work is required even to clarify the issues involved.

*Other Factors*    Several other aspects of the mental states of psychotic patients have been implicated in delusional action. Shore (1979) reported that flattening of affect allowed the schizophrenic patient to severely injure himself as a consequence of his delusion. Other authors (Greilsheimer & Groves, 1979; Waugh, 1986) have also reported flattening of affect in association with self-harm based on delusions, and Mullen (1988) has argued that "emotional blunting" is associated with violence in schizophrenia. Hafner and Boker (1973), however, in their large study of mentally abnormal offenders, found that only a small proportion of schizophrenic offenders had flatness of affect. Some of the issues involved have been discussed in the section covering drive, motivation, and affect. The degree of systemization of delusional beliefs was found by Hafner and Boker to be related to violent behavior, and several less methodologically sound studies, reviewed by Krakowski et al. (1986), have reached similar conclusions. The presence of hallucinations or perceptual changes in cases where delusions of jealousy and poisoning are associated with violence has been referred to by

Shepherd (1961), Mowat (1966), and Varsamis, Adamson, and Sigurdson (1972). In mania, Schipkowensky (1968) has invoked the "pathologically increased social connection of the manic" to explain what he regards as a very low incidence of violence in these patients (quoted by Krakowski et al., 1986). Psychodynamic factors are important concomitants of delusionally motivated self-harm according to Maclean and Robertson (1976), who state that "castration fears, failure to resolve oedipal conflicts, repressed homosexual impulses, severe guilt and self punishment are ubiquitous in such cases." Other authors describe such theories as unwarranted generalization (Tapper et al., 1979) or subjective (Sweeney & Zamecnik, 1981); the debate here has echoes of a more general one concerning the relevance of psychodynamic theory to psychiatry.

## Conclusions Regarding the Literature

This section has reviewed the theoretical basis for action, pointing to the reappearance of beliefs as important causes of action after a period during which more behaviorist explanations held sway. Recent explanations have been described in which action is seen as caused by a combination of belief and desire and triggered by factors such as noticings. It has been argued that these concepts correspond to some of the findings of psychiatric research. Desire may well correspond to psychiatric concepts of motivation, drive, and inclination and noticing find likely equivalents in the field of perceptual changes, perhaps influenced by other cognitive aspects of psychosis. The correspondence is far from exact, however, while the details of how desires and beliefs are triggered by noticings to form the intention to act have not been clarified for healthy subjects, let alone for patients suffering from psychosis. As Fulford (1989) has pointed out, avenues of research in this area are legion and underexplored.

An improved understanding of the likelihood of delusional beliefs being acted upon would help psychiatrists assess the risk to the psychotic patient and others. To this end, it would be advantageous to be able to attribute risk either to the belief itself or to other features of the patient's psychosis. Unfortunately, most of the studies quoted here rely on a violent or otherwise spectacular act for their case ascertainment. There is a clear need for more broadly based studies of delusional action if this understanding of the risk of delusional action is to be approached.

In 1941, Aubrey Lewis wrote:

> Patients often do not act in accordance with their delusional beliefs, especially when these are fleeting or chronic. . . . But this is, on the whole, unusual in the early or acute stages of the illness: a patient will then act on his beliefs violently or in terror; he may go to the police or be driven to suicide. (p. 1189)

Lewis alludes to two factors that have been discussed here—namely, the chronicity of delusions and their emotional context. It seems that research could also usefully measure such aspects of delusional beliefs as conviction and preoccupation, and quantify the behavioral correlates of these components. Measurement of the behavioral correlates of other aspects of psychosis, such as insight and affective incongruity, also seems likely to be of value. It was in the light of these considerations that the research described in the next section was designed.

# The Present Study

## The Method

We screened all psychotic patients admitted to a general psychiatric hospital in South London, and identified 98 who were suffering from at least one non-mood-congruent delusion. Fifteen either refused to participate in the study or were too thought disordered to do so, leaving us with a study population of 83. Using a reliable instrument, the Present State Examination (PSE; Wing, Cooper, & Sartorius, 1974), we obtained a description of their psychiatric phenomenology. Some suffered from more than one delusion; these subjects were asked which was most important to them. The next stage involved detailed measurement of the phenomenology of this delusion, henceforth referred to as the *principal belief*. This was done using the Maudsley Assessment of Delusions Schedule (MADS), a standardized interview covering various aspects of phenomenology. These were: (1) the degree of conviction with which the belief was held; (2) the evidence that supported the beliefs; (3) the associated affect; (4) the actions that (in the subject's own view) resulted; (5) the degree of preoccupation; (6) the systematization; and (7) the level of insight present. The MADS is described in Appendix 12A, and the development of the scale has been described (Taylor et al., 1994). Finally, a description of the subject's behavior was obtained from informants; this description was obtained blind to the results of the interview with the patient.

There were three stages to the analysis of our data. First, we estimated the frequency with which actions based on delusions occurred. This was done both for actions as described by the subjects themselves and for actions described by informants. When subjects described their own actions, we allowed them to assess the link with a delusion themselves, asking whether the principal belief led them to do anything. When informants rated action, we used the consensus judgment of a panel of experts to determine whether that action was or was not the result of a delusion. Second, we tried to establish whether any of the various categories of delusion mentioned in the previous section were particularly associated with action. Third, we tried to establish whether any of the more subtle elements of phenomenology, measured using the MADS, were similarly associated with action. Of particular interest in the context of this book was the assessment of the role of insight. David (1990) identified three elements to the phenomenon, each of which was addressed by our methodology. An awareness of being ill is covered by items such as, "Are you psychologically unwell in any way?" "Is there anything wrong with your nerves?" and "Do you think that seeing a psychiatrist might help you?" A willingness to accept treatment was examined by such items as, "Do you think that medication would help you in any way?" And an ability to relabel abnormal experiences was tested in the same way that David has suggested—namely, by rating the subject's response to a contradiction of his or her belief, a contradiction couched in hypothetical terms.

## The Quantity and Quality of Acting on Delusions

*Self- and Informant-Reported Delusional Action*    The prevalences of self-reported delusional action are listed in table 12.1. Sixty percent of the sample reported at least one delusional action and 20% claimed three or more.

TABLE 12.1 Prevalence of Specific Self-Reported Delusional Actions

|  | "Yes" | (%) |
|---|---|---|
| Have you written to anyone? | 10 | (13) |
| Have you tried to stop X happening? | 27 | (35) |
| Have you tried to protect yourself in any way? | 19 | (25) |
| Have you ever tried to escape what is happening? | 13 | (17) |
| Have you ever broken anything because of this? | 15 | (19) |
| Have you hit anyone because of this? | 14 | (18) |
| Have you tried to harm yourself because of X? | 11 | (14) |
| Have you tried to move or leave your house (area) because of X? | 9 | (12) |
| Has X stopped you from meeting friends? | 28 | (36) |
| Has X stopped you from watching TV or | 22 | (29) |
| listening to the radio? | 28 | (33) |
| Has X stopped you from eating or drinking anything? | 15 | (19) |
| Has X stopped you from using transport? | 14 | (18) |
| Has X stopped you from going to work? | 12 | (15) |
| Has X stopped you from taking medication? | 6 | (8) |
| Has X stopped you from going to the hospital or your doctor on an outpatient basis? | 4 | (5) |

Latent class analysis (see Everitt, 1986) was used to study the underlying distribution of these actions. Table 12.2 gives the final parameter values for the three classes generated; each value represents the probability of a positive response on a given action for each of the three classes.

The first class gave high probabilities on combinations involving either no action at all or any single action, with the exception of protect and escape. It also included responses involving two behaviors, of which one was writing. This class we have labeled "none or single action." All the combinations with high probabilities of membership of the second class contained various combinations of hitting and breaking objects, together with any other action. This we have labeled "aggressive action." The third class consisted largely of combinations of behavior involving stopping, protecting, escaping, and moving. A single response of escaping, and to a lesser extent protecting, had high

TABLE 12.2 Latent Class Analysis of Self-Reported Delusional Action

|  | Class 3 (Defensive) | Class 1 (None or single action) | Class 2 (Aggressive and/or self-harm) |
|---|---|---|---|
| Action |  |  |  |
| Write | 0.14 | 0.12 | 0.08 |
| Stop | 0.13 | 0.45 | 0.59 |
| Protect | 0.05 | 0.74 | 0.56 |
| Escape | 0.00 | 0.23 | 0.63 |
| Break | 0.17 | 0.70 | 0.00 |
| Hit | 0.10 | 1.00 | 0.00 |
| Self-harm | 0.07 | 0.54 | 0.14 |
| Move | 0.04 | 0.46 | 0.18 |
| Number | 13 | 61 | 9 |
| (Percentage) | 15.7% | 73.5% | 10.8% |

probabilities of belonging to this class, which we have labeled "defensive action." Frequencies of each category are listed in Table 12.2.

On the basis of information given to us by informants, half of our subjects were rated as having either definitely or probably acted on their principal belief in the month prior to admission. This figure rose to 77% when behavior based on any delusion was rated from the same information. No association was found between self- and informant-reported delusional action.

Two examples of lack of congruence are given. A 22-year-old woman believed that people were trying to harm her using occult powers, but denied doing anything as a result. Her parents, on the other hand, reported that she had assaulted her sister, climbed out of a window to escape her persecutors, and gone to the police station to complain about her parents' use of diabolic powers. An opposite example was a 30-year-old woman who believed people in her neighborhood were imposters. She described asking them who they really were and also visits to other neighborhoods looking for new accommodation. However, her sister had not observed any unusual behavior concerning the neighbors, or any attempts to leave the area. Instead, the sister said that the subject would buy food only in certain shops and ate food only for diabetics, although she was not a diabetic. She was classified as a nonactor by informant report because none of the informant-observed actions could be linked to her mental state as revealed by the PSE.

*Categories of Delusion Associated with Action*    Attempts were made to link the content of delusion with both self-reported and observer-reported actions. For this purpose, only those delusions reported by more than 10% of the sample were studied further. Thus excluded were delusions of depersonalization, subcultural delusions, delusions of jealousy, and delusions concerning physical appearance. Looking first at the latent class-derived classification of self-reported acting on delusions, we found that the presence of delusions of catastrophe was significantly associated with the subject's being classified as an aggressive actor. There was a similar but weak trend for passivity experiences. There was no association between membership in any of the three classes of self-reported delusional action and the presence of delusions of reference, delusional memories, religious delusions, delusions of jealousy, persecutory delusions, grandiose delusions, delusions of guilt, or sexual delusions.

Turning to the consensus-derived judgments based on informant-reported action, we found that delusions of catastrophe were significantly associated with lack of action on the principal belief. Furthermore, there was a strong association between delusions of catastrophe and lack of action on any belief. There was a suggestion that delusions of guilt are negatively associated with delusional action, and a similar negative association was obtained if grandiose delusions were present. There was no relationship, either positive or negative, between passivity delusions and action, and IQ had no apparent effect. The presence of persecutory delusions, on the other hand, was associated with probable and definite delusional action.

Certain cautions are necessary when interpreting these findings. Although significant statistical associations were found between the presence of delusions of catastrophe and passivity delusions, on the one hand, and lack of action, on the other, the proportion of the sample with each delusion was small. Seventeen percent had delusions of catastrophe and 19% passivity delusions. Nevertheless, we have identified a class of abnormal beliefs that seem to inhibit acting on delusions. It is important to differentiate, however, between the presence of a delusion associated with delusional action in general and action based on that delusion in particular. The results described above show that the presence of certain delusions inhibit delusional action in general, not that certain delusions are more likely to be directly acted upon. To address this issue we analyzed specific associations between the type of principal belief and the action. Only persecutory and passivity delusions occurred with sufficient frequency for this to be done. Using the consensus ratings, persecutory delusions were significantly more likely to be acted upon than all other principal beliefs, but passivity delusions were no more likely to be acted upon than all other delusions.

*Phenomenology of Delusions That Are Acted Upon*    When behavior was rated by informants, no association was found between aspects of delusional phenomenology and action. In assessing the phenomenological correlates of action when that action is defined by the patient, the sample was divided using the latent class analysis described above. Patients who failed to act on their delusions or who acted very little (nonactors) were compared to those who acted in an aggressive or defensive manner (actors). Action based on delusions was associated with delusional phenomenology in two areas. First, acting was associated with being aware of evidence that supported the belief and with having actively sought out such evidence; it was also associated with a tendency to reduce the conviction with which a belief was held when that belief was challenged using a hypothetical contradiction. Second, acting was associated with feeling sad, frightened, or anxious as a consequence of the delusion. None of the other elements of phenomenology examined—namely, the degree of conviction with which a belief was held, its systematization, or the degree of preoccupation that it provoked—were associated with action. Nonsignificant trends toward an association with action were noted for some items relating to insight ("Are you psychologically unwell?", "Do you think that medication might help you?") but not for others ("Do you think that seeing a psychiatrist might help you?," "How far do you think others share your belief?").

As part of the testing of the MADS, all subjects were reinterviewed three to five days after collection of the data presented above. The same questions were asked concerning the phenomenology of the principal belief. The data from this second interview were analyzed to test for associations with delusional action. The associations with action were maintained for the affective features. With regard to the ability to identify information supporting the delusional belief, actively seeking such information and the response to a hypothetical contradiction of the delusion, the associations with acting were not maintained. An attempt was also made to compare the two groups of actors identified by latent class analysis—namely, those who acted predominantly aggressively and those whose actions were generally defensive. The numbers were small (9 and 14), and no significant differences were noted between the two groups.

## Our Results in Light of Previous Work

The methods we chose had a number of limitations. First, with regard to the material collected from informants, it is reasonable to assume that informants were unaware of at least some delusional action. Other possible causes of false negatives were that informants might describe only actions they considered relevant to the subject's illness, although this was reduced by using a standardized interview containing a checklist of actions. False positives were also possible. With the occasional exception, informants were not trained observers of unusual behaviors. They may have reported some that did not occur, perhaps to precipitate admission. All interviews took place after admission, however, and it was emphasized that the information obtained would not be communicated to the clinical team or recorded in the notes.

Second, with regard to the information obtained from the subject, it is possible that some behavior was not admitted to, perhaps because it was considered either too trivial or too embarrassing. The reverse is equally possible—that the subject was more likely to reveal both beliefs and actions to a neutral observer than to a member of his or her family. Indeed, one of the most robust findings of the study was the lack of congruence between the subjects' assessments of action and those of the informants.

Methodological problems are also apparent in the manner in which abnormal beliefs were linked to abnormal behavior. Some delusions were, by their nature, almost impossible to link with actions. For example, the principal belief identified for one subject was "thoughts are put into my mind from spaces in the air." It is difficult to think of any behavior that could logically be linked to this belief, so although the subject had shown a number of unusual behaviors, which may have been linked in the subject's mind to his beliefs, as these links were not accessible to an outside observer, the subject was classified as a nonactor. These problems notwithstanding, we have described delusional action in a general psychiatric population. We have investigated which categories of delusion are more likely to be associated with action, and identified some of the phenomenological correlates of that action.

What are the implications of our study? The previous finding of an association between violent behavior in the mentally disordered and passivity experiences (Taylor, 1985) led us to hypothesize a relationship between passivity experiences and self-reported delusional action. This was not confirmed, however, nor was an association found for informant-observed actions. This may reflect sample differences between the studies, since violent behavior was considerably less frequent in the current study than in that conducted by Taylor. We had also reasoned that the perceptual abnormalities associated with passivity experiences give additional "proof" of the correctness of the delusional intuition. This may be correct, but was not a risk factor for delusional action. Again, however, it is possible that passivity delusions are not risk factors for the nonviolent behavior typical of our sample, but are associated with serious violence.

The finding of an association between delusions of catastrophe and self-report of aggressive action was surprising and unexpected. Furthermore, delusions of catastrophe were significantly negatively related to informant-observed delusional action. We cannot explain why delusions of catastrophe should have apparently opposite effects on self- and informant-reported behavior and, unless replicated, cannot exclude a type 1 error. Turning to the consensus judgments made on the basis of informant-reported action, we report that persecutory delusions were the sole phenomenological feature associated with delusional action in general. Although this is intuitively comprehensible, we were surprised that the association did not extend to passivity delusions, and we also did not predict that certain delusions (catastrophe and, perhaps, guilt) would protect against action. Observable delusional action is more likely in the presence of persecutory delusions and less likely in the presence of delusions of guilt and grandiose delusions.

It should be emphasized that these results do not mean that acting upon grandiose or delusions of guilt is unlikely, but that delusional action as a consequence of any belief becomes less likely if the subject experiences either grandiose or delusions of guilt. We are able to conclude only that persecutory delusions per se are more likely to be acted on than other types of delusion.

The discrepancy between self-report and information from informants was maintained with regard to the phenomenological correlates of a delusion being acted upon. Thus, when the testimony of informants was used to define action, there was no association between aspects of delusional phenomenology and the likelihood of that delusion being acted upon. This contrasts with the positive findings noted when action is defined by the subject himself. Action is a more likely consequence of a delusional belief if the subject can identify evidence in support of that belief; this finding, as we have seen, is not simply a reflection of intellectual function. It is consistent with the view of McGinn (1979), discussed earlier, that action is based on a combination of desires and beliefs and is triggered by *noticings*, internal or external cues which precipitate action. The findings of the study suggest that these noticings are far from a passive experience; action is rendered much more likely where a subject actively seeks evidence to confirm or refute his or her belief. The findings also raise the possibility that some acting on delusional beliefs may be the result of the subject's testing his or her beliefs in an attempt to confirm or refute them. This interpretation would in turn be supported by the finding that acting on a delusion is more likely when the subject is able to countenance evidence that contradicts that belief.

The finding that emotions such as unhappiness, fear, and anxiety, when found as a consequence of a delusion, are associated with action is consistent with Bleuler's (1924) view, discussed in the second section of this chapter, that action is largely a consequence of affectivity. The willingness of patients who act on their delusions to countenance hypothetical contradiction of their delusional beliefs is perhaps surprising; it might have been expected that patients who ignored contradiction would be more likely to act. It is consistent, however, with the findings that conviction and systematization are not associated with action and with the suggestion that action is more likely when beliefs are questioned and evidence is sought to confirm or refute them.

Previous studies have found an association between the ability to countenance a hypothetical contradiction and recovery from delusions. Brett-Jones, Garety, and Hemsley (1987) found this in subjects being treated with psychotropic medication; Chadwick and Lowe (1990) found that drug-resistant subjects who were able to countenance a contradiction to their delusional beliefs responded better to cognitive behavioral therapy than those who were not so able. They also found that noticing actual evidence contradictory to the belief was associated with recovery. We have found that a positive response to a hypothetical contradiction is associated with acting on delusional beliefs. These findings raise the possibility that acting on delusional beliefs, particularly where the action is designed to test out the validity of the belief, is itself related to recovery; this issue is worthy of further investigation.

That the associations between the ability to identify information supporting a delusional belief and acting on that belief were not maintained when the subjects were reinterviewed three to five days later may suggest that the questions used to elicit this information were unreliable. The interrater reliability was good, however, and the findings are consistent with each other. It is more likely that the ability to identify information supporting a delusional belief is a genuine but transient element of the phenomenology of delusional action. The affective connotations on a belief, on the other hand, would seem to be more stable over time. It is possible that an affect-laden delusional belief is acted upon only when the subject perceives certain information that seems to bear out that belief; again, this is consistent with the theoretical work of McGinn (1979). There remains the question of the degree to which these associations are independent of phenomenological categories based on the content of the delusion. When the presence of persecutory content was controlled for, the associations described above were maintained. The results suggest that the associations we have described are independent of phenomenological categories based on content. One exception may concern feeling frightened as a result of a delusion, which is associated with action for delusions of persecution but not for other delusions.

Of the negative findings relating to the phenomenological correlates of acting on delusions, the effect of conviction has already been mentioned. The lack of an association between action and elation may shed some light on the apparent low incidence of violence in manic patients (see Schipkowensky, 1968). The lack of an association between systematization and insight, on the one hand, and action, on the other, might be considered surprising in view of previous findings (Hafner & Boker, 1973; Roback & Abramowitz, 1979). Methodological differences make direct comparisons with these studies difficult. Hafner and Boker's study was limited to very serious offender patients, and Roback and Abramowitz used only general measures of behavior and did not attempt to measure behavior arising as a consequence of specific delusional beliefs. As mentioned in the discussion of methodology, recent writing on the subject of insight has included description of a number of phenomenological dimensions (David, 1990). The nonsignificant trends that we report suggest that some of these dimensions (e.g., the ability to recognize illness) are more strongly associated with action than others (e.g., the ability to relabel as abnormal unusual mental events).

## Conclusions

We have found that actions based on delusional beliefs are more common than had previously been recognized. This was the case whether action was measured using self-report or information from informants. Half of the sample reported that they had acted at least once in accordance with their delusions. Violent behavior in response to delusions was uncommon. Information provided by informants suggested that some aspects of the behavior of half the sample were probably or definitely congruent with the content of their delusions. We have also identified some phenomenological correlates of acting on delusions. In particular, acting is more likely when the subject is aware of evidence that supports his or her belief and with affect-laden delusions. Further research could usefully test these associations in a prospective study. Research on larger patient populations may also be able to identify phenomenological differences in the delusional beliefs of aggressive and defensive actors.

*Notes*

1. The team was led by Dr. Pamela Taylor and consisted of ourselves, Drs. John Cutting, Graham Dunn, Philippa Garety, Don Grubin, Mrs. Katarzyna Ray, and Dr. Alison Reed. The project was funded by a grant from the John D. and Catherine T. MacArthur Foundation and Dr. Wessely was a recipient of a Research Fellowship from the Wellcome Foundation. At the time this chapter was written Dr. Buchanan was the recipient of a Research Fellowship from the Special Hospitals Service Authority. That part of the chapter which reviews some theoretical considerations has been published previously (Buchanan, 1993).

## Appendix

### *Maudsley Assessment of Delusions Schedule and measures of interrater reliability*

The complete instrument takes the form of a semistructured interview and associated instructions. Interrater reliability was measured as part of the testing of the instrument. Where more than two ratings were available for an item, the interrater reliability is described as a weighted Kappa coefficient; where only two ratings were available, it is described as an unweighted Kappa.

| Item | Number of Ratings Available | Interrater Reliability |
|---|---|---|
| 1. Conviction | | |
| How sure are you about X? | 5 | 0.84 |
| 2. Belief Maintenance Factors | | |
| Can you now explain why you continue to think that X is so? | | |
| Has anything happened since the idea first came to you? | | |
| a. Events or states since formation | 2 | 1.0 |
| b. Events or states in last week | 2 | 0.78 |
| c. Internal state maintaining belief (e.g., mood, abnormal experience) | 2 | 0.59 |
| d. External events maintaining beliefs | 2 | 0.75 |
| Do you at present (or have you in the past month) looked for any evidence or information either to confirm your view or to test whether it may be mistaken? | 2 | 0.73 |
| Asking you to think about it now, can you think of anything at all that has happened that goes against your belief? | 2 | 0.75 |
| When you think about it now, is it at all possible that you are mistaken about X? | 2 | 0.91 |
| 3. Affect Relating to Chosen Belief | | |
| How does that belief make you feel? Does it make you feel: | | |
| a. Elated? | 2 | 0.71 |
| b. Unhappy, miserable, depressed? | 2 | 0.88 |
| c. Terrified, frightened? | 2 | 0.92 |
| d. Anxious, tense? | 2 | 0.83 |
| e. Angry? | 2 | 0.92 |

*(continued)*

| Item | Number of Ratings Available | Interrater Reliability |
|---|---|---|
| 4. Action | | |
| Does X make you do anything in particular? | | |
|   a. Have you talked to anyone about X? | 3 | 0.77 |
|   b. Have you written to anyone? | 3 | 1.0 |
|   c. Have you tried to stop X from happening? | 3 | 0.91 |
|   d. Have you tried to protect yourself in any way? | 3 | 0.75 |
|   e. Does X make you lose your temper? | 3 | 0.79 |
|   f. Have you ever broken anything because of this? | 3 | 0.94 |
|   g. Have you felt like hitting someone because of it? | 3 | 0.87 |
|   h. Have you hit anyone because of it? | 3 | 0.81 |
|   i. Do you know the person or people you have or may have harm(ed)? | 3 | 0.79 |
|   j. Have you tried to harm yourself or harmed yourself accidentally because of X? | 3 | 0.91 |
|   k. Have you tried to move or leave your house because of X? | 3 | 0.86 |
|   l. Have other changes resulted? | 3 | 0.59 |
| For Those Hearing Voices Only: | | |
| Do the voices tell you to do anything? | 3 | 1.0 |
| Do you have to obey? | 3 | 0.85 |
| Do you do anything to escape them? | 3 | 1.0 |
| Has X stopped you from doing things you would normally have done? | | |
| Has X stopped you from meeting friends? | 3 | 0.72 |
| Has X stopped you from watching TV? | 3 | 0.91 |
| Has X stopped you from eating or drinking anything? | 3 | 0.82 |
| Has X stopped you from using transport? | 3 | 0.78 |
| Has X stopped you from going to work? | 3 | 0.70 |
| Has X stopped you from taking medication? | 3 | 0.65 |
| Has X stopped you from going to the hospital or your doctor on an outpatient basis? | 3 | 0.79 |
| Is there anything else that X has stopped you from doing? | 3 | 1.0 |
| 5. Preoccupation | 5 | 0.62 |
| 6. Systematization | 4 | 0.58 |
| 7. Insight | | |
| How far do you think others share your beliefs? | 5 | 0.88 |
| Do you ever discuss your ideas with others? | 2 | 0.83 |
| Do you ever have arguments about your beliefs? | 5 | 0.89 |
| Earlier I asked you whether or not you felt others shared your belief about X. I'd like to clarify whether you feel that other people also believe X—either openly or perhaps without talking about it? | 3 | 0.78 |
| What would have to happen to make you think that you might be wrong about X? | 3 | 0.62 |
| Do you think that seeing a psychiatrist might help you (has helped you) in any way? | 3 | 0.79 |
| Do you think that medication might help you (has helped you) in any way? How? | 4 | 0.90 |
| How much have you discussed X with your doctor and the nurses on the ward? | 3 | 0.71 |

| Item | Number of Ratings Available | Interrater Reliability |
|---|---|---|
| Are you psychologically unwell in any way? Is there anything wrong with your nerves? | 3 | 0.84 |
| Let me suggest something hypothetical to you—something that does not fit with your view and you could tell me how you think you would react. | 4 | 0.90 |
| If the Behavior or Act Injured or Could Have Injured Someone, or Caused Damage to Property: | | |
| Looking back on (the behavior X), do you now feel that you were justified, or were you wrong to do what you did? | 3 | 0.68 |
| If the Behavior or Act Was Against the Law: | | |
| Was (the behavior of X) against the law? | 3 | 0.19 |
| If the Act Involved Personal Danger or Risk (e.g., arrest): | | |
| How dangerous was (the behavior of X)? Would you take the same risk again? | 3 | 0.40 |
| Why do you feel that (the people involved) responded to you in the way they did? Were they right to do so? | 3 | 1.0 |

### References

Abrams, R., & Taylor, M. A. (1976). Catatonia. *Archives of General Psychiatry, 33,* 579–581.

Albert, D. M., Burns, W. P., & Scheie, H. G. (1965). Severe orbitocranial foreign-body injury. *American Journal of Opthalmology, 60,* 1109–1111.

Anaclerio, A. M., & Wicker, H. S. (1970). Self induced solar retinopathy by patients in a psychiatric hospital. *American Journal of Opthalmology, 69,* 731–736.

Anderson, E., & Trethowan, W. (1973). *Psychiatry* (3rd ed.). London: Bailliere, Tindall.

Austin, J. L. (1956–7). A plea for excuses. Proceedings of the Aristotelian Society 57, 1–30. Reprinted in A. R. White (Ed.), *The philosophy of action* (pp. 19–42). Oxford: Oxford University Press.

Bach-y-Rita, G. (1974). Habitual violence and self mutilation. *American Journal of Psychiatry, 131,* 1018–1020.

Bach-y-Rita, G., & Veno, A. (1974). Habitual violence: A profile of 62 men. *American Journal of Psychiatry, 131,* 1015–1017.

Bartko, G., Herczeg, I., & Zador, G. (1988). Clinical symptomatology and drug compliance in schizophrenic patients. *Acta Psychiatrica Scandinavica, 77,* 74–76.

Bauman, E. (1971). Schizophrenic short-term memory: A deficit in subjective organisation. *Canadian Journal of Behavioral Science, 3,* 55–65.

Beilin, L. M. (1953). Genital self-mutilation by mental patients. *Journal of Urology, 70,* 648–655.

Beilin, L. M. & Gruenberg, J. (1948). Genital self mutilation by mental patients. *Journal of Urology, 59,* 635–641.

Bemporad, J. R. (1967). Perceptual disorders in schizophrenia. *American Journal of Psychiatry, 123,* 971–976.

Blacker, K., & Wong, N. (1963). Four cases of autocastration. *Archives of General Psychiatry, 8,* 169–176.

Bleuler, E. (1911/1950). *Dementia praecox oder die Gruppe der Schizophrenien* (J. Zinkin, Trans.). New York: International University Press.

Bleuler, E. (1924). *Textbook of Psychiatry* (A. A. Brill, Trans.). New York: Macmillan.

Bowden, P. (1990). De Clerambault syndrome. In R. Bluglass & P. Bowden (Eds.), *Principles and practice of forensic psychiatry* (pp. 821–822). Edinburgh: Churchill Livingstone.

Brett-Jones, J., Garety, P. A., & Hemsley, D. (1987). Measuring delusional experiences: A method and its application. *British Journal of Clinical Psychology, 26,* 257–265.

Brodsky, M. (1963). Interpersonal stimuli as interference in a sorting task. *Journal of Personality, 31,* 517–533.

Buchanan, A. (1993). Acting on delusion: A review. *Psychological Medicine, 23,* 123–134.

Buchanan, A., Reed, A., Wessely, S., Garety, P., Taylor, P., Grubin, D., & Dunn, G. (1993). Acting on delusions. II: The phenomenological correlates of acting on delusions. *British Journal of Psychiatry, 163,* 77–81.

Campbell, K. (1970). *Body and mind.* New York: MacMillan.

Campion, J., Cravens, J. M., Rotholc, A., Weinstein, H. C., Covan, F., & Alpert, M. (1985). A study of 15 matricidal men. *American Journal of Psychiatry, 142,* 312–317.

Chadwick, P., & Lowe, C. (1990). The measurement and modification of delusional beliefs. *Journal of Consulting and Clinical Psychology, 58,* 225–232.

Christodoulou, G. N. (1978). Syndrome of subjective doubles. *American Journal of Psychiatry, 135,* 249–251.

Cleveland, S. E., Fisher, S., Reitman, E. E., & Rothaus, P. (1962). Perception of body size in schizophrenia. *Archives of General Psychiatry, 7,* 277–285.

Cook, M., & Simukonda, F. (1981). Anhedonia and schizophrenia. *British Journal of Psychiatry, 139,* 523–525.

Crane, D. L. (1976). More violent Capgras. *American Journal of Psychiatry, 133,* 1350.

Cravens, J. M., Campion, J., Rotholc, A., Covan, F., & Cravens, R. A. (1985). A study of 10 men charged with patricide. *American Journal of Psychiatry, 142*(9), 1089–1092.

Crowder, J. E., Gross, C. A., Heiser, J. F., & Crowder, A. M. (1979). Self-mutilation of the eye. *Journal of Clinical Psychiatry, 40,* 420–423.

Cutting, J. (1985). *The psychology of schizophrenia.* Edinburgh: Churchill Livingstone.

David, A. (1990). Insight and psychosis. *British Journal of Psychiatry, 156,* 798–808.

Davidson, D. (1971). Mental events. In L. Foster & J. W. Swanson (Eds.), *Experience and theory* (pp. 79–101). London: Duckworth.

de Clerambault, C. G. (1942). Les Psychoses passionelles. In *Oeuvres Psychiatriques* (pp. 315–322). Paris: Presses Universitaires de France.

De Pauw, K. W., & Szulecka, T. K. (1988). Dangerous delusions. *British Journal of Psychiatry, 152,* 91–96.

D'Orban, P. T., & O'Connor, A. (1989) Women who kill their parents. *British Journal of Psychiatry, 154,* 27–33.

Dougherty, F. E., Bartlett, E. S., & Izard, C. E. (1974). Responses of schizophrenics to expressions of the fundamental emotions. *Journal of Clinical Psychology, 30,* 243–246.

Enoch, M. D., Trethowan, W. H., & Barker, J. C. (1967). *Some Uncommon psychiatric syndromes.* Bristol: John Wright.

Everitt, B. (1986). Finite mixture distributions as models for group structure. In A. Lovie (Ed.), *New developments in statistics for psychology and the social sciences* (pp. 113–128). Methuen: London.

Feffer, M. H. (1961). The influence of affective factors on conceptualization in schizophrenia. *Journal of Abnormal and Social Psychology, 63,* 588–596.

Fish, F. (1974). *Fish's clinical psychopathology* (M. Hamilton, Ed.). Bristol: Wright.

Fishbain, D. A. (1987). The frequency of Capgras delusions in a psychiatric emergency service. *Psychopathology, 20,* 42–47.

Frith, C. D. (1987). The positive and negative symptoms of schizophrenia reflect impairments in the perception and initiation of action. *Psychological Medicine, 17,* 631–648.

Frith, C. D., & Done, D. J. (1989). Experiences of alien control in schizophrenia reflect a disorder in the central monitoring of action. *Psychological Medicine, 19,* 359–363.

Fulford, K. W. M. (1989). *Moral theory and medical practice.* Cambridge: Cambridge University Press.

Garety, P. A., & Helmsley, D. R. (1987). Characteristics of delusional experience. *Archives of Psychiatry and Neurological Sciences, 236,* 294–298.

Gibbens, T. C. N. (1958). Sane and insane homicide. *Journal of Criminal Law, Criminology and Police Science, 49,* 110–115.

Gillies, H. (1965). Murder in the West of Scotland. *British Journal of Psychiatry, 111,* 1087–1094.

Goldstein, R. L. (1987). More forensic romances: de Clerambault's syndrome in men. *Bulletin of the American Academy of Psychiatry and the Law, 15*(3), 267–274.

Gorin, M, (1964). Self-inflicted bilateral enucleation. *Archives of Opthalmology, 72,* 225–226.

Green, C. M. (1981). Matricide by sons. *Medicine, Science and the Law, 21,* 207–214.

Greilsheimer, H., & Groves, J. C. (1979). Male genital self-mutilation. *Archives of General Psychiatry, 36,* 441–446.

Guthrie, E. R. (1952). *The psychology of learning.* New York: Harper.

Hafner, H., & Boker, W. (1973). *Crimes of violence by mentally abnormal offenders.* Cambridge: Cambridge University Press.

Harrow, M., Grinker, R. R., Holzman, P. S., & Kayton, L. (1977). Anhedonia and schizophrenia. *American Journal of Psychiatry, 134,* 794–797.

Hartmann, H. (1925). Self-mutilation. *Jahrbuch fur Psychiatrie und Neurologie, 44,* 31; abstracted in *Archives of Neurology and Psychiatry, 15,* 384–386.

Haslam, J. (1823). *Sketches in Bedlam.* London: Sherwood, Jones.

Hull C. L. (1943). *Principles of behavior.* New York: Appleton-Century-Crofts.

Hull, C. L. (1951). *Essentials of Behaviour.* New Haven: Yale University Press.

Hunter, W. J. (1930). *Human Behavior.* Chicago: University of Chicago Press.

Hutchesson, E. A., & Volans, G. N. (1989). Unsubstantiated complaints of being poisoned. *British Journal of Psychiatry, 154,* 34–40.

Huq, S. F., Garety, P. A., & Hemsley, D. R. (1988). Probabilistic judgments in deluded and non deluded subjects. *Quarterly Journal of Experimental Psychology, 40A*(4), 801–812.

Iscoe, I., & Veldman, D. J. (1963). Perception of an emotional continuum by schizophrenics, normal adults and children. *Journal of Clinical Psychology, 19,* 272–276.

Jaspers, K. (1963). *General psychopathology* (J. Hoenig & M. Hamilton, Trans.). Manchester: Manchester University Press.

Jones, I. H. (1965). Observations on schizophrenic stereotypies. *Comprehensive Psychiatry, 6,* 323–335.

Jonsson, C-O., & Sjostedt A. (1973). Auditory perception in schizophrenia: A second study of the intonation test. *Acta Psychiatrica Scaninavica, 49,* 588–600.

Kant, O. (1927). Beitrage zur Paranoiaforschung. 1. Die objektive Realitatsbedeutung des Wahns. *Zeitschrift fur die gesamte Neurologie und Psychiatrie, 108,* 625–644.

Kendler, K. S., Glazer, W. M., & Morgenstern, H. (1983). Dimensions of delusional experience. *American Journal of Psychiatry, 140,* 466–469.

Kraines, S. H. (1957). *Mental depressions and their treatment.* New York: Macmillan.

Krakowski, M., Volavka, J., & Brizer, D. (1986). Psychopathology and violence: A review of literature. *Comprehensive Psychiatry 27*(2), 131–148.

Kraupl Taylor, F. (1983). Descriptive and developmental phenomena. In M. Shepherd & O. L. Zangwill (Eds.) *Handbook of psychiatry, vol. 1* (pp. 59–94). Cambridge: Cambridge University Press.

Krechevsky, I. (1932). "Hypotheses" in rats. *Psychological Review, 39,* 516–532.

Kushner, A. W. (1967). Two cases of autocastration due to religious delusions. *British Journal of Medical Psychology, 40*, 293–298.

Lanzkron, J. (1963). Murder and insanity: A survey. *American Journal of Psychiatry, 119*, 754–758.

Leff, J., Kuipers, L., Berkowitz, R., Everlein-Vries, R., & Sturgeon, D. (1982). A controlled trial of social intervention in the families of schizophrenic patients. *British Journal of Psychiatry, 141*, 121–134.

Levin, H. S., & Benton, A. L. (1977). Facial recognition in "pseudoneurological" patients. *Journal of Nervous and Mental Diseases, 164*, 135–138.

Lewis, A. J. (1941). Psychological medicine. In F. W. Price (Ed.), *A textbook of the practice of medicine* (pp. 1804–1893). London: Oxford University Press.

Lewis, N. D. C. (1928). The psychobiology of the castration reaction. *Psychoanalytic Review, 15*, 174–209, 304–323.

Lin, I. F., Spiga, R., & Fortsch, W. (1979). Insight and adherence to medication in chronic schizophrenics. *Journal of Clinical Psychiatry, 40*, 430–432.

Lyketsos, G. C., Paterakis, P., Beis, A., & Lyketsos, C. G. (1985). Eating disorders in schizophrenia. *British Journal of Psychiatry, 146*, 255–261.

McGinn, C. (1979). Action and its explanation. In N. Bolton (Ed.), *Philosophical problems in psychology* (pp. 20–42). London: Methuen.

Maclean, G., & Robertson, B. (1976). Self enucleation and psychosis. *Archives of General Psychiatry, 33*, 242–249.

Maas, R. L., Prakash, R., Hollender, M. H., & Regan, W. (1984). Double parricide—matricide and patricide: A comparison with other schizophrenic murders. *Psychiatric Quarterly, 56*(4), 286–290.

Mawson, D. (1985). Delusions of poisoning. *Medicine, Science and the Law, 25*(4), 279–287.

Mayer-Gross, W., Slater, E., & Roth, M. (1960). *Clinical psychiatry.* London: Cassell.

Mendez, R., Keily, W. F., & Morrow, J. W. (1972). Self emasculation. *Journal of Urology, 107*, 981–985.

Merskey, H. (1980). *Psychiatric illness* (3rd ed.). London: Balliere, Tindall.

Milgram, N. A. (1960). Cognitive and empathic factors in role-taking by schizophrenic and brain-damaged patients. *Journal of Abnormal Psychology, 60*, 219–224.

Miller, F. T., & Chabrier, L. A. (1988). Suicide attempts correlate with delusional content in major depression. *Psychopathology, 21*, 34–37.

Mintz, I. L. (1964). Autocannibalism: A case study. *American Journal of Psychiatry, 120*, 1017.

Mowat, R. (1966). *Morbid jealousy and murder.* London: Tavistock.

Mowrer, O. H. (1960). *Learning theory and behavior.* New York: John Wiley.

Mullen, P. E. (1979). The mental state and states of mind. In P. Hill, R. Murray, & A. Thorley (Eds.), *Essentials of postgraduate psychiatry* (pp. 3–36). London: Grune and Stratton.

Mullen, P. E. (1988). Violence and mental disorder. *British Journal of Hospital Medicine, 40*, 460–463.

Papineau, D. (1978). *For science in the social sciences.* London: MacMillan.

Papineau, D. (1990). To every purpose under heaven. *Sunday Correspondent,* May 6.

Planansky, K., & Johnston, R. (1977). Homicidal aggression in schizophrenic men. *Acta Psychiatrica Scandinavica, 55*, 65–73.

Reich, S. S., & Cutting, J. (1982). Picture perception and abstract thought in schizophrenia. *Psychological Medicine, 12*, 91–96.

Roback, H. B., & Abramowitz, S. I. (1979). Insight and hospital adjustment. *Canadian Journal of Psychiatry, 24*, 233–236.

Robertson, G., & Taylor, P. J. (1985). Some cognitive correlates of schizophrenic illness. *Psychological Medicine, 15*, 81–98.

Rollin, H. R. (1977). McNaughton's madness. in D. J. West & A. Walk (Eds.), *Daniel McNaughton: His trial and the aftermath* (pp. 91–99). Gaskell: Ashford.

Romanik, R. L., & Snow, S. (1984). Two cases of Capgras' syndrome. *American Journal of Psychiatry, 141,* 720.

Rosen, D. H., & Hoffman, A. M. (1972). Focal suicide: Self-enucleation by two young psychotic individuals. *American Journal of Psychiatry, 128,* 1009–1012.

Schipkowensky, N. (1968). Affective disorders: Cyclophrenia and murder. *International Psychiatry Clinics, 5,* 59–75.

Shakow, D. (1950). Some psychological features of schizophrenis. In M. L. Reymert (Ed.), *Feelings and emotions* (pp. 383–390). New York: McGraw Hill.

Shepherd, H. (1961). Morbid jealousy: A psychiatric symptom. *Journal of Mental Science, 107,* 687–753.

Shore, D. (1979). Self-mutilation and schizophrenia. *Comprehensive Psychiatry, 20*(4), 384–387.

Shore, D., Anderson, D. J., & Cutler, N. R. (1978). Prediction of self-mutilation in hospitalized schizophrenics. *American Journal of Psychiatry, 135,* 1406–1407.

Shore, D., Filson, C. R., & Johnson, W. E. (1988). Violent crime arrests and paranoid schizophrenia: The White House case studies. *Schizophrenia Bulletin, 14,*(2), 279–281.

Shore, D., Filson, C. R., Johnson, W. E., Rae, D. S., Muehrer, P., Kelley, D. J., Davis, T. S., Waldman, I. N., & Wyatt, R. J. (1989). Murder and assault arrests of White House cases: Clinical and demographic correlates of violence subsequent to civil commitment. *American Journal of Psychiatry, 146*(5), 645–651.

Shubsachs, A. P. W., & Young, A. (1988). Dangerous delusions: The "Hollywood phenomenon." *British Journal of Psychiatry, 152,* 722.

Silva, J. A., Leong, G. B., Weinstock, R., & Boyer, C. L. (1989). Capgras syndrome and dangerousness. *Bulletin of the American Academy of Psychiatry and the Law, 17*(1), 5–14.

Slater, E., & Roth, M. (1969). *Clinical psychiatry,* 3rd ed. London: Bailliere.

Spence, K. W. (1956). *Behavior theory and conditioning.* New Haven: Yale University Press.

Spiegel, D. E., Gerard, R. M., Grayson, H. M., & Gengerelli, J. A. (1962). Reactions of chronic schizophrenic patients and college students to facial expressions and geometric forms. *Journal of Clinical Psychology, 18,* 396–402.

Standage, K. F., Moore, J. A., & Cole, M. G. (1974). Self-mutilation of the genitalia by a female schizophrenic. *Canadian Psychiatric Association Journal, 19,* 17–20.

Sweeney, S., & Zamecnik, K. (1981). Predictors of self-mutilation in patients with schizophrenia. *American Journal of Psychiatry, 138*(8), 1086–1089.

Tapper, C. M., Bland, R. C., & Danyluk, L. (1979). Self inflicted eye injuries and self-inflicted blindness. *Journal of Nervous and Mental Disease, 167*(5), 311–314.

Taylor, C. (1964). *The Explanation of Behaviour.* London: Routledge.

Taylor, P. J. (1985). Motives for offending among violent and psychotic men. *British Journal of Psychiatry, 147,* 491–498.

Taylor, P., Garety, P., Buchanan, A., Reed, A., Wessely, S., Ray, K., Dunn, G., & Grubin, D. (1994). Delusions and violence. In J. Monahan & H. Steadman (Eds.), *Violence and mental disorder* (pp. 161–182). Chicago: University of Chicago Press.

Taylor, P., Mahendra, B., & Gunn J. (1983). Erotomania in males. *Psychological Medicine, 13,* 645–650.

Tomison, A. R., & Donovan, W. M. (1988). Dangerous delusions: The "Hollywood phenomenon." *British Journal of Psychiatry, 153,* 404–405.

Tenzer, J. A., & Orozco, H. (1970). Traumatic glossectomy. *Oral Surgery, 30,* 182–184.

Turner, J. B. (1964). Schizophrenics as judges of vocal expressions of emotional meaning. In J. R. Davitz (Ed.), *The communication of emotional meaning* (pp. 129–142). New York: McGraw-Hill.

Van Putten, T., Crumpton, E., & Yale, C. (1976). Drug refusal in schizophrenia and the wish to be crazy. *Archives of General Psychiatry, 33,* 1443–1446.

Varsamis, J., Adamson, J. D., & Sigurdson, W. F. (1972). Schizophrenics with delusions of poisoning. *British Journal of Psychiatry, 121,* 673–675.

Vaughn, C. E., & Leff, J. P. (1976). The influence of family and social factors on the course of psychiatric illness. *British Journal of Psychiatry, 129,* 125–137.

Virkkunen, M. (1974). On arson committed by schizophrenics. *Acta Psychiatrica Scandinavica, 50,* 152–160.

Watson, C. G., Jacobs, L., & Kucala, T. (1979). A note on the pathology of anhedonia. *Journal of Clinical Psychology, 35,* 740–743.

Waugh, A. C. (1986). Autocastration and biblical delusions in schizophrenia. *British Journal of Psychiatry, 149,* 656–659.

Weckowicz, T. E., & Sommer, R. (1960) Body image and self concept in schizophrenia. *Journal of Mental Science, 106,* 17–39.

Weinstock, R. (1976). Capgras syndrome: A case involving violence. *American Journal of Psychiatry, 133,* 855.

Wessely, S. (1993). Violence and psychosis. In C. Thompson & P. Cohen (Eds.), *Violence: Basic and clinical science* (pp. 119–134). London: Butterworth-Heinemann.

Wessely, S., Buchanan, A., Reed, A., Cutting, J., Everitt, B., Garety, P., & Taylor, P. (1993). Acting on delusions. I: Prevalence. *British Journal of Psychiatry, 163,* 69–76.

Westmermyer, J., & Serpass, A. (1972). A third case of self-enucleation. *American Journal of Psychiatry, 129,* 484.

Wing, J. K., Cooper, J. E., & Sartorius, N. (1974). *Measurement and classification of psychiatric symptoms.* Cambridge: Cambridge University Press.

Witherspoon, C., Feist, F., Morris, R., & Feist, R. (1989). Ocular self-mutilation. *Annals of Opthalmology, 21,* 255–259.

Yang, H., Brown, G., & Magargal, L. (1981). Self-inflicted ocular mutilation. *American Journal of Opthalmology, 91,* 658–663.

## 13

E. FULLER TORREY

# Violent Behavior by Individuals with Serious Mental Illness

## The Role of Treatment Compliance and Insight

The perception of an association between violent behavior and serious mental illness is a major cause of stigma affecting individuals with these disorders. Advocates attempting to decrease stigma frequently claim that seriously mentally ill individuals are no more violent than the general population. Studies bearing on this question are reviewed in this chapter. As shall be seen, this review reveals that although the vast majority of seriously mentally ill individuals are not more dangerous than the general population, recent studies suggest that a subgroup is more dangerous. Noncompliance with medication and substance abuse are common in this subgroup, indicating that these factors may be important predictors of future violence. Relevant to the focus of this chapter are data that indicate that poor insight into mental disorder is strongly associated with noncompliance, and denial is a common feature of substance abuse. The role poor insight may play in the prediction of violence is discussed after a review of existing literature on violence in the seriously mentally ill. Until the problem of dangerousness among this subgroup of patients is understood, it will be difficult to substantially decrease stigma against individuals with these illnesses.

## Historical Context

The idea that some individuals with serious mental illnesses may become violent was prevalent throughout the 19th century. In 1857, for example, Dr. John Gray published an analysis of 49 cases of attempted or completed homicide committed by seriously mentally ill patients whom he had treated (Gray, 1857). Dr. Emil Kraepelin, in his 1919 treatise on schizophrenia, observed that "in certain circumstances the impulsive

269

actions of the patients may become extraordinarily dangerous" (Kraepelin, 1919/1971). In movies, the stereotype of individuals with mental illnesses as homicidal maniacs can be found as early as *The Maniac Cook* in 1909 (Hyler, Gabbard, & Schneider, 1993).

Studies have shown that this stereotype has continued to be widespread. In a 1980 survey of college students' beliefs about individuals with schizophrenia, Wahl (1987) found that 52% of them believed that "aggression, hostility, [and] violence" were common or very common attributes while only 9% said these attributes were uncommon or very uncommon. A 1987 study of residents of Ohio revealed that perceived dangerousness was the single most important attribute in creating a negative and stigmatized status for mentally ill individuals (Link, Cullen, Frank, & Wozniak, 1987).

The media have both reflected and propagated this stereotype. Day and Page (1986), in a study of Canadian newspapers between 1977 and 1984, found that the traits of dangerousness and unpredictability were commonly attributed to individuals with serious mental illnesses. Other recent studies have found that newspaper stories tend to specifically link mental illness to crime, and that such stories are more likely placed on the front page (Wahl, 1992). One study of prime-time television revealed that dangerousness and unpredictability were commonly attributed to TV characters who were mentally ill (Wahl, 1982), while another study found that 72% of mentally ill characters on TV dramas were portrayed as violent (Signorelli, 1989). Movies linking mental illness to violence have continued to be popular over the years; examples of this genre have included *Psycho, Repulsion, Friday the 13th, Halloween, Nightmare on Elm Street,* and more recently *Silence of the Lambs* and *Single, White Female.*

Stigmatization and negative stereotypes are major problems for both individuals with serious mental illnesses and their families. They limit the availability of housing, jobs, social programs, and even psychiatric care; indeed, some individuals with a serious mental illness say that the stigma is worse than the disease itself. For this reason, the National Alliance for the Mentally Ill (NAMI) and the National Stigma Clearinghouse under the New York State Alliance for the Mentally Ill (AMI) have made concerted efforts in recent years to combat the stigma and negative stereotype connected to serious mental illnesses. The link between serious mental illnesses and violent behavior has also been questioned by some writers who assert that "a mentally ill person is not significantly more likely than anyone else to be violent" (Trafford, 1988). Since the association between serious mental illnesses and violent behavior is crucial to destigmatizing these illnesses, it is important to examine the available data regarding this association.

## Studies of Violent Behavior by Individuals with Serious Mental Illnesses

The incidence of violent behavior among individuals with serious mental illnesses has been examined by studying five different groups: (1) individuals who are arrested; (2) psychiatric inpatients; (3) psychiatric outpatients; (4) families with seriously mentally ill members; and (5) seriously mentally ill individuals identified by surveys of the general population. Each of these groups contributes a different perspective to the problem.

## Individuals Who Are Arrested

The arrest rate of seriously mentally ill individuals has traditionally been the most commonly used measure of their dangerousness. Studies carried out in 1922, 1930, 1938, and 1945 all found "that mentally ill persons had a lower arrest rate than the general population" (Brown, 1985, p. 133) and led to the oft-quoted claim that mentally ill individuals are no more dangerous than other people. One possible reason this was true at the time is that most seriously mentally ill individuals were confined to psychiatric hospitals for much of their adult lives.

Since the advent of deinstitutionalization in the 1960s, studies of seriously mentally ill individuals have found their arrest rate to be substantially higher than that of the general population. A 1992 survey of 1,391 U.S. jails reported that 7.2% of inmates had manifest symptoms of schizophrenia or bipolar disorder (Torrey, Stieber, & Ezekiel). Methodologically, the best studies of mentally ill individuals in jails were carried out by Teplin (1990) in Chicago (6.4% of jail admissions had schizophrenia, mania, or major depression) and by Guy, Platt, & Zwerling (1985) in Philadelphia (14.4% of jail admissions had schizophrenia or mania); most other studies have reported results falling between these estimates (Torrey et al., 1992). Studies of state prisons have also reported that inmates with schizophrenia and bipolar disorder constitute a substantial minority of the population; in a review of these studies, Jemelka, Trupin, and Chiles (1989) concluded "that 10 to 15 percent of prison populations have a major *DSM-III-R* thought disorder or mood disorder and need the services usually associated with severe or chronic mental illnesses" (pp. 483–484).

Arrest rates alone, however, are not good indexes of violent behavior because the majority of people are arrested for nonviolent offenses. This is especially true for seriously mentally ill individuals, among whom arrests for misdemeanors such as trespassing and disorderly conduct are very common (Torrey et al., 1992). A study in Alaska found that "only 28 percent of the arrests of referred schizophrenic patients were for violent crimes" (Phillips, Wolf, & Coons, 1988). The Alaskan study also estimated that 1% of all persons with schizophrenia in Alaska are arrested for violent crimes each year (Phillips et al., 1988, p. 609).

Lamb and Grant (1982) carried out studies in the Los Angeles County Jail of the types of crimes committed by seriously mentally ill individuals. Among 96 male inmates referred for psychiatric evaluation, 43 had been charged with misdemeanors and 53 with felonies; among the latter, 27 of the men (28% of the total group) had been charged with violent crimes (9 armed robbery, 8 assault with a deadly weapon, 4 murder, 2 assault on a peace officer, 2 felony assault, and 2 rape). A similar study of 97 female inmates referred for psychiatric evaluation found that 60 had been charged with misdemeanors and 37 with felonies, including 17 (18% of the total group) with violent crimes (Lamb & Grant, 1983).

Another approach to this problem is to study the psychiatric status of individuals who have been charged with particular types of violent crimes. Martell and Dietz (1992) identified 36 individuals who had pushed or tried to push other people in front of subway trains in New York City. Of the 36 individuals, 25 were referred for psychiatric evaluation and data were available on 20 of these. Among the 20, the diagnostic breakdown was as follows: 14 schizophrenia (8 of them had the paranoid subtype), 1 schizoaffective disorder, 1 bipolar disorder, 3 psychosis not otherwise specified, and 1 antisocial personality disorder. Except for one episode that took place during an attempted robbery, "all of the motives reported by these offenders reflected psychotic symptoms" (p. 474). Thus, individuals with serious mental illnesses appear to be responsible for a majority of cases of this particular type of violent crime.

### Psychiatric Inpatients

Numerous studies have been done on violent acts committed by mentally ill persons prior to admission, during the course of hospitalization, and following discharge from psychiatric hospitals. The first and second types of studies are of limited usefulness because violent acts are a major selection criteria for psychiatric hospital admission and because psychiatric ward personnel and policies may influence the number of violent acts committed by patients. Studies of discharged patients are more useful, and in fact should err on the side of minimizing the problem, since patients are usually not discharged until they are considered to no longer be potentially violent.

Several studies of individuals discharged from psychiatric hospitals have been carried out since deinstitutionalization. Studies up to 1979 were reviewed by Rabkin (1979), who concluded that "over the past 20 years, mental patients discharged from public facilities as a group have total arrest rates for all crimes that equal or exceed public rates with which they have been compared. Arrest and conviction rates for the subcategory of violent crimes were found to exceed general population rates in every study in which they were measured."

A more recent study by Klassen and O'Connor (1990) of male psychiatric patients who had a history of past violent behavior reported that 25 to 30% of them became violent again within one year after discharge. Another recent study by Steadman found "that 27 percent of released male and female patients report at least one violent act within a mean of four months after discharge" (Monahan, 1992, p. 515). Shore, Filson, and Rae (1990), in a study of hospitalized White House cases (individuals, usually with schizophrenia, who present themselves at the White House to see the president for delusional reasons), reported that following discharge, subjects with a history of prior arrests had a threefold higher rate of subsequent arrests for murder, assault, or robbery than subjects without prior arrests or a control population. Similar findings emerged from a Swedish study of 644 individuals with schizophrenia who were followed for 15 years following their initial psychiatric hospitalization, during which time they committed four times more violent offenses than a nonpsychiatrically ill control population (Lindquist & Allebeck, 1990). Studies such as these led the late Dr. Saleem Shah, of the National Institute of Mental Health, to write in 1990 that "almost every large study since the sixties has found that persons with histories of mental hospitalization (typically in public sector facilities) tend to have subsequent arrest rates higher than those for the general population" (Shah, 1990, p. 21).

### Psychiatric Outpatients

In addition to the postdischarge studies of psychiatric inpatients cited above, three studies of violent behavior among psychiatric outpatients have been carried out. In the first,

TABLE 13.1  Summary of Link et al. (1992) Study of Violent Behavior

| | Percentage of Individuals Exhibiting This Behavior | |
| --- | --- | --- |
| | Weapon Use in Past 5 Years | "Hurting Someone Badly" (Lifetime) |
| Nonpsychiatric residents | 2.7 | 5.4 |
| Psychiatric patients | | |
| First contact | 2.1 | 18.8** |
| Repeat Contact | 12.9** | 11.7 |
| Former patients | 11.1* | 16.7* |

*$p < .05$
**$p < .01$

Bartels, Drake, Wallach, & Freeman (1991), in New Hampshire, rated 133 outpatients diagnosed with schizophrenia on a five-point scale as follows: (1) no hostility; (2) irritability and argumentiveness; (3) verbally threatening behavior or mild object-directed aggression; (4) destruction of property or interpersonal assault without harm; and (5) assaultiveness with potential for actual harm. Of the 133 outpatients, 3 were rated as level 5, 14 as level 4, 24 as level 3, 28 as level 2, and 64 as level 1, having no hostility. Higher levels of hostility were significantly correlated with being male and with having a diagnosis of schizoaffective disorder. There was also a strong correlation between hostility and medication compliance; 71% of the outpatients rated at levels 4 and 5 had problems with medication compliance compared to only 17% of those rated at level 1 ($p < 0.001$). Furthermore, higher levels of hostility strongly predicted rehospitalization of the individual within one year ($p = 0.002$).

Another U.S. study of violent behavior in psychiatric outpatients was reported by Link, Andrews, and Cullen (1992) in New York. They compared 186 outpatients and 46 inpatients with 521 community residents who had not received any psychiatric care. Methodologically, the study is probably the best for violent behavior in psychiatric patients that has been done to date, with the groups matched on a wide variety of demographic characteristics and violent behavior measured in multiple ways (arrests, hitting others, fighting, weapon use, and "hurting someone badly"). The psychiatric patients were further divided into first-contact patients who had begun treatment within the past year, repeat treatment patients who had begun treatment more than a year previously and who were currently being treated, and former patients who had been treated in the past but not within the previous year.

The psychiatric patients were found to have engaged in significantly more violent behavior than the nonpsychiatric community residents. For the two most important indicators of violence, the results are summarized in table 13.1 and show that the psychiatric patients living in the community were 2 to 3 times more likely to have used a weapon or to have hurt someone badly compared to other community residents. Assessing demographic and socioeconomic variables, Link et al. found that none of them accounted for the differences in violent behavior between the two groups. The only variable that did account for the differences was the current level of psychotic symptoms—that is, the sicker the patients, the more likely they were to have exhibited violent behavior.

Similar findings were reported in a recent English study of 538 individuals with schizophrenia living in the Camberwell district of London. As controls, the researchers used individuals with psychiatric diagnoses other than schizophrenia and matched for age and sex with the study group. Compared to the controls, males with schizophrenia were found to have a 3.9 times greater risk and females with schizophrenia a 5.3 times greater risk for conviction for assault and serious violence (Wessely, et al., 1994).

The potential for violence by outpatients with serious mental illnesses is a threat that is also familiar to mental health professionals who work with such patients. In recent years, there have been several assaults on professionals by seriously mentally ill outpatients, including at least three that were fatal (Psychiatrist killed, 1985; Doctor stabbed, 1993; Dillon, 1992).

### Families with a Seriously Mentally Ill Member

In 1990, an extensive study was carried out by the National Alliance for the Mentally Ill of 1,401 families with a seriously mentally ill family member (Steinwachs, Kasper, & Skinner, 1992). In almost all cases, the ill family member had been diagnosed with schizophrenia, bipolar disorder, or major depression. The researchers reported that within the preceding year, 10.6% of the seriously mentally ill individuals had physically harmed another person and another 12.2% had threatened to harm another person. There was a marked sex difference for threatening harm (24.9% of males and 12.5% of females), but surprisingly little sex difference for actually harming someone (11.9% of males and 9.5% of females). An earlier survey of NAMI families had found that "over one-third of the families reported that their ill relative was assaultive and destructive in the home either sometimes or frequently" (Hatfield, 1990, p. 33).

The results of the NAMI surveys are consistent with other reports of violence by individuals with serious mental illnesses against family members. Straznickas, McNeil, & Binder (1993) reported that among psychiatric hospital admissions who had physically attacked someone within the preceding two weeks, family members had been the object of the assault 56% of the time. A similar study by Tardiff (1984) reported that family members had been the object of the assault 65% of the time. Previous surveys of problems encountered by families with a seriously mentally ill relative living at home have also reported threatening or assaultive behavior to be a common problem (Runions & Prudo, 1983).

The results of the NAMI surveys are also consistent with anecdotal reports of violence against family members by seriously mentally ill individuals (Acker & Fine, 1989; Richardson, 1990; Phillips, 1991). A frequent theme in these accounts is the association between the violence and the mentally ill individual's refusal to take medication; for example, "Jane Doe," in a *New York Times* article entitled "My Brother Might Kill Me," said that her brother's "last several attacks" all took place "following his refusal to take his medication" (Doe, 1987, p. 13). As has been described in the chapters by Drs. Amador and McEvoy, such noncompliance is common in patients who lack insight into having a mental disorder. The psychological as well as physical trauma that these family members sustain when faced with a relative who has no insight and who refuses to take medication was summarized by one mother who had been the recipient of an attack:

The thought of being attacked and physically harmed by another is frightening in itself, but when the attacker is your own flesh and blood, it is additional, unspeakable trauma upon trauma as your whole being sways between love and fear. (Dearth, Labenski, & Mott, 1986, p. 74)

## Seriously Mentally Ill Individuals Identified by Surveys of the General Population

Two studies have been done of violent behavior among individuals with serious mental illnesses who were identified by surveys of the general population. As such, the individuals in these studies were not selected in any way by treatment criteria or by having been arrested. The first was the American five-site Epidemiological Catchment Area (ECA) program carried out between 1980 and 1983 by the National Institute of Mental Health (Swanson, et al., 1990). Violence in the survey was assessed with four criteria: (1) hitting or throwing things at one's wife, husband, or partner; (2) hitting one's child hard enough to cause bruises or injury; (3) physical fighting with others, and (4) using a weapon such as a stick, knife, or gun in a fight. A major shortcoming of the study was the lack of rating of severity of the violent behavior—that is, hitting someone with a stick and killing someone with a gun were rated equally.

The results, summarized in table 13.2, show that individuals who have serious mental illnesses and are living in the community report having been violent within the previous year much more frequently than individuals who have no mental disorder. The frequency with which individuals with schizophrenia reported having used a weapon in a fight (21.5 times more than individuals with no psychiatric disorder) is especially noteworthy. In addition, the study found that almost one third of the individuals with schizophrenia or schizophreniform disorder also met diagnostic criteria for drug or alcohol abuse or dependence, and that these individuals had a much higher rate of reported violence than did those without this cofactor. Individuals with drug or alcohol abuse or dependence but without a serious mental illness had higher rates of reported violence than did individuals with serious mental illness alone.

The other random community survey of violent behavior among seriously mentally ill individuals was carried out in Sweden (Hodgins, 1992). The subjects included all individuals born in Stockholm in 1953 and still living there 30 years later. The category

TABLE 13.2  Violence Among Individuals with Serious Mental Illnesses in ECA Survey

| | Percent Positive Response Within Past Year | | | | |
| --- | --- | --- | --- | --- | --- |
| Diagnosis | Number | Partner | Hit Child | Physical Fight w/ Others | Used Weapon |
| No psychiatric disorder | 7,870 | 0.6 | 0.1 | 0.8 | 0.4 |
| Serious mental illness | | | | | |
| Schizophrenia or schizophreniform | 114 | 5.3 | 0.8 | 6.9 | 8.6 |
| Bipolar disorder | 30 | 5.3 | 2.1 | 0 | 0 |
| Major depression | 282 | 5.2 | 1.2 | 4.8 | 5.0 |

of violent crimes included all offenses involving the use of threat of physical violence (for example, assault, rape, robbery, unlawful threat, and molestation). The category of major mental disorder included schizophrenia, paranoid states, major affective disorders, and other psychoses. Men with major mental disorders were found to be 4.2 times more likely to have been convicted of a violent crime and women with major mental disorders were found to be 27.5 times more likely to have been convicted of a violent crime than men and women with no psychiatric diagnoses.

## Media Accounts of Violent Behavior by Individuals with Serious Mental Illnesses

In addition to the objective studies reviewed above, it is useful to examine media accounts of violent behavior by individuals with serious mental illnesses. Although the media do not use scientific methodology in the selection of its subjects, coverage reflects events in the community and also shapes public opinion about these events. As Steadman (1981) has noted: "What the public knows about how the mentally ill behave is for the most part garnered from newspaper reports, television and radio news, and television dramatizations" (p. 311).

Isolated examples of media coverage of mentally ill individuals who commit violent acts can be found throughout the 20th century. Among the most highly publicized episodes in the years following the Second World War were the 13 murders committed by Howard Unruh in Camden, New Jersey, in 1949 (Yoder, 1950); the 13 murders committed by Herbert Mullin in the San Francisco Bay area in 1972 (Lunde & Morgan, 1980); and the multiple spree of rapes, robberies, and murders of Joseph Kallinger ("The Shoemaker") in the Philadelphia area in 1974 (Schreiber, 1983). All three men were diagnosed with schizophrenia.

In recent years, however, reports of violence by seriously mentally ill individuals have become commonplace. A highly publicized example of such reports for each year since 1980 follows:

1980    In New York, Dennis Sweeney, diagnosed with paranoid schizophrenia, killed Congressman Allard Lowenstein, whom Sweeney believed was causing his auditory hallucinations (Margolick, 1992).

1981    In Washington, D.C., John Hinckley, diagnosed with schizophrenia, shot President Reagan and three others (Hinckley & Hinckley, 1985).

1982    In Tokyo, a pilot for Japan Air Lines, responding to auditory hallucinations, crashed an airliner into Tokyo Bay (Pilot-test system, 1983).

1983    In California, Michael Miller, a young man with schizophrenia who was the son of President Reagan's tax attorney, killed his mother (Tax lawyer's son, 1983).

1984    In California, Henry Lucas, a drifter who had been diagnosed with schizophrenia, was charged with the murder of 36 women (Gorney, 1984).

1985    In Philadelphia, Sylvia Seegrist, diagnosed with schizophrenia, killed three people and wounded seven others in a shooting spree in a shopping mall (Massacre, 1985).

1986    In New York, Juan Gonzalez, diagnosed with schizophrenia, killed two and wounded nine others on the Staten Island ferry in an attack with a sword (Sullivan, 1986).

1987    In Michigan, Bartley Dobben, diagnosed as psychotic, killed his two young sons by putting them into a foundry ladle (Suspect's ills, 1987).

1988    In Chicago, Laurie Dann, diagnosed with schizophrenia, killed one child and wounded five others in an attack in a school classroom (Eggington, 1991).

1989    In Louisville, Joseph Wesbecker, diagnosed with bipolar disorder, killed seven coworkers and wounded 13 others (Smothers, 1989).

1990    In Atlanta, James Brady, diagnosed with schizophrenia and who believed he was being controlled by a machine in his body, killed one and wounded four in a shooting spree in a shopping center (Long, 1990).

1991    In California, Philip Jablonski, diagnosed with schizophrenia and with past convictions for rape and murder, killed four more women within seven months following his release from prison (Furillo, 1991).

1992    In New York, Larry Hogue, diagnosed with chronic psychosis and drug abuse, was involuntarily hospitalized after attempting to injure residents of a Manhattan neighborhood (Lyall, 1993).

1993    In Alabama, Eileen Janezic, diagnosed with bipolar disorder, was charged with the murder of a minister and the shooting of another man. At the time of her arrest she was carrying the "Satanic Bible" (Bell, 1993).

These examples include only incidents in which seriously mentally ill individuals attacked other people. They do not include nonassault cases such as Randall Husar, who in 1986 smashed with a hammer the glass case holding the Constitution and the Bill of Rights in Washington, D.C. (Anderson, 1986), or Stephen Blumberg, who in 1990 was arrested in Iowa for stealing approximately 11,000 rare books from libraries (Maraniss, 1990), or Patrick Lee Frank, who in 1992 was indicted for setting 20 church fires in Tennessee and Florida (Drifter indicted, 1992). All three men had been diagnosed with schizophrenia. Nor do they include other highly publicized but less serious assaults, such as the man "muttering about earthquakes and revelations" who, without warning, punched Senator John Glenn during a 1989 public tree-planting ceremony (Castenada, 1989, p. B1).

In reviewing these and other media accounts of violent acts by individuals with serious mental illness, three aspects stand out. First, most of the perpetrators of the violent acts had previously been under psychiatric care. Indeed, in many cases, the seriously mentally ill individual had been evaluated and released by a psychiatrist within days or even hours of the act. Second, seriously mentally ill women appear to commit almost as many violent acts as do seriously mentally ill men; this is in sharp contrast to violent acts committed by nonmentally ill individuals, for which men are responsible for the vast majority. Third, media accounts of violent acts by mentally ill individuals appear to have increased in frequency since approximately 1980, and seem to be continuing to increase. Such an increase would be consonant with many of the studies discussed previously, including one study that specifically reported an increasing incidence of violent behavior by mentally ill individuals (Karras & Otis, 1987).

It is, of course, not possible to quantify violent acts by individuals with serious mental illnesses from media sources, since an unknown percentage of such acts come to media attention. In an effort to assess the frequency of those that do, however, the author collected all such examples reported in a single newspaper (*Washington Post*) covering the Washington, D.C., metropolitan area of approximately 3 million people for one year (1992). They included the following:

- Jayant Vatz, diagnosed with bipolar disorder and responding to "a thousand voices," pleaded guilty to the murder of his father and stepmother (Marcus, 1992, p. B1).
- Sandra Moneymaker, said to have "severe depression with psychotic features," was found innocent by reason of insanity in the killing of her two sons (Woman who killed, 1992, p. C6).
- Kathlynn Najeera, suffering from "acute paranoid schizophrenia," was found insane and committed to a mental hospital after she intentionally drove her car into and killed a 10-year-old boy on a bicycle (Duggan, 1992, p. D10).
- Brian Bechtold, diagnosed with paranoid schizophrenia, was said to be legally insane at the time he killed his mother and father (Man who said, 1992).
- Alan Newman, arrested and suspected of being responsible for five homicides, had previously been found to be "acutely psychotic" and "characteristically quite disturbed" by a psychiatrist (Jennings & Heath, 1992, p. D1).
- Hadden Clark, who killed a young woman in her home, had been twice diagnosed with schizophrenia (Jennings, 1992).

Insofar as these reports are representative of the population of the country, there would have been a total of approximately 500 similar incidents reported by newspapers in the United States in 1992.

## Discussion

It is a well-documented fact that America is a violent society; of the 19 million crime victimizations reported in 1990, nearly one third of them involved violence (Reiss & Roth, 1993). Within this broad landscape of violence, the contribution of seriously mentally ill individuals to the total picture is not large. This stands in contrast to less violent societies such as Iceland, in which only 47 homicides were committed over 80 years, but individuals with serious mental illnesses were responsible for 13 (28%) of them (Petersson & Gudjonsson, 1981). Alcohol and drug abusers in the United States are, as a group, much more violent than are individuals with serious mental illnesses.

The studies reviewed above verify that the vast majority of individuals with serious mental illnesses are not violent and not more dangerous than the general population. A subgroup of such individuals, however, is more dangerous and the data suggest that this may be an increasing problem. The fact that "27 percent of released male and female [psychiatric] patients report at least one violent act within a mean of four months after discharge" (Monahan, 1992, p. 515), that 8.6% of individuals with schizophrenia living in the community had used a weapon in a fight within the preceding year (Swanson et al., 1990), and that 10.6% of individuals with serious mental illnesses had physically harmed another person within the preceding year (Steinwachs et al., 1992), should be of concern to all mental health professionals. As summarized by Dr. John Monahan after his review of such studies: "The data that have recently become available, fairly read, suggest the one conclusion I did not want to reach . . . there appears to be a relationship between mental disorder and violent behavior" (Monahan, 1992, p. 519). Since there are by conservative estimates approximately 2.5 million individuals with schizophrenia and bipolar disorder in the United States, the total number of violent acts being committed by these individuals is of great concern.

Insofar as there is a relationship between violent behavior and a subgroup of individuals with serious mental illnesses, then the public stereotype that links violence to mental illness is based on reality and not merely stigma. As such, present attempts to combat this stereotype by campaigns of public education will fail until the problem of violent behavior is addressed. Lagos, Perlmutter, and Saexinger (1977) noted this fact as early as 1977, in an article entitled "Fear of the Mentally Ill: Empirical Support for the Common Man's Response." In 1981, Steadman similarly observed that "recent research data on contemporary populations of ex-mental patients supports these public fears [of dangerousness] to an extent rarely acknowledged by mental health profession-als. . . . It is [therefore] futile and inappropriate to badger the news and entertainment media with appeals to help destigmatize the mentally ill" (Steadman, 1981, p. 314). In a similar vein, Monahan recently added: "The data suggest that public education pro-grams by advocates for the mentally disordered along the lines of 'people with mental illness are no more violent than the rest of us' may be doomed to failure. . . . And they should: the claim, it turns out, may well be untrue" (Monahan, 1992, p. 519). Cur-rently, then, the average citizen may ride to work on a bus with a poster proclaiming that mentally ill individuals are not dangerous while simultaneously reading that day's newspaper headline that says in effect that some of them are dangerous.

Since violent acts by individuals with serious mental illnesses are carried out by only a small minority, are there indicators from the studies suggesting which individuals these are likely to be? One strong predictor of potential violence that is applicable to everyone is the person's history of violent behavior. A second strong predictor also applicable to everyone is concurrent alcohol or drug abuse. Among individuals with serious mental illnesses, concurrent alcohol or drug abuse may be an even stronger predictor of violent behavior because many individuals experience an exacerbation of their symptoms while abusing alcohol or drugs. Although no data were available to address the question of whether drug abusing mentally ill individuals also lack insight into their illness, such a relationship seems feasible, given the high incidence of denial seen in substance abusers. The role of insight in the prediction of violence is discussed further below, particularly with respect to the issue of noncompliance with prescribed medication.

A third factor that appears to be an important predictor of violent behavior in seri-ously mentally ill individuals is noncompliance with medication. It is known that peo-ple who are mentally ill do not take medication for a variety of reasons, including lack of insight, medication side effects, and a poor doctor-patient relationship. It is also known that individuals with serious mental illnesses have a high rate of failure to take medication; in one study, only 50% of them were still taking prescribed antipsychotic medication one year following hospital discharge (Weiden, Dixon, & Frances). Indi-viduals who do not take prescribed medication appear to be much more likely to com-mit violent acts. For example, in the Bartels et al. (1991) study of psychiatric outpa-tients, "71 percent of the violent patients . . . had problems with medication compliance, compared with only 17 percent of those without hostile behaviors" (p. 166) and the correlation was highly statistically significant ($p < 0.001$). Similarly, in a study of inmates in a state forensic hospital, Smith (1989) found a highly significant correlation ($p < 0.001$) between the failure to take medication and having committed violent acts in the community. Another measure of the failure to take prescribed antipsychotic medication is the continuing presence of prominent psychotic symptoms, since taking medication reduces such symptoms in most cases. In the Link et al. (1992) study of seriously mentally ill individuals living in the community, psychotic symptoms were highly correlated with fighting ($p < 0.001$) and with hitting others ($p < 0.01$) and were "the only variable that accounts for differences in levels of violent/illegal behavior between patients and never-treated community residents" (p. 201). A similar association of psychotic symptoms and violent acts was reported by Dr. Pamela Taylor in her English study of 121 men with psychosis who had committed crimes. She concluded that "over 80 percent of the offenses of the psychotic [men] were probably attributable to their illness. . . . " (p. 497). Within the psychotic group, those driven to offend by their delusions were most likely to have been seriously violent, and psychotic symptoms probably accounted directly for most of the very violent behavior" (Taylor, 1985, p. 491). Studies of psychiatric inpatients have also consistently shown correlations between insufficient medication and increased violent behavior (Yesavage, 1982; Weaver, 1983; Smith, 1989).

At an anecdotal level, there is support for believing that the failure to take medication is an important predictor for violent behavior in individuals with serious mental illnesses. Phrases such as "he had gone a long time without his medication" [when he killed his mother] (Baltimore man, 1990, p. D3) and "his daughter was not taking her medication at the time of the slaying" [of her mother] (Crofton woman, 1990, p. D3) recur regularly in newspaper accounts of such violent acts. The data, then, suggest that individuals with serious mental illnesses are not more dangerous than the general population *when they are taking their antipsychotic medication*. However, when they are not taking their medication, some of them *are* more dangerous.

The fact that many individuals with serious mental illnesses do not take the medication prescribed to control their psychotic symptoms is not unexpected. The brain—the organ which we use for insight and appreciation of our needs—is the same organ whose function is impaired by schizophrenia and bipolar disorder. In fact, recent studies have indicated that schizophrenia patients with unawareness of illness perform more poorly than those with awareness on measures of frontal lobe functioning (see chapters 1, 7, and 15). Other studies have shown insight to be severely impaired in many seriously mentally ill individuals. For example, a study by David (1992) in London found that 47% of inpatients with psychosis scored poorly on a measure of insight. A more recent study by Amador et al. (1994) in New York reported that nearly 60% of 221 patients with schizophrenia had "moderate to severe unawareness of having a mental disorder" (p. 823). Amador et al. (1991) also reviewed studies relating insight to medication compliance and reported that the bulk of the evidence supports a direct relationship between the two (p. 122). In chapter 14 of this volume, the relationship between insight into illness and compliance with treatment is discussed at length. Calling lack of insight the core problem of mentally ill homeless individuals, the *Wall Street Journal* said that "that problem, simply put, is that the mentally ill require treatment which they are incapable of seeking for themselves" (Psychosis, 1990, p. 15).

Taken together, these data suggest that lack of insight may play a significant role in predicting the violence of patients with severe mental illnesses. Over and above any relationship to noncompliance with prescribed medication, it is possible that such deficits in self-awareness could also lead to breakdowns in self-monitoring and modulation of affect (e.g., anger and fear). Without an intact capacity to self-monitor effectively, self-control of violent impulses may become difficult. To date, there have been no published studies investigating the relationship between insight into illness and violent behaviors in the severely mentally ill. Clearly, this issue will need to be examined in future work if we are to gain a better understanding of violence in such individuals.

In addition to history of violence, concurrent substance abuse, and medication noncompliance, previous studies have suggested other possible predictors of violence in individuals with serious mental illnesses. Delusions, especially those in which persons believe that someone or something has taken control of their mind, have been found to be correlated with violent behavior in studies in England (Taylor, Mullen, & Wessely, 1993). Neurological impairment in mentally ill individuals is also found more commonly in those who are violent (Krakowski et al., 1989), and there has been speculation that some violent mentally ill individuals may have a form of epilepsy that has not been diagnosed. Command hallucinations are also frequently cited as predictors of violent behavior.

Is it possible to predict which seriously mentally ill individuals will become violent? Studies done in the 1970s reported that mental health professionals were unable to predict violence in their patients at more than a chance level. A recent reanalysis of those studies by Apperson, Mulvey, and Lidz (1993) demonstrated flawed methodology in many of the earlier studies, while Lidz, Mulvey, and Gardner (1993) concluded that "clinical judgment has been undervalued in previous research" (p. 1010). Utilizing all the predictive factors enumerated above, it may be possible to predict violent behavior in seriously mentally ill individuals at a clinically useful level. An important longitudinal study of risk assessment in individuals with serious mental illnesses is currently under way in Pittsburgh, PA, Worcester, MA, and Kansas City, MO, funded by the MacArthur Foundation, but will not be completed until 1995 (Monahan & Steadman, in press).

Finally, it should be remembered that violent behavior by individuals with serious mental illnesses is merely one aspect of a larger problem: the failure of public psychiatric services and deinstitutionalization. Other aspects of this problem include the large number of seriously mentally ill individuals among the homeless (Torrey, 1988), the large number of seriously mentally ill individuals in jails and prisons (Torrey et al., 1992; Jemelka et al., 1989), and the revolving door of psychiatric hospital readmissions, through which 30% of discharged patients are readmitted to the hospital within 30 days following discharge (Davidson, 1991), with some individual patients accumulating over 100 readmissions (Geller, 1992).

The fact that some seriously mentally ill individuals, especially those who are not taking prescribed medications (who probably lack insight), are more prone to acts of violence has important implications for mental health services. Many such acts are theoretically preventable with good medication compliance and assertive case management; under such conditions one Canadian study reported a comparatively low incidence of violent acts by discharged patients with serious mental illnesses (Lafave, Pinkney, & Gerber, 1993). These data suggest that, if medication compliance can be increased, then the risk for violent acts can be reduced. As several chapters in the present volume discuss, increased insight into illness is one of the best, if not the best, predictor of compliance with prescribed treatments. Poor insight, because it is so strongly associated with noncompliance with treatment, may also be a characteristic of individuals prone to violence. As such, increased insight should mitigate against violent behaviors in the seriously mentally ill.

*Acknowledgments*    Parts of this manuscript were previously published in *Hospital and Community Psychiatry*. Reprinted here with permission.

*References*

Acker, J., & Fine, M. J. (1989). Families under siege: A mental health crisis. *Philadelphia Inquirer*, September 10–14 (5 parts), pp. 1A–10A.

Amador, X. F., Andreasen, N. C., Flaum, M., Strauss, D. H., Yale, S. A., Clark, S., & Gorman, J. M. (1994). Awareness of illness in schizophrenia, schizoaffective and mood disorders. *Archives of General Psychiatry, 51*, 826–836.

Amador, X. F., Strauss, D. H., Yale, S. A. (1991). Awareness of illness in schizophrenia. *Schizophrenia Bulletin, 17*, 113–132.

Anderson, J. W. (1986). Man smashes constitution case. *Washington Post*, October 11, pp. A1, B2.

Apperson, L. J., Mulvey, E. P., & Lidz, C. W. (1993). Short-term clinical prediction of assaultive behavior: Artifacts of research methods. *American Journal of Psychiatry, 150*, 1374–1379.

Baltimore man charged in mother's slaying. (1990). *Washington Post*, December 27, p. D3.

Bartels, J., Drake, R. E., Wallach, M. A., & Freeman, D. H. (1991). Characteristic hostility in schizophrenic outpatients. *Schizophrenia Bulletin, 17*, 163–171.

Bell, C. (1993). Shooting suspect's bond is $250,000. *Huntsville Times*, September 5, p. B1.

Brown, P. (1985). The transfer of care: Psychiatric deinstitutionalization and its aftermath. London: Routledge and Kegan Paul.

Castenada, R. (1989). Sen. Glenn assaulted. *Washington Post*, October 26, p. B1.

Crofton woman found guilty in mother's slaying. (1990). *Washington Post*, September 28, p. D3.

David, A., Buchanan, A., Reed, A., Almeida, O. (1992). The assessment of insight in psychosis. *British Journal of Psychiatry, 161*, 599–602; and personal communication with Dr. David.

Davidson, R. (1991). A mental health crisis in Illinois. *Chicago Tribune*, December 9, p. 18.

Day, D. M., & Page, S. (1986). Portrayal of mental illness in Canadian newspapers. *Canadian Journal of Psychiatry, 31*, 813–816.

Dearth, N., Labenski, B. J., Mott, E. M., & Pellegrini, L. M. (1986). *Families helping families: Living with Schizophrenia*. New York: W. W. Norton.

Dillon, S. (1992). Social workers: Targets in a violent society. *New York Times*, November 18, pp. A1, B6.

Doctor stabbed by patient. (1993). *Lafayette Advertiser*, April 10, p. A2.

Doe, J. (1987). My brother might kill me. *New York Times*, May 6, p. 13.

Drifter indicted in church fires. (1992). *Washington Post*, February 14, p. A19.

Duggan, P. (1992). P.G. woman ruled insane in bike death. *Washington Post*, May 5, p. D10.

Egginton, J. (1991). *Day of fury*. New York: William Morrow.

Furillo, A. (1991). Why a killer was set free. *San Francisco Examiner*, July 24, pp. A1, A10.

Geller, J. L. (1992). A report on the "worst" state hospital recidivists in the U.S. *Hospital and Community Psychiatry, 43*, 904–908.

Gorney, C. (1984). Anatomy of a killer. *Washington Post*, October 11, pp. B1, B6.

Gray, J. P. (1857). Homicide in insanity. *American Journal of Insanity, 14*, 119–143.

Guy, E., Platt, J. J., Zwerling, I., & Bullock, S. (1985). Mental health status of prisoners in an urban jail. *Criminal Justice and Behavior, 12*, 29–53.

Hatfield, A. B. (1990). *Family education in mental illness*. New York: Guilford Press, p. 33, citing a study by R. W. Swan and M. R. Lavitt, Patterns of adjustment to violence in families of the mentally ill. Elizabeth Wisna Research Center, Tulane University School of Social Work, New Orleans.

Hinckley, J., & Hinckley, J. A. (1985). *Breaking points*. Grand Rapids, MI: Chosen Books.

Hodgins, S. (1992). Mental disorder, intellectual deficiency, and crime. *Archives of General Psychiatry, 49*, 476–483.

Hyler, S. E., Gabbard, G. O., & Schneider, I. (1993). Movie madness. *Journal of the California Alliance for the Mentally Ill, 4*, 4–7.

Jemelka, R., Trupin, E., & Chiles, J. A. (1989). The mentally ill in prisons. *Hospital and Community Psychiatry, 40*, 481–485.

Jennings, V. T. (1992). Family trouble plagued alleged Bethesda killer. *Washington Post*, November 15, p. B1.

Jennings, V. T., & Heath, T. (1992). Gun that killed 4 was stolen in VA: Suspect has history of violence, psychosis. *Washington Post*, October 14, p. D1.

Karras A., & Otis, D. B. (1987). A comparison of inpatients in an urban state hospital in 1975 and 1982. *Hospital and Community Psychiatry, 38*, 963–967.

Klassen, D., & O'Connor, W. (1990). Assessing the risk of violence in released mental patients: A cross-validation study. *Psychological Assessment: A Journal of Consulting and Clinical Psychology, 1*, 75–81.

Kraepelin, E. (1919/1971). *Dementia praecox and paraphrenia*. Huntington, NY: Robert E. Krieger.

Krakowski, M. I., Convit, A., Jaeger, J., Shang, L., Volavka, J. (1989). Neurological impairment in violent schizophrenic inpatients. *American Journal of Psychiatry, 146*, 849–853.

Lafave, H. G., Pinkney, A. A., & Gerber, G. J. (1993). Criminal activity by psychiatric clients after hospital discharge. *Hospital and Community Psychiatry, 44*, 180–181.

Lagos, J. M., Perlmutter, K., & Saexinger, H. (1977). Fear of the mentally ill: Empirical support for the common man's response. *American Journal of Psychiatry, 134*, 1134–1137.

Lamb, H. R., & Grant, R. W. (1982). The mentally ill in an urban county jail. *Archives of General Psychiatry, 39*, 17–22.

Lamb, H. R., & Grant, R. W. (1983). Mentally ill women in a county jail. *Archives of General Psychiatry, 40*, 363–368.

Lidz, C. W., Mulvey, E. P., & Gardner, W. (1993). The accuracy of predictions of violence to others. *Journal of American Medical Association, 269*, 1007–1011.

Lindquist, P., & Allebeck, P. (1990). Schizophrenia and crime. A longitudinal follow-up of 644 schizophrenics in Stockholm. *British Journal of Psychiatry, 157*, 345–350.

Link, B. G., Andrews, H., Cullen, F. T. (1992). The violent and illegal behavior of mental patients reconsidered. *American Sociological Review, 57*, 275–292.

Link, B. G., Cullen, F. T., Frank, J., Wozniak, J. F. (1987). The social rejection of former mental patients: Understanding why labels matter. *American Journal of Sociology, 92*, 1461–1500.

Long, K. (1990). James Brady: A life in search of himself. *Atlanta Constitution*, May 22, pp. A1, A13.

Lunde, D. T., & Morgan, J. (1980). *The die song*. New York: WW Norton.

Lyall, S. (1993). Danger of mentally ill homeless to be re-evaluated in New York. *New York Times*, January 22, pp. A1, B2.

Man who said he killed parents may be sent to mental hospital. (1992). *Washington Post*, August 5, p. D3.

Maraniss, D. (1990). The complete collector. *Washington Post*, April 1, pp. A1, A23.

Marcus, E. (1992). Man pleads guilty in deaths of father, stepmother. *Washington Post*, February 1, p. B1.

Margolick, D. (1992). Lowenstein killer moves toward freedom. *New York Times*, November 1, pp. 49, 54.

Martell, D. A., & Dietz, P. E. (1992). Mentally disordered offenders who push or attempt to push victims onto subway tracks in New York City. *Archives of General Psychiatry, 49*, 472–475.

Massacre at the mall. (1985). *Washington Post*, November 2, p. A12.

Monahan, J. (1992). Mental disorder and violent behavior. *American Psychologist, 47*, 511–521.

Monahan, J., & Steadman, H. J. (in press). Toward a rejuvenation of risk assessment research. In J. Monahan & H. Steadman (Eds.), *Violence and mental disorder: Developments in risk assessment.* Chicago: University of Chicago Press.

Petersson, H., & Gudjonsson, G. H. (1981). Psychiatric aspects of homicide. *Acta Psychiatrica Scandinavica, 64*, 363–372.

Phillips, B. J. (1991). No one to ease his demon grip. *Philadelphia Inquirer*, July 23, p. 17.

Phillips, M. R., Wolf, A. S., & Coons, D. J. (1988). Psychiatry and the criminal justice system: Testing the myths. *American Journal of Psychiatry, 145*, 605–610.

Pilot-test system assailed. (1983). *Newsday*, May 18, p. 38.

Psychiatrist killed by patient. (1985). *American Medical News*, August 16, p. 17

Psychosis and civil rights. (1990). *Wall Street Journal*, September 28, p. 15.

Rabkin, J. (1979). Criminal behavior of discharged mental patients: A critical appraisal of the research. *Psychological Bulletin, 86*, 1–27.

Reiss, A. J., & Roth, J. A. (1993). *Understanding and preventing violence.* Washington, DC: National Academy Press.

Richardson, D. (1990). Dangerousness and forgiveness. *Journal of the California Alliance for the Mentally Ill, 2*, 4–5.

Runions, J., & Prudo, R. (1983). Problem behaviors encountered by families living with a schizophrenic member. *Canadian Journal of Psychiatry, 28*, 383–386.

Schreiber, F. R. (1983). *The shoemaker: The anatomy of a psychotic.* New York: New American Library.

Shah, S. A. (1990). Violence and the mentally ill. *Journal of the California Alliance for the Mentally Ill, 2*, 20–21.

Shore, D., Filson, C. R., Rae, D. S. (1990). Violent crime arrest rates of White House case subjects and matched control subjects. *American Journal of Psychiatry, 147*, 746–750.

Signorelli, N. (1989). The stigma of mental illness on television. *Journal of Broadcasting and Electronic Media, 33*, 325–331.

Smith, L. D. (1989). Medication refusal and the rehospitalized mentally ill inmate. *Hospital and Community Psychiatry, 40*, 491–496.

Smothers, R. (1989). Disturbed past of killer of 7 is unraveled. *New York Times*, September 16, p. 10.

Steadman, H. J. (1981). Critically reassessing the accuracy of public perceptions of the dangerousness of the mentally ill. *Journal of Health and Social Behavior, 22*, 310–316.

Steinwachs, D. M., Kasper, J. D., & Skinner, E. A. (1992). *Family perspectives on meeting the needs for care of severely mentally ill relatives: A national survey.* Arlington, VA: National Alliance for the Mentally Ill.

Straznickas, K. A., McNeil, D. E., & Binder, R. L. (1993). Violence toward family caregivers by mentally ill relatives. *Hospital and Community Psychiatry, 44*, 385–387.

Sullivan, R. (1986). Doctors had tried to hospitalize suspect in slashing on ferryboat. *New York Times*, November 11, pp. A1, B3.

Suspect's ills are described. (1987). *Washington Post*, November 29, p. A20.

Swanson, J. W., Holzer, C. E., Ganju, V. K., & Jono, R. T. (1990). Violence and psychiatric disorder in the community: Evidence from the Epidemiologic Catchment Area surveys. *Hospital and Community Psychiatry, 41*, 761–770.

Tardiff, K. (1984). Characteristics of assaultive patients in private hospitals. *American Journal of Psychiatry, 141*, 1232–1235.

Tax lawyer's son committed. (1983). *New York Times*, May 9, p. 15.

Taylor, P. (1985). Motives for offending amongst violent and psychotic men. *British Journal of Psychiatry, 147*, 491–498.

Taylor, P. J., Mullen, P., & Wessely, S. (1993). Psychosis, violence and crime. In J. Gunn & P. J. Taylor (Eds.), *Forensic psychiatry: Clinical, legal and ethical issues* (pp. 330–371). London: Butterworth and Heinemann.

Teplin, L. A. (1990). The prevalence of severe mental disorder among male urban jail detainees: Comparison with epidemiologic catchment area program. *American Journal of Public Health, 80*, 639–669.

Torrey, E. F. (1988). *Nowhere to go: The tragic odyssey of the homeless mentally ill*. New York: Harper and Row.

Torrey, E. F., Stieber, J., Ezekiel, J., Wolfe, S. M., Sharfstein, J., Noble, J. H., and Flynn, L. M. (1992). *Criminalizing the seriously mentally ill: The abuse of jails as mental hospitals*. Washington, DC: National Alliance for the Mentally Ill and Public Citizen's Health Research Group.

Trafford, A. (1988). For the mentally ill, another stigma. *Washington Post*, January 5, p. A17.

Wahl, O. F. (1987). Public vs. professional conceptions of schizophrenia. *Journal of Community Psychology, 15*, 285–291.

Wahl, O. (1992). Mass media images of mental illness: A review of the literature. *Journal of Community Psychology, 20*, 343–352.

Wahl, O. F., Roth, R. (1982). Television images of mental illness: Results of a metropolitan Washington media watch. *Journal of Broadcasting, 28*, 599–605.

Weaver, K. E. (1983). Increasing the dose of antipsychotic medication to control violence. Letter, *American Journal of Psychiatry, 140*, 1274.

Weiden, P. J., Dixon, L., & Frances, A. (1991). Neuroleptic compliance in schizophrenia. In C. Tamminga & C. Schulz (Eds.), *Advances in neuropsychiatry and psychopharmacology*, Vol. 1: Schizophrenia research. New York: Raven Press.

Wessely, S. C., Castle, D., Douglas, A. J., & Taylor, P. J. (in press). The criminal careers of incident cases of schizophrenia. *Psychological Medicine, 24*(2), 483–502, 1994, May.

Woman who killed sons found insane. (1992). *Washington Post*, February 25, p. C6.

Yesavage, J. A. (1982). Inpatient violence and the schizophrenic patient: An inverse correlation between danger-related events and neuroleptic levels. *Biological Psychiatry, 17*, 1331–1337.

Yoder, R. M. (1950). The strange case of Howard Unruh. *Saturday Evening Post*, September 16, pp. 24–25.

# PART V

# Clinical
# Implications
# of
# Poor Insight

# 14

JOSEPH P. MCEVOY

# The Relationship Between Insight in Psychosis and Compliance with Medications

*It appears that the psychiatric patients who would benefit most by systematic medication are often seriously remiss. (Klein et al., 1974)*

Schizophrenia is a terrible illness. It most commonly strikes people at a young age. It severely limits their potential to work and support themselves, to marry, and to have satisfying relationships. If untreated, it pushes its victims to the sidelines of existence, where they waste their lives attending to hallucinatory perceptions or preoccupied with mistaken beliefs. Acute exacerbations of schizophrenia bring immediate dangers to afflicted patients themselves, pain and hardship to their families, and steep financial costs to society. It is a chronic disease and, especially if untreated, may follow a deteriorating, dilapidated course (Wyatt, 1991).

Effective treatments are available for schizophrenia. Classical antipsychotic drugs resolve exacerbations and forestall relapse. New therapeutic agents (e.g., clozapine, risperidone, and others) appear to offer greater therapeutic efficacy and have more benign side effects. With early (i.e., as soon as possible after the initial psychopathology appears) treatment of first psychotic episodes, the likelihood of good recovery approaches 90% (Lieberman et al., 1992). In contrast, if patients remain untreated over prolonged periods of active illness, or repeatedly stop their medications and relapse, they take longer to respond to treatment when it is initiated and they respond less fully (Wyatt, 1991).

Yet clinicians almost never see patients with schizophrenia who complain of having a terrible illness, or who actively seek treatment for its ravages. Rather, "among chronic schizophrenics, failure to comply with prescribed drug schedules is the most common reason for hospital readmission" (Caton, 1984, p. 76).

In this chapter, we will present evidence that lack of insight in psychosis leads to noncompliance with medications. First, we will review the studies that provide valid estimates of the prevalence of medication noncompliance among patients with schizo-phrenia. Subsequently, we will examine the often flawed conceptual frameworks within which patients consider their need for medications, and determine how these flawed frameworks relate to noncompliance. Finally, we will propose strategies, sup-ported by the available evidence, that may enhance compliance and thereby minimize the devastation wrought by this disease.

## Do Patients with Schizophrenia Take Their Medications?

In this section we will address only those studies that include an external validating measure of compliance—that is, either urine colorimetric tests or receipt of long-acting injectable antipsychotic drugs.

### Studies that Utilize Urine Colorimetric Tests

The Forrests (1961) developed colorimetric tests that could detect the presence of the original phenothiazine antipsychotic drugs and their metabolic products in the urines of patients who had recently been taking these drugs. Although the tests have limita-tions (they can detect only very recent noncompliance), they offer advantages over patient self-report or pill counts. Only completely negative urine tests will be utilized as indicators of noncompliance in this review.

On the basis of extensive work with these urine tests, the Forrests (1961, p. 301) conclude that "spot checks as well as systematic testing of hospital populations show that at least 5 percent to 15 percent of patients in institutions successfully 'cheek' their drugs." This 5 to 15% noncompliance rate among inpatients is confirmed by reports from other authors who have studied the problem. Neve (1958) found negative urines in 6 (10%) of 56 inpatients for whom chlorpromazine had been prescribed; in all 6 cases the patients either admitted to noncompliance when confronted or quickly developed positive urines when switched from tablets to liquid concentrate given under close supervision. Hare and Willcox (1967) found negative urines in 6% of inpatients and in 15% of less well-supervised day hospital patients for whom chlorpro-mazine or imipramine was prescribed. Wilson and Enoch (1967) found negative urines in 16% of 50 inpatients with schizophrenia supposedly taking chlorpromazine tablets; these patients' urines all converted to positive when the medication orders were switched from tablets to liquid concentrate. Irwin, Weitzel, and Morgan (1971) found that 7% of closed-ward patients, but 32% of less supervised open-ward patients, had negative urines despite prescribed chlorpromazine or thioridazine. These authors also note:

> Another interesting group consisted of 27 inpatients who were permitted to leave the hos-pital during the Christmas holiday for two to four weeks. Urine specimens were obtained when these patients returned to the hospital. Urinary testing indicated that 13 of 23 patients (57%) had not taken chlorpromazine as prescribed. (p. 1633)

We may expect that outpatients, who are largely without medical supervision, will have even higher rates of noncompliance. Indeed, Willcox, Gillan, and Hare (1965) found negative urines in 32% of 22 outpatients with schizophrenia for whom chlorpro-

TABLE 14.1 The Relationships between Level of Supervision and Compliance (Urine Colorimetric Tests)

| Study | Number (%) with Negative Urines |
|---|---|
| Hare and Willcox (1967) | |
| Inpatients | 7/120 (6%) |
| Day patients | 4/27 (15%) |
| Outpatients | 42/125 (33%) |
| Irwin et al. (1971) | |
| Locked ward | 5/67 (7%) |
| Open ward | 6/19 (32%) |
| Outpatients | 14/40 (35%) |

mazine was prescribed. McClellan and Cowan (1970) reported a surprisingly low 8% rate of negative urines among 286 outpatients for whom chlorpromazine and/or imipramine was prescribed. Irwin et al. (1971) report that 35% of outpatients had negative urines despite prescribed phenothiazines.

When the rates of negative urines are compared across patient groups at a single institution (see table 14.1), "the principal factor governing patient intake of medication appeared to be the amount of direct patient supervision" (Irwin et al., 1971, p. 1631).

### Studies Utilizing Long-Acting Intramuscular Preparations

Whether or not a patient comes to clinic to receive his or her injection of long-acting antipsychotic is another objective measure of compliance. Johnson and Freeman (1972) twice surveyed the attendance registers at four outpatient clinics in their geographical region to determine the percentages of patients who had failed to appear for recently scheduled injections of long-acting antipsychotic medication. Noncompliance rates ranged from 7 to 27%, with a mean of 17%.

Carney and Sheffield (1976) reported on 418 patients treated with long-acting injectable antipsychotic medications (fluphenazine enanthate, fluphenazine decanoate, or flupenthixol decanoate) for, on average, two to three years. The rates at which patients were withdrawn from treatment with these drugs ranged from 23 to 43%. Only 5 to 7% of patients were listed as uncooperative. The remainder were withdrawn primarily because of extrapyramidal side effects. It is possible that the willingness of these clinicians to discontinue injectable medications when extrapyramidal side effects became distressing kept "uncooperativeness" to a minimum.

Even in highly selected populations of patients who agree to participate in long-term follow-up studies of treatment with long-acting injectable antipsychotic medications, substantial rates of noncompliance are present. Sixteen of 44 (36%) patients missed at least one injection during the one-year study of Falloon, Watt, and Shepherd (1978), despite regular visits in the patients' homes by community nurses. Given the high level of support and supervision in this trial, only 2 (5%) of these patients persisted in their refusal of medications to the point of relapse.

Quitkin, Rifkin, Kane, Ramos-Lorenzi, and Klein (1978) also listed noncompliance as a reason for withdrawal from study in 8 of 30 (27%) chronic schizophrenic patients treated with fluphenazine decanoate and followed prospectively for one year.

### Studies in Which Patients Control Their Own Pharmacotherapy

Two studies are available in which matched groups of patients were randomly assigned to either receive their medications in a standard, supervised manner or to be in charge of taking their own medications. Both studies include external validating measures of compliance.

Klein, Lynn, Axelrod, and Dluhy (1974) studied 40 inpatients for whom chlorpromazine and/or imipramine was prescribed. Twenty of these patients were randomly assigned to open wards where they were responsible for taking their own medications. The other 20 remained on a locked ward where their medications were administered by a nurse. Urine tests were negative in only 7.5% of the patients who received their medications from nurses, but were negative in 40% of those patients responsible for taking their own medications. It is noteworthy that half of the patients in both groups received instruction from the nursing staff as to the nature, uses, dosage, and side effects of their medications. This instruction did not increase compliance.

Chien (1975) studied 47 chronically ill patients with schizophrenia who resided in cooperative apartments in the community. All were stabilized on biweekly injections of fluphenazine enanthate 37.5 mg IM. These patients were randomly assigned to one of three treatment strategies: the first group continued to receive fluphenazine enanthate 37.5 mg IM Q 2 wks as originally prescribed by the physician; the second group selected the frequency of injections themselves; the third group received placebo injections Q 2 wks. At the end of one year, 13 of 15 patients (87%) who were switched to placebo had deteriorated sufficiently to be removed from the study—that is, failed. Only 2 of 16 patients (12%) receiving the physician-regulated fluphenazine injections failed. In contrast, 6 of 16 (37%) of the self-regulated patients failed. However, 5 of the 6 failures in the self-regulated group (i.e., 32% of that group) simply stated they did not need any medication during the first week of the study and rapidly deteriorated to the point of removal from the study within the first 6 months. The remaining patients in the self-regulated group took, on average, about half the originally prescribed number of injections (i.e., extended their dosing interval to Q 4 wks). Perhaps because of the high dose originally prescribed, these patients did well.

### Summary of Compliance Studies

When patients with schizophrenia are responsible for taking their own *pills* (e.g., when they are outpatients), one third to one half of them will be noncompliant at any given time. This medication noncompliance may be temporary or fluctuating in individual patients. Weiden et al. (1991) report that although 48% of their patients became noncompliant for at least one week over a year of follow-up, only 30 to 40% were noncompliant at any given assessment interval.

The rates at which patients fail to take *injections* of long-acting antipsychotic medications are slightly lower (15–35%). The use of long-acting injectable preparations

may facilitate supervision (see section on ways to increase compliance), thereby limiting noncompliance. However, the samples studied in programs of treatment with
long-acting injectable preparations may be biased by the refusal of highly noncompliant patients to participate.

Rates of medication compliance appear to be powerfully influenced by the level of
supervision in differing treatment situations. However, there also appear to be differences intrinsic to patients that may determine whether they comply. Approximately
50% of patients will take their medications as prescribed with little or no support
required. An additional 35% of patients will comply if provided with supervision and
support. The remaining 15% of patients will do anything they can to avoid taking medications under any circumstances, and may require coercion to remain compliant.

Later in this chapter we will consider some of the practical (e.g., access and cost)
and pharmacological (discomforting side effects) reasons why patients may fail to take
their medications, but first we will focus on how patients conceptualize themselves,
specifically in terms of their need for medications.

## Patients' Conceptual Frameworks Regarding Medication

What are the conceptual frameworks within which patients with schizophrenia consider their need for medications?

### General Populations of Patients with Schizophrenia

Parkes, Brown, and Monck (1962) followed a group of 68 patients with schizophrenia
for whom antipsychotics were prescribed at index discharge. Twenty-seven of the 68
(40%) stopped their medication within two months of leaving hospital. When asked
why, all claimed that they did not need drugs.

Serban and Thomas (1974) surveyed 516 patients with chronic schizophrenia at the
time of their discharge from an index hospitalization. Although 69% of these patients
stated they believed regular use of medications would be helpful in treating their illness, only 29% stated that they took their medications regularly when outpatients.

Soskis (1978) compared 25 inpatients with schizophrenia who were receiving
antipsychotics with 15 medical inpatients receiving medication for a variety of serious medical illnesses. Only 4% of the schizophrenic patients acknowledged a diagnosis of schizophrenia, and only 32% included any concepts related to mental illness
in their explanation as to why they were receiving medications. In contrast, 40% of
the medical patients knew their diagnoses, and 87% included accurate concepts as to
what was wrong in explaining their need for medications. Although both schizophrenic and medical patients gave generally positive assessments of how helpful the
medications had been for them, 44% of the schizophrenic patients (in contrast to
only 7% of the medical patients) said they would stop medications if they had the
choice. Both groups were more likely to say they would take medications the more
they reported that medications helped them ($r = .54$, $p < .01$ for schizophrenic
patients; $r = .57$, $p < .05$ for medical patients). The patients with schizophrenia were
also less likely to say they would take medications the more they reported awareness
of side effects ($r = .42$, $p < .05$).

McEvoy, Aland, Wilson, Guy, and Hawkins (1981) studied 45 chronically hospitalized schizophrenic patients. Although 98% of these patients were aware they were taking medications, only 47% reported any present need for medications, and only 44% believed they would need medication in the future. A small but significant positive correlation ($r = .32$, $p < .05$) existed between the patients' beliefs that they had a mental illness and their reported need for medications.

Thompson (1988) studied a group of 65 young adult chronic psychiatric patients, nearly all of whom had diagnoses of schizophrenia. These patients were asked to characterize "the typical adult in the community," "the typical hospitalized mental patient," and themselves on a 20-item semantic differential. Two thirds ($n = 43$) of these patients described themselves as much more like typical members of the community than like mental patients. Although members of this subgroup reported less psychological distress than those in the subgroup who described themselves as mental patients, they also reported less compliance with medications and they more frequently required hospitalization.

### Medication Refusers

A small proportion of patients with schizophrenia actively refuse treatment. Reporting on a mixed diagnostic group of patients assigned to one of several classes of pharmacotherapy, Raskin (1961) found that refusers had little faith in their clinicians and readily acknowledged their hostility to treatment.

Serban and Thomas (1974) noted that, at the time of discharge, 19% of their chronic schizophrenia patients stated that they would not take medications as outpatients under any circumstances.

Van Putten (1974) reported that 12% of the chronic schizophrenic patients he followed in an outpatient clinic adamantly refused to take medication at all, and equated the drugs with poison. Discomforting extrapyramidal side effects—in particular, akathisia—were significantly associated with reluctance to take medications. This author stated that "even mild EPI is difficult to bear on a maintenance basis."

In a later study, Van Putten, Crumpton, and Yale (1976) acknowledged that extrapyramidal side effects were not a complete explanation. He contrasted 29 habitual drug refusers with 30 drug compliers at the end of hospitalizations during which "medication was adjusted so that each patient experienced either none or minimal extrapyramidal side effects." At the time of discharge, after all patients had been treated, albeit involuntarily if necessary, with antipsychotic medications, the initial medication refusers were *still* rated as significantly more ill and less cooperative than the medication-compliant patients.

Appelbaum and Guthiel (1980) examined occurrences of medication refusal on a 40-bed inpatient ward that had 56 admissions over the three months of study. Refusal, as defined in this study, "required an affirmative act beyond mere nonappearance at the medication room door, i.e., either explicit verbal rejection of the medications or a failure to respond to a direct approach by a member of the ward staff." Most of these episodes of refusal were brief and quickly resolved by clarifications about the medications. However, in 10 patients (18% of all admissions), refusals were recurrent or persistent, and refusals interfered with treatment in 5 patients. Eight of these 10 patients were schizophrenic, with either "prominent paranoid elements in their illnesses which appeared to motivate their refusal," or "deep-seated delusional beliefs about their medications" (p. 344). The authors argued that these delusion-based refusals must be conceptualized as manifestations of the illness, rather than as an exercising of civil rights, or else these patients would not receive needed care.

When new regulations in California required that all patients sign informed-consent forms prior to treatment with antipsychotic medications, Marder et al. (1983) studied 15 schizophrenic patients admitted on a *voluntary* basis who subsequently refused to sign consent for treatment, and compared these patients to 15 nonrefusing patients. The refusers were rated as significantly more ill on the Brief Psychiatric Rating Scale (BPRS; Overall & Gorham, 1962). They were rated as having less insight into their illness, less confidence in staff, and a more impaired understandings of the rationale for treatment. The authors note that many of the refusing patients appeared bewildered and confused by the consent form, and they were often unable to explain their refusal. They often refused to participate in other ward activities as well, and this negativism and perplexity seemed to be intrinsic components of their psychopathology.

This same group (Marder, Swann, et al., 1984) reported that 15 of 31 (48%) *involuntarily* committed patients would refuse medication if they had the choice. Refusers had higher psychosis ratings on the BPRS, and higher ratings for mood elevation. They had significantly less confidence in the staff, showed less acknowledgment of their illness, had less understanding of the rationale for treatment, and were less likely to believe that medications helped them, relative to nonrefusers. After treatment was administered to these patients, despite their objections, their psychopathology diminished. Significant improvements occurred in their confidence in the ward staff and their understanding of the rationale for treatment, but not in their acknowledgment of illness. Six of the 12 initial refusers who were still available for interview at the end of two weeks no longer wished to refuse medication.

Irwin et al. (1985) interviewed 33 sequentially admitted patients with schizophrenia, and found that only 5 (15%) would prefer to refuse treatment. Neither acknowledgment of illness, factual understanding about the medications, nor prior experience of extrapyramidal side effects predicted consent vs. refusal. Rather, patients' perceived benefits from prior antipsychotic treatment most powerfully predicted willingness to consent.

Hoge et al. (1990) found that 103 (7.2%) of the 1,434 psychiatric patients admitted to four acute inpatient units in state-operated mental health facilities in Massachusetts over a six-month period refused treatment with antipsychotic medication. On admission, refusers had significantly higher psychosis ratings than compliant patients, and significantly less acknowledgment of illness and need for treatment. Refusers were significantly more likely to have refused medications in the past as well. During the index hospitalization, refusers were more likely to require seclusion or restraint and had longer hospitalizations than treatment acceptors.

## Patients with Coexisting Organic Impairment

Geller (1982) surveyed 281 very chronic patients at a state psychiatric hospital. Only 8% of these patients could correctly name at least one medication they were taking *and* accurately report its dosing schedule and its intended effect. Of the patients who could give understandable verbal responses to the questions, fewer than 50% opined that the medications they were taking helped them in any way. Not surprisingly, longer length of stay and diagnoses of dementia or mental retardation each independently contributed to the likelihood that patients would have no understanding of their medications.

Macpherson, Double, Rowlands, and Harrison (1993) reported on a similar chronically institutionalized group of 100 patients randomly selected from the population of a long stay hospital. The mean age of these patients was 63 years, with a range from 24 to 89 years. Only 23 of these patients could correctly name at least one of their medications. Ten patients showed some understanding of the intended therapeutic action of the medication, with 5 of these 10 also being among those who could name a medication. Thus, a total of 28 of the 100 patients could *either* name a medication they were taking *or* tell something about its method of therapeutic action. Of note, only 36 of these 100 patients could accurately give their age to within one year. Patients who knew their age were significantly more likely to understand the therapeutic action of their medications.

*Summary of Patients' Views*    When we query general populations of patients with schizophrenia about their need for treatment, 30 to 50% of them report that they do not need medications or would stop taking them if that option was readily available, (Parkes et al., 1962; Soskis, 1978; McEvoy et al., 1981, Thompson 1988). Fewer than half acknowledge that they have a mental illness (Soskis 1978; McEvoy et al., 1981; Thompson, 1988). Those patients who do not see themselves as ill, or who report no need for medications, are less likely to report compliance with medications (Soskis, 1978; McEvoy et al., 1981 Thompson, 1988).

Up to 20% of patients with schizophrenia may openly and clearly refuse to take medications; as expected, among the "enriched" population of newly involuntarily committed patients the portion of refusers approaches 50%. It is almost tautologic to note that refusers are more hostile and have less confidence in the staff caring for them. It is important to understand that the decision process leading to refusal takes place in a mind altered by psychopathology. Certainly at the time of refusal, and perhaps even after treatment (Van Putten et al., 1976), refusers evidence higher levels of psychopathology than patients who agree to medications.

Among chronically hospitalized patients in whom there is clear evidence of cognitive compromise (e.g., age disorientation), understanding of medications is markedly limited, and we cannot expect compliance in such patients unless they are completely supervised.

## Insight as Predictor of Compliance

Does acknowledgment of illness and need for medication predict that patients will take their medications?

### The Available Studies

The studies reviewed in this section reflect wide variations in how acknowledgment of illness and need for medication were rated and in how compliance was determined.

TABLE 14.2    The Relationship Between Insight and Compliance (Lin et al., 1979)

| Group | Number in group | Percentage adherent |
|---|---|---|
| I+B+R+ | 12 | 58 |
| I+B+R− | 11 | 45 |
| I+B− | 8 | 25 |
| I−B+ | 26 | 23 |
| I−B− | 43 | 16 |

From Lin et al. (1979).

Nonetheless, consistent themes emerge. Lin, Spiga, and Fortsch (1979) studied a group of 100 patients with schizophrenia shortly after their release from index hospitalizations. Patients were scored as having insight (I+) if they answered yes to *any* of the following three questions that referred back to their recent inpatient stay:

1. Do you think you had to be in the hospital?
2. Do you think you had to see a psychiatrist?
3. Do you think you had to see a doctor?

Only 31 patients were I+, and 69 I−. Patients were scored as perceiving benefit from treatment (B+) if they responded affirmatively to the question, While you were in the hospital, did the medication do you any good? (49 patients were B+, 51 B−). Of the 23 patients who both had insight and perceived benefit from treatment, 12 also perceived a relationship between mental problems and a benefit from treatment (I+B+R+). Patients whose claims to have faithfully taken their medications could be corroborated by family or aftercare staff were judged as adherent to medications (M+, $n = 26$). The other 74 patients were considered M−. As can be seen in table 14.2, there was a progressive decline in likelihood of adherence moving from the I+B+R+ group to groups with progressively less acknowledgment of illness and need for treatment. Unfortunately, larger percentages of patients are found in these latter groups. Fourteen of 31 patients (45%) who had insight were medication adherent, in contrast to 12 of 69 (17%) patients without insight (Chi square = 7.19, $p < .01$). Eighteen of 49 (36%) patients who perceived benefit from treatment were medication adherent, in contrast to 8 of 51 (15%) who did not perceive benefit (Chi square = 4.71, $p < .0.05$).

Bartko, Herczeg, and Zador (1988) developed two 4-point scales for assessing lack of feeling of illness (the patient denies being ill either spontaneously or when interviewed) and lack of insight into illness (the patient fails to acknowledge his or her emotional state and behavior assessed as pathologic by the physician, and does not perceive the necessity of treatment). Fifty-eight patients with schizophrenia were rated on these scales at the time of their discharge from an index hospitalization. All of these patients were treated with long-acting depot antipsychotics, and followed over one year of aftercare. Thirty-two of the 58 patients (55%) became noncompliant over the follow-up, as evidenced by missed appointments or deliberate discontinuation of medications. Baseline ratings of lack of feeling of illness and lack of insight into illness were significantly higher in those patients who noncomplied than in compliant patients.

McEvoy, Apperson, et al. (1989) administered an 11-item Insight and Treatment Attitudes Questionnaire (ITAQ) to 46 patients with schizophrenia at index discharge. Two to three years after these patients were discharged, two research associates independently reviewed these patients' aftercare records and interviewed all available clinicians who were familiar with these patients' courses and outcomes. At 30-day follow-up, 75% of patients were compliant, but only 53% remained compliant over the total duration of follow-up; 61% of patients were rehospitalized at least once. Multivariate tests revealed that the presence of an assertive individual in the patient's aftercare environment who supported the patient's continuation in treatment was significantly associated with outcome. In particular, patients with such an individual supporting their involvement in aftercare were significantly more likely to be compliant with treatment 30 days after discharge and over the long-term follow-up. The association between insight and outcome approached statistical significance, $F(10, 66) = 1.95; p = .053$. In particular, patients with more insight were significantly less likely to be readmitted over the course of follow-up, and there was a trend for patients with more insight to be compliant with treatment 30 days after discharge. The contributions to outcome of an assertive individual in the aftercare environment and the patient's level of insight appeared to be independent.

The finding by McEvoy, Apperson, et al. (1989) that lack of insight is associated with rehospitalization supports the earlier reports of Heinrichs, Cohen, and Carpenter (1985) that early insight, defined as "a patient's ability, during the early phase of a decompensation, to recognize that he or she is beginning to suffer a relapse of his or her psychotic illness," predicts that a decompensation can be successfully resolved on an outpatient basis, without need for rehospitalization.

Weiden et al. (1991) followed 72 patients, 85% of whom had schizophrenia, after an index hospitalization. Forty-eight percent of these patients became noncompliant with medications for at least one week over a year of follow-up. Baseline features of patients that were significantly associated with noncompliance included denial of illness, perceived coercion, and perceived stigma. In contrast, baseline features significantly associated with compliance included perceived good relationship with the physician, perceived benefit from medications, and fear of future relapse.

Buchanan (1992) measured insight in 61 patients with schizophrenia prior to their discharge from an index hospitalization by asking 6 questions:

1. Do you think that you have been unwell during this admission?
2. Do you think that you will become ill again?
3. Did treatment help?
4. Will you take treatment after you discharge?
5. Will you ever get back to your old self?
6. Why were you in the hospital?

Compliance over the ensuing two years of follow-up was assessed by inspection of records and by analysis of urine. Fifty-nine percent of patients were compliant at the end of one year, and 51% at the end of two years. Affirmative responses to question 3 (a belief that medication had helped during the admission) and question 4 (a stated willingness to take treatment after discharge) were significantly positively associated with compliance over the follow-up. A history of compliance with treatment prior to the index hospitalization and voluntary status during the index hospitalization were also significantly associated with compliance over follow-up.

McEvoy, Freter, Merrit, and Apperson (1993) prospectively followed 24 outpatients with schizophrenia over a year of follow-up. These patients, as a group, were relatively insightful and were engaged in highly active aftercare programs. Only 3 of these patients required rehospitalization over the year of follow-up, precluding comparison between rehospitalized and not rehospitalized patients using standard statistical tests. However, the mean scores of the 3 rehospitalized patients were outside the 95% confidence limits for the 21 not rehospitalized patients on two of the baseline measures: rehospitalized patients had lower baseline insight scores (15.3 vs. 19.2, SEM 1.4) and fewer years since their first hospitalization (1.3 vs. 9.7, SEM 1.4).

### Insight Predicts Compliance

The percentages of patients remaining compliant with treatment in these studies ranged from a low of 26% over one year (Lin et al., 1979) to a high of 51% over two years (Buchanan, 1992). Acknowledgment of illness (Lin et al., 1979; Weiden et al., 1991; Heinrichs et al., 1985; Bartko et al., 1988) and/or benefit from medications (Lin et al., 1979; McEvoy, Apperson, et al., 1989, McEvoy et al., 1993; Buchanan, 1992) was significantly associated with compliance and avoidance of rehospitalization across all the available studies.

In the second section of this chapter we found that approximately one third to one half of patients with schizophrenia will noncomply with medications if given the opportunity. In the third section, we presented evidence that approximately one third to one half of patients with schizophrenia deny they are ill or need treatment. In this section, we have demonstrated the link that those patients who deny their illness or need for treatment are significantly more likely to be among the group who noncomply.

## Ways to Increase Compliance

What can be done to increase the likelihood that patients with schizophrenia will take their medications?

### Practical Issues

For general medical patients, longer times between referral and actual appointment (Haynes, 1979a, b) and longer waiting times at clinic before actually being seen (Blackwell, 1976) are associated with diminished likelihood of continuation in treatment. We may expect that delays in service delivery will similarly reduce compliance in patients with mental illness. In fact, immediate responsiveness may be required to adequately address the needs of patients with serious mental illness (Cohen, 1993).

Cost can limit access to treatment among the poor (Haynes, 1976). Davis, Estess, Simonton, and Gonda (1977) have reported significantly higher dropout rates among self-pay patients with schizophrenia, relative to those on public support.

## Pharmacologic Issues

More complex pharmacologic treatments, both in terms of the number of drugs prescribed and the frequencies at which they must be taken, are associated with diminished compliance (Haynes, 1979a, b; Dunbar & Agras, 19809). Fortunately, the most commonly prescribed antipsychotic and antiparkinson agents can be taken once daily.

It is very likely that distressing extrapyramidal side effects contribute to noncompliance (Falloon et al., 1978; Hogan, Awad, & Eastwood, 1983; Seltzer, Roncari, & Garfinkle, 1988). In many (Marder, Van Putten, et al., 1984; Van Putten, Marder, & Mintz, 1990; McEvoy, Hogarty & Steingard, 1991) but not all (Rifkin, Doddi, Karajgi, Borenstein, & Wachspress, 1990) *acute treatment studies* prospectively comparing different doses of antipsychotics, significantly more patients dropped out of study in the higher dose groups complaining of distressing side effects. In outpatient *maintenance studies* comparing long-acting injectable medications (the blood and brain levels of which cannot be altered by the patients who receive them) with oral medications (the levels of which patients may surreptitiously lower by partial noncompliance), significantly higher rates of termination owing to "toxicity" are reported with the injectable preparations (Rifkin, Quitkin, et al., 1977; Falloon et al., 1978). We may recall that among the patients reported by Chien (1975; see second section, this chapter) who could self-regulate their fluphenazine enanthate injections, the 10 of 16 who remained on treatment halved their doses. Side effects of medication were the most common reasons (35%) for refusal of medications in the study of Hoge et al. (1990).

Weiden et al. (1991) have made the important point that old extrapyramidal side effects (EPSE) that were very distressing may, although now remote in time, have left a lingering distaste for medications.

As noted in the second section of this chapter, rates of documented noncompliance appear to be lower in patients treated with long-acting injectable antipsychotic medications than in patients receiving pills (see also Kane & Borenstein, 1985). Perhaps the most important way in which long-acting injectable preparations support compliance is by making noncompliance openly apparent when it occurs (Johnson & Freeman, 1972). Clinicians do not observe patients taking or not taking pills at home, however, they do know when patients fail to appear for their injections. The information that a patient has not taken an injection is useful, however, only if family, friends, or clinical staff go out and attempt to reengage the patient in treatment.

## Support, Supervision, Coercion

The studies reviewed in the second section of this chapter document that compliance with medication can be progressively increased to levels greater than 90% by progressively increasing supervision by staff, but that compliance falls to levels approaching 50% in unsupervised outpatients for whom pills are prescribed.

Supervision of outpatients by family members or friends can enhance compliance (Willcox et al., 1965; Reilly, Wilson, & McClinton, 1969; McEvoy, Apperson, et al., 1989; Buchanan, 1992). Parkes et al. (1962) reported that it made a great difference whether the taking of the drug was supervised: 14 (82%) of the 17 patients whose drug administration was supervised by a relative or a friend took their drugs as ordered, compared with 26 (46%) of the 56 nonsupervised. (p. 975)

Supervision need not be unpleasant. In an inpatient study (McEvoy, Freter, et al., 1989), we were impressed by the many patients who consistently responded no when asked if they were ill or needed treatment, but who expressed a clear willingness to take medications in the hospital. When we asked them to explain this pattern of response, they generally noted how pleasant the nurses were, and that it was a routine and not a bother. Others have reported improved compliance when they offered free lunches at the clinic on the days that injections were given (Cassino, Spellman, Heiman, Shupe, & Sklebar, 1987).

All too often, coercive (as opposed to supportive) forms of supervision must be brought to bear after patients have failed to comply with medications, have become actively psychotic, and have become dangerous to themselves or others. The available evidence suggests that the patients who most resist treatment and require coercion show little or no improvement in acknowledgment of illness and need for treatment even when they are forcibly treated, despite the fact that their psychopathology diminishes significantly (Marder, Swann, et al., 1984; McEvoy, Applebaum, Apperson, Geller, & Freter, 1989). Therefore, it seems foolish to expect that after discharge these patients will continue on treatment when the choice is again theirs in the outpatient setting. Unfortunately, the outpatient commitment laws in many states, and the procedures for enduring outpatient follow-up of resistant patients in many mental health centers, are not adequate at the present time to assure that such patients take their prescribed medications outside of hospital.

## Can Insight Be Improved?

This question requires much more study. Methods for directly improving insight through psychoeducation and cognitive rehabilitation are currently under investigation (described in detail elsewhere in this book), with the hope that improvements in insight will translate into improvements in treatment compliance. However, given the limited improvements in insight and treatment compliance produced by stark learning experiences such as repeated involuntary commitments and hospitalizations, it may be that these techniques will prove only partially successful.

Interestingly, in the general medical literature, "there appears to be no relationship between patients' knowledge of their disease or its therapy and their compliance with the associated treatment regimen" (p. 36), nor is there a correlation between patients' intelligence or educational achievement and compliance (Haynes, 1976). Most authors (Soskis, 1978; Hogan et al., 1983; Irwin et al., 1985) report no relationship between schizophrenic patients' abstract knowledge about the illness and compliance. Klein et al. (1974) and Boczkowski, Zeichner, and DeSanto (1985) reported no improvement in compliance among patients given education about the illness.

On a more optimistic note, Boczkowski et al. (1985) found a behavioral tailoring (BT) approach to result in significantly higher levels of compliance than psychoeducation on control interventions. The BT approach is described as follows:

The investigator helped each participant tailor his prescribed regimen so that it was better adapted to his personal habits and routines. This involved identifying a highly visible location for placement of medications and pairing the daily medication intake with specific routine behavior of the participant. Each participant was given a self-monitoring spiral calendar, which featured a dated slip of paper for each dose of the neuroleptic. The participant was instructed to keep the calendar near his medications and to tear off a slip each time he took a pill. (p. 668)

Seltzer, Roncari, and Garfinkel (1980) combined didactic information about the nature of schizophrenia and its pharmacological treatment with a behavioral component that reinforced drug-taking behavior. The latter intervention may have been the more important component in producing improved compliance in the treated group.

### Ways to Increase Compliance

A number of simple, commonsense procedures appear capable of improving compliance in patients with serious mental illness. (It is striking how rarely they are applied.) These include seeing patients quickly when they need to be seen, avoiding complicated medication schedules, protecting patients from having to pay the full costs of expensive medications, and avoiding distressing side effects.

There is no evidence that abstract understanding about schizophrenia or the pharmacological mechanisms of antipsychotic medications is associated with greater compliance, and those studies that attempted to improve patients' understanding of their illness and its treatment showed no improvement in compliance (Klein et al., 1974; Boczkowski et al., 1985).

There is compelling evidence that patients who state that they personally are ill and/or need treatment are more compliant. I am not aware of studies that have tested an approach that strives to directly change patients' self-images to one more acknowledging of illness and need for treatment. It appears that greater acknowledgment of illness is associated with higher levels of depression, and such an approach should be taken cautiously.

It appears that behavioral compliance may be achievable independently of expressed insight, through behavioral programs that incorporate medication compliance into patients' daily routines and provide consistent rewards for taking medications.

## Conclusions

The degree to which a patient with schizophrenia acknowledges that he or she has a serious mental illness and needs treatment (insight) has consistently been found to predict how readily that individual will seek, or at least cooperate with, treatment. Patients with low levels of insight, whether measured at discharge from an index hospitalization or in the outpatient setting, are less likely to comply with treatment and more likely to require hospitalization during follow-up care. Low levels of insight are common in schizophrenia and, as Weiden et al. (1991) state, "it seems that public health planning for the outpatient treatment of schizophrenia should *assume* that most patients become noncompliant to their maintenance neuroleptic regiment" (p. 294).

Methods for directly improving insight through psychoeducation and cognitive rehabilitation are currently under investigation (described in detail elsewhere in this book), with the hope that improvements in insight will translate into improvements in treatment compliance. However, until such techniques are demonstrated to be successful, clinicians must expect the continued necessity to bring treatment to a substantial percentage of schizophrenic patients who do not believe they need it, and who certainly do not actively seek it. We need to follow up the positive studies (e.g., Boczkowski, et al., 1985), which suggest that we bypass the provision of abstract knowledge and instead directly incorporate simple medication taking behaviors into patients' daily routines and reward patients for compliance.

Many schizophrenic patients will, despite having little insight, go along with treatment that is brought to them. The presence of an effective individual (family member, rest-home supervisor, outreach worker, etc.) in the patient's aftercare environment, who urges the patient to stay in treatment, may assist in compliance. Research is needed to determine how to educate and assist such individuals in the patient's aftercare environment so that they can most effectively support compliance.

In contrast to their limited acknowledgment of the benefits of treatment, patients with schizophrenia are well aware of the distressing side effects (extrapyramidal side effects, sexual dysfunction, etc.) associated with antipsychotic medications. Studies to determine whether pharmacologic strategies that produce less EPSE and sexual dysfunction result in improved compliance have yet to be done. Long-acting intramuscular forms of neuroleptic (e.g., fluphenazine decanoate or haloperidol decanoate) permit closer monitoring of compliance than oral forms.

A small percentage of patients actively resist treatment. Presently available evidence suggests that such patterns of deficient insight and noncompliance are fairly stable over time. If repeatedly noncompliant patients become dangerous when actively ill, caregivers may attempt to enforce treatment through prolonged inpatient commitment or through outpatient commitment. Unfortunately, the outpatient commitment laws in many states, and the procedures for enduring follow-up of such patients in many mental health centers, are not adequate at the present time to ensure that such patients take their prescribed medications outside of hospital.

Thus, those who wish to care for patients with schizophrenia must realize that, in many cases, treatment cannot simply be. Rather, all too often we must *influence* our patients to accept treatment. Much research is needed to determine how we can most effectively, and least intrusively, exert this influence to enhance compliance and preempt relapse.

*References*

Appelbaum, P. S., & Gutheil, T. G. (1980). Drug refusal: A study of psychiatric inpatients. *American Journal of Psychiatry, 137*(3), 340–346.

Bartko, G., Herczeg, I., & Zador, G. (1988). Clinical symptomatology and drug compliance in schizophrenic patients. *Acta Psychiatrica Scandinavica, 77,* 74–76.

Blackwell, B. (1976). Treatment adherence. *British Journal of Psychiatry, 129,* 513–531.

Boczkowski, J. A., Zeichner, A., & DeSanto, N. (1985). Neuroleptic compliance among chronic schizophrenic outpatients: An intervention outcome report. *Journal of Consulting and Clinical Psychology, 53*(5), 666–671.

Buchanan, A. (1992). A two-year prospective study of treatment compliance in patients with schizophrenia. *Psychological Medicine, 22*, 787–797.

Carney, M. W. P., & Sheffield, B. F. (1976). Comparison of antipsychotic depot injections in the maintenance treatment of schizophrenia. *British Journal of Psychiatry, 129*, 476–481.

Cassino, T., Spellman, N., Heiman, J., Shupe, J., & Sklebar, H. J. (1987). Invitation to compliance: The Prolixin brunch. *Journal of Psychosocial Nursing and Mental Health Services, 25*, 15–19.

Caton, C. (1984). *Management of chronic schizophrenia.* New York: Oxford University Press.

Chien, C. P. (1975). Drugs and rehabilitation in schizophrenia. In M. Greenblatt (Ed.), *Drugs in combination with other therapies* (pp. 13–34). New York: Grune & Stratton.

Cohen, N. L. (1993). Stigmatization and the "noncompliant" recidivist. *Hospital and Community Psychiatry, 44*(11), 1029.

Davis, K. L., Estess, F. M., Simonton, S. C., & Gonda, T. A. (1977). Effects of payment mode on clinic attendance and rehospitalization. *American Journal of Psychiatry, 134*(5), 576–578.

Falloon, I., Watt, D. C., & Shepherd, M. (1978). A comparative controlled trial of pimozide and fluphenazine decanoate in the continuation therapy of schizophrenia. *Psychological Medicine, 8*, 59–70.

Forrest, F. M., Forrest I. S., & Mason, A. S. (1961). Review of rapid urine tests for phenothiazine and related drugs. *American Journal of Psychiatry, 118*, 300–307.

Geller, J. L. (1982). State hospital patients and their medication: Do they know what they take? *American Journal of Psychiatry, 139*(5), 611–615.

Hare, E. H., & Willcox, D. R. C. (1967). Do psychiatry inpatients take their pills? *British Journal of Psychiatry, 113*, 1435–1439.

Haynes, R. B. (1976). A critical review of the "determinants" of patient compliance with therapeutic regimens. In R. B. Haynes & D. L. Sackett (Eds.), *Compliance with therapeutic regimens* (pp. 27–39). Baltimore: Johns Hopkins University Press.

Haynes, R. B. (1979a). Determinants of compliance: The disease and the mechanics of treatment. In R. B. Haynes, D. W. Taylor, & D. L. Sackett (Eds.), *Compliance in health care* (pp. 49–63). Baltimore: Johns Hopkins University Press.

Haynes, R. B. (1979b). Strategies for improving compliance: A methodological analysis and review. In R. B. Haynes, D. W. Taylor, & D. L. Sackett (Eds.), *Compliance in health care* (pp. 121–143). Baltimore: Johns Hopkins University Press.

Heinrichs, D. W., Cohen, B. P., & Carpenter, W. T. (1985). Early insight and the management of schizophrenic decompensation. *Journal of Nervous and Mental Disease, 173*, 133–138.

Hogan, T. P., Awad, A. G., & Eastwood, R. (1983). A self-report scale predictive of drug compliance in schizophrenics: Reliability and discriminative validity. *Psychological Medicine, 13*, 177–183.

Hoge, S. K., Appelbaum, P. S., Lawlor, T., Beck, J. C., Litman, R., Greer, A., Gutheil, T. G., & Kaplan, E. (1990). A prospective, multi-center study of patients' refusal of antipsychotic medication. *Archives of General Psychiatry, 47*, 949–956.

Irwin, D. S., Weitzel, W. D., & Morgan, D. W. (1971). Phenothiazine intake and staff attitudes. *American Journal of Psychiatry, 127*(12), 1631–1635.

Irwin, M., Lovitz, A., Marder, S. R., Mintz, J., Winslade, W. J., Van Putten, T., & Mills, M. J. (1985). Psychotic patients' understanding of informed consent. *American Journal of Psychiatry, 142*(11), 1351–1354.

Johnson, D. A. W., & Freeman, H. (1972). Long acting tranquilizers. *The Practitioner, 208*, 395–400.

Kane, J. M. (1985). Compliance issues in outpatient treatment. *Journal of Clinical Psychopharmacology, 5*(3), 22S–27S.

Kane, J. M., & Borenstein, M. (1985). Compliance in the long-term treatment of schizophrenia. *Psychopharmacology Bulletin, 21*(1), 23–27.

Klein, R. H., Lynn, E. J., Axelrod, H., & Dluhy, J. (1974). Self-administration of medication by psychiatric inpatients. *Journal of Nervous and Mental Disease, 158*(6), 450–455.

Lieberman, J. A., Alvir, J. M. J., Woerner, M., Degreef, G., Bilder, R. M., Ashtari, M., Bogerts, B., Mayerhoff, D. I., Geisler, S. H., Loebel, A., Levy, D. L., Hinrichsen, G., Szymanski, S., Chakos, M., Koreen, A., Borenstein, M., & Kane, J. M. (1992). Prospective psychobiology in first-episode schizophrenia at Hillside Hospital. *Schizophrenia Bulletin, 18*(3), 351–371.

Lin, I. F., Spiga, R., & Fortsch, W. (1979). Insight and adherence to medication in chronic schizophrenics. *Journal of Clinical Psychiatry, 40,* 430–432.

MacPherson, R., Double, D. B., Rowlands, R. P., & Harrison, D. M. (1993). Long-term psychiatric patients' understanding of neuroleptic medication. *Hospital and Community Psychiatry, 44*(1), 71–73.

Marder, S. R., Mebane, A., Chien, C. P., Winslade, W. J., Swann, E., & Van Putten, T. (1983). A comparison of patients who refuse and consent to neuroleptic treatment. *American Journal of Psychiatry, 140*(4), 470–472.

Marder, S. R., Swann, E. Winslade, W. J., Van Putten, T., Chien, C. P., & Wilkins, J. N. (1984). A Study of Medication Refusal by Involuntary Patients. *Hospital and General Psychiatry, 35*(7), 724–726.

Marder, S. R., Van Putten, T., Mintz, J., McKenzie, J., Lebell, M., Faltico, G., & May, P. R. A. (1984). Costs and benefits of two doses of fluphenazine. *Archives of General Psychiatry, 41,* 1025–1029.

McClellan, T. A., & Cowan, G. (1970). Use of antipsychotic and antidepressant drugs by chronically ill patients. *American Journal of Psychiatry, 126*(12), 1771–1773.

McEvoy, J. P., Aland, J., Wilson, W. H., Guy, W., & Hawkins, L. (1981). Measuring chronic schizophrenic patients' attitudes towards their illness and treatment. *Hospital and Community Psychiatry, 32*(12), 586–588.

McEvoy, J. P., Appelbaum, P. S., Apperson, L. J., Geller, J. L., & Freter, S. (1989). Why must some schizophrenic patients be involuntarily committed? The role of insight. *Comprehensive Psychiatry, 30*(1), 13–17.

McEvoy, J. P., Apperson, L. J., Appelbaum, P. S., Ortlip, P., Brecosky, J., Hammill, K., Geller, J. L., & Roth, L. (1989). Insight in schizophrenia: Its relationship to acute psychopathology. *Journal of Nervous and Mental Disease, 177*(1), 43–47.

McEvoy, J. P., Freter, S., Everett, G., Geller, J. L., Appelbaum, P., Apperson, L. J., & Roth, L. (1989). Insight and the clinical outcome of schizophrenic patients. *Journal of Nervous and Mental Disease, 177*(1), 48–51.

McEvoy, J. P., Freter, S., Merrit, M., & Apperson, L. J. (1993). Insight about psychosis among outpatients with schizophrenia. *Hospital and Community Psychiatry, 44*(9), 883–884.

McEvoy, J. P., Hogarty, G. E., & Steingard, S. (1991). Optimal dose of neuroleptic in acute schizophrenia. *Archives of General Psychiatry, 48,* 739–745.

Neve, H. K. (1958). Demonstration of Largactil (chlorpromazine hydrochloride) in the urine. *Journal of Mental Science, 104,* 488–490.

Overall, J. E., & Gorham, D. R. (1962). BPRS: The Brief Psychiatric Rating Scale. In W. Guy (Ed.), *ECDEU assessment manual for psychopharmacology,* rev. ed. (pp. 157–169). Rockville, MD: National Institute of Mental Health.

Parkes, C. M., Brown, G. W., & Monck, E. M. (1962). The general practitioner and the schizophrenic patient. *British Medical Journal, i,* 972–976.

Quitkin, F., Rifkin, A., Kane, J., Ramos-Lorenzi, J. R., & Klein, D. F. (1978). Long-acting oral vs. injectable antipsychotic drugs in schizophrenics. *Archives of General Psychology, 35,* 889–892.

Raskin, A. (1961). A comparison of acceptors and resistors of drug treatment as an adjunct to psychotherapy. *Journal of Consulting Psychology, 25*(4), 366.

Reilly, E. L., Wilson, W. P., & McClinton, H. K. (1967). Clinical characteristics and medication history of schizophrenics readmitted to the hospital. *International Journal of Neuropsychiatry*, 85–90.

Rifkin, A., Doddi, S., Karajgi, B., Borenstein, M., & Wachspress, M. (1991). Dosage of haloperidol for schizophrenia. *Archives of General Psychiatry, 48,* 166–170.

Rifkin, A., Quitkin, F., Rabiner, C. J. (1977). Fluphenazine decanoate, oral fluphenazine and placebo in remitted schizophrenics. *Archives of General Psychiatry, 34,* pp. 43–47.

Seltzer, A., & Hoffman, J. B. (1980). Drug compliance of the psychiatric outpatient. *Canadian Family Physician, 11,* 10–15.

Seltzer, A., Roncari, I., & Garfinkel, P. (1980). Effect of patient education on medication compliance. *American Journal of Psychiatry, 25,* 638–645.

Serban, G., & Thomas, A. (1974). Attitudes and behaviors of acute and chronic schizophrenic patients regarding ambulatory treatment. *American Journal of Psychiatry, 131*(9), 991–995.

Soskis, D. A. (1978). Schizophrenic and medical inpatients as informed drug consumers. *Archives of General Psychiatry, 35,* 645–647.

Streicker, S. K., Amdur, M., & Dincin, J. (1986). Educating patients about psychiatric medications: Failure to enhance compliance. *Psychosocial Rehabilitation Journal, 4,* 15–28.

Thompson, E. H., Jr. (1988). Variation in the self-concept of young adult chronic patients: Chronicity reconsidered. *Hospital and Community Psychiatry, 39*(7), 771–775.

Van Putten, T. (1974). Why do schizophrenic patients refuse to take their drugs? *Archives of General Psychiatry, 31,* 67–72.

Van Putten, T., Crumpton, E., & Yale, C. (1976). Drug refusal in schizophrenia and the wish to be crazy. *Archives of General Psychiatry, 33,* 1443–1446.

Van Putten, T., Marder, S. R., & Mintz, J. (1990). A controlled dose comparison of haloperidol in newly admitted schizophrenic patients. *Archives of General Psychiatry, 47,* 754–758.

Weiden, P. J., Dixon, L., Frances, A., Appelbaum, P., Haas, G., & Rapkin, B. (1991). Neuroleptic noncompliance in schizophrenia. In C. A. Tamminga & S. C. Schulz (Eds.), *Advances in Neuropsychiatry and Psychopharmacology* (pp. 285–296). New York: Raven Press.

Willcox, D. R., Gillan, R., & Hare, E. H. (1965). Do psychiatric outpatients take their drugs? *British Medical Journal, ii,* 790–792.

Wilson, J. D., & Enoch, M. D. (1967). Estimation of drug rejection by schizophrenic inpatients, with analysis of clinical factors. *British Medical Journal, 113,* 209–211.

Wyatt, R. J. (1991). Neuroleptics and the natural cause of schizophrenia. *Schizophrenia Bulletin, 17*(2), 325–350.

# 15

PAUL H. LYSAKER

MORRIS D. BELL

# Impaired Insight in Schizophrenia

## Advances from Psychosocial Treatment Research

Lack of insight or unawareness of illness has long been observed in individuals with schizophrenia (Wilson, Ban & Guy, 1986; Greenfield, Strauss, Bowers, & Mandelkern, 1989). It represents a puzzling phenomenon in which patients, despite all evidence to the contrary, appear not to know they are ill and behave in a manner grossly inconsistent with their own best interests. For example, such a patient may tell his clinicians he has no symptoms, enjoys life, and needs no medication despite the fact that he lives in perpetual fear of an anonymous assassin, has no friends, is unable to work, and appears sleepless, unkempt, and malnourished.

While research has confirmed that lack of insight is associated with medication noncompliance and poorer treatment outcome (e.g., Bartko, Herczeg, & Zador, 1988; Heinrichs, Cohen, & Carpenter, 1985; Lin, Spiga, & Fortsch, 1979; McEvoy, Applebaum, Geller, & Freter, 1989), the issue of its etiology and treatment have only recently begun to receive systematic attention. Regarding etiology, there are currently two prominent theories about the causes of impairments in insight. One hypothesis suggests that lack of insight is a coping strategy that patients employ to help them recover from schizophrenia (McGlashan, Levy, & Carpenter, 1975). For example, a patient may find that denying that she was ever ill, rather than trying to integrate that information into her self concept, makes it less complicated to return to her job and assume the rule of a "regular" worker. Denial that there was anything wrong in this case is hypothesized to be in the service of facilitating her return to normalcy, even though this denial may mean that she neglects to take the needed medication, resulting in a greater likelihood of relapse.

An alternative hypothesis is that poor insight in schizophrenia stems from enduring cognitive impairments similar to those experienced by neurology patients with anosognosia (Amador, Strauss, Yale, & Gorman, 1991). Support for the second hypothesis has come from several sources. Factor analytic studies of symptom rating scales have found that impaired insight clusters with symptoms of cognitive impairment such as stereotyped thinking and cognitive disorganization (Bell, Lysaker, Goulet, Milstein, & Lindemeyer, in press; Kay & Sevy, 1990). Additionally, a recent study by Young, Davila, and Scher (1993) has reported significant correlations between performance on neuropsychological testing and ratings of unawareness of illness.

Because poor insight is associated with poorer medication compliance and poorer outcome, it becomes important both clinically and from a research standpoint to evaluate the potential of various treatments to improve insight. Little is known, however, as to whether various treatments can increase awareness of illness. This may be due in part to the fact that treatment research seldom includes improvement in insight as an outcome variable. When insight has been included as an outcome variable, it appears to remain unchanged despite concurrent improvements in other acute symptoms (McEvoy, Apperson, et al., 1989). This suggests that standard psychiatric treatments aimed at resolving acute symptoms do not substantially affect insight. The question of whether other treatments, such as psychosocial treatment, might be effective has not been addressed.

## The Relevance of Psychosocial Treatment Research

Psychosocial treatment research affords several unique opportunities to explore the etiology and treatment of impairment in insight: (1) we can study the insight of subjects in a post-acute phase of illness when long-term deficits are no longer obscured by acute symptom exacerbations; (2) we can assess compliance with all aspects of treatment, not just medication; (3) we can explore the links between insight and functional impairments at work; and (4) we can directly examine the effects of psychosocial treatment on the level of insight.

In this chapter we will present findings from our psychosocial treatment research relevant to the understanding of the etiology of impaired insight in schizophrenia and its responsiveness to treatment. Specifically, we will present findings that suggest: (1) lack of insight is associated with poorer compliance with rehabilitation; (2) lack of insight is associated with greater functional impairment in a therapeutic work program; (3) lack of insight is associated with a stable pattern of neuropsychological deficits; and (4) neuropsychological deficits are associated with lesser degrees of improvement in insight following participation in psychosocial rehabilitation.

## Measurement of Insight

In each of the studies described below, unawareness of illness was measured using the insight and judgment item on the Positive and Negative Syndrome Scale (PANSS; Kay, Fiszbein, & Opler, 1987). The PANSS is a 30-item rating scale completed by clinically trained research staff at the conclusion of chart review and a semistructured interview. It offers three rationally derived categories: positive symptoms, which should not be present in a normal mental status (e.g., hallucinations and delusions); negative symptoms, representing behaviors which should be present in a normal mental status but are not (e.g., blunted affect and emotional withdrawal); and general symptoms, which are common across categories of psychopathology (e.g., anxiety, lack of insight, and depression).

The PANSS lack of insight and judgment item, which is contained in the general symptoms scale, incorporates three dimensions of insight (awareness of the symptoms of the disorder, the consequences, and the need for treatment) into a single global rating made along a 7-point scale. A rating of 1 indicates good to excellent insight, while 2 indicates minor or nonclinically significant impairments in insight. A rating of 3 suggests that the subject is aware of his or her illness and the need for medication, but underestimates the seriousness of some aspects. A 4 suggests fluctuating awareness of present illness and substantially limited awareness of the need for treatment, while a rating of 5 indicates an acknowledgment of past symptoms but a denial of present ones. Ratings of 6 or 7 indicate a continual denial of past and/or present disturbances. Although we use the term *insight*, we recognize that this cognitive capacity is composed of multiple aspects. As such, when describing our studies, insight refers only to those aspects assessed by the aforementioned PANSS item. Good interrater reliability for this item was found for raters in our studies (intraclass $r = .74$; Bell, Lysaker, Goulet, Milstein, & Lindemeyer, 1994).

## Impaired Insight and Compliance with Rehabilitation

While the associations between impaired insight and medication noncompliance are well documented, research has not examined whether impaired insight is related to compliance with other forms of treatment, including psychosocial treatments. To explore this issue, we examined the association between insight measured by the PANSS insight and judgment item and the number of weeks in which 47 subjects worked during the first month (i.e., 5 weeks) of a six-month rehabilitation program.

All subjects qualified for a diagnosis of either schizophrenia or schizoaffective disorder using the structured interview for *DSM-III-R* (SCID, Spitzer, Williams, Gibbon, & First, 1989). Subjects were predominantly unmarried white males with an average age of 40 years, a high school education, and a mean of 10 lifetime hospitalizations. All subjects were receiving some form of concurrent treatment at the time of work placement: 28 were outpatients, 15 were living in a halfway house program, and 14 were inpatients.

Work placements were assigned one week following a comprehensive psychosocial evaluation that included a measurement of insight using the PANSS insight and judgment scale. Efforts were made to assign subjects to work placements consistent with their previous work history and current interests. While the staff who arranged work placements were not blind to the PANSS ratings, assignment was made without reference to the symptom measures. Work placements included working at the West Haven V.A. Medical Center alongside regular employees at sites such as the escort service, laundry, pharmacy, electrical shop, and medical administration.

Correlations between insight and the number of weeks worked (i.e., the number of weeks in which subjects worked at least four hours at their assigned placement) revealed that poorer levels of insight were associated with fewer weeks worked ($r = .37$).

This finding suggests that subjects with impaired insight experienced difficulties complying with the most basic requirements of vocational rehabilitation (i.e., attendance at the work site).

This finding parallels the link observed between impairments in insight and medication noncompliance and suggests that noncompliance with treatment may be an associated feature of poor insight. Previously, noncompliance with medication has been attributed to a willful desire to avoid the effects of medication. In studies of medication compliance, subjects may have refused medication because they disputed its need or feared troubling side effects. In this study, however, all subjects voiced a desire to work from the onset, and there are no comparable noxious side effects of work. It appears, therefore, that impairment in insight may be associated with a generalized difficulty following through with treatment, possibly due to deficits in self-monitoring.

## Impaired Insight and Functional Impairment at Work

There are at least two reasons to hypothesize that insight may be related to functional impairments at work. First, because patients with impaired insight might deny problems with work in the same way that they deny their illness, they may be unable to detect their own errors. They might, for example, be unable to accept the criticism or help they may need to improve their work performance. They may also have poor relationships with coworkers because of their tendency to deny any threatening or uncomfortable realities.

A second reason to hypothesize that insight is related to functional impairments at work is that neurological impairments that may underlie impaired insight are likely to limit the capacity to work and the ability to process and respond to social cues and complex interpersonal communications. If a person cannot comprehend that he has an illness due to generalized difficulties processing information, he may also have grave difficulties working and forming positive relationships with others at the work site.

To explore this issue, we examined the work performance of a subset of the subjects described above who worked during the fifth week of their initial five-week period ($n = 37$). It was decided to examine work performance in the fifth week of work, rather than earlier, because we reasoned that by then subjects would have settled into stable work patterns and underlying deficits and strengths would have emerged. The subset of 37 subjects studied in this analysis had demographics similar to the 47 described above.

To assess work performance, the Work Personality Profile (WPP, Bolton & Roesseler, 1986) was used. The WPP is a work performance inventory completed after direct observation and supervisor interview that generates five factor analytically derived scores: task orientation (staying focused on one's work tasks); social skills (showing interest in coworkers); work motivation (working at routine jobs without resistance; work conformance (following rules and regulations); and personal presentation. Coefficient alpha ranging from .83 to .91 for factor scores are reported by the authors. Examination of interrater reliability for this measure, using a subsample of 24 patients, found interclass correlations ranging from .80 to .95.

As predicted, poorer insight was found to be related to functional impairment at work. Higher ratings of impaired insight predicted poorer rating of social skills ($r = .37$, $p < .05$) and personal presentation ($r = .33$, $p < .05$) on the WPP. This suggests that for patients in a post-acute phase of illness, those with impaired insight had greater difficulty getting along with others and behaving in a socially appropriate fashion at work. Specifically, these patients may appear disinterested in others and rarely initiate or respond to conversation with their coworkers. They may also have had difficulty dressing appropriately and refraining from making irrelevant comments.

## Insight and Performance on Neuropsychological Testing over Time

As noted earlier, research has supported the hypothesis that cognitive deficits underlie impaired insight in schizophrenia. In particular, Young et al. (1993) have reported finding a significant relationship between poorer performance on the Wisconsin Card Sorting Test (WCST) and a measure of unawareness of illness. They found that a discriminant analysis produced a linear combination of WCST scores that could correctly categorize over three fifths of their subjects as either aware or unaware of their illnesses. To similarly test whether impairments in insight were related to poorer WCST performance and to test whether these deficits are stable over time, we compared the performance of 92 subjects on three administrations of WCST over a period of one year (Lysaker & Bell, 1994).

The WCST (Heaton, 1981) is a commonly administered neuropsychological test sensitive to diffuse cognitive deficits and fixed frontal lobe deficits in schizophrenia

TABLE 15.1 Characteristics of Subjects with Impaired and Unimpaired Insight

|  | Intact Insight (N = 63) | Impaired Insight (N = 29) |
|---|---|---|
| Age | $42 \pm 8^a$ | $46 \pm 11$ |
| Education | $13 \pm 2$ | $13 \pm 2$ |
| IQ | $107 \pm 13$ | $97 \pm 13^*$ |
| Lifetime psychiatric hospitalizations | $10 \pm 9$ | $7 \pm 6$ |
| Years at longest full-time job | $3 \pm 4$ | $5 \pm 6$ |
| PANSS scores |  |  |
| Positive | $20 \pm 5$ | $19 \pm 6$ |
| Negative | $16 \pm 5$ | $18 \pm 6$ |
| General | $37 \pm 7$ | $38 \pm 6$ |
| Sex |  |  |
| Female | $4^b$ | 2 |
| Male | 59 | 27 |
| Ethnicity |  |  |
| African American | 17 | 9 |
| Latino | 1 | 2 |
| White | 45 | 18 |
| Treatment status |  |  |
| Outpatient | 45 | 20 |
| Halfway house | 11 | 3 |
| Inpatient | 7 | 6 |

[a]mean ± 1 standard deviation
[b]frequency
*Between groups difference $p < .01$

(Robinson et al., 1980; Braff et al., 1991). It asks subjects to sort cards that vary according to number, color, and shape of objects according to a matching principle, of which the subject is not informed. For example, the subject may be asked to correctly sort a card containing a single green cross to one of the following 4 key cards: a card with one red triangle, a card with two green stars, a card with three yellow crosses or a card with four blue circles. In the case where the matching principle is color, the card must be paired with the key card containing two green stars. In the case where the matching principle is number, the card must be paired with the key card with one red triangle. In the case where the matching principle is shape, the card must be paired with the key card with three yellow crosses. The matching principle shifts unannounced after ten correct responses. The three WCST scores examined in this study were: nonperseverative errors, which is the number of errors in which a subject incorrectly responds using various response patterns; perseverative errors, which is the number of errors in which a subject continuously responds incorrectly using the same response pattern; and categories completed, which is the number of times a subject scores 10 consecutive correct items.

If neuropsychological deficits underlie impairments in insight, then one would expect subjects with impaired insight to demonstrate a pattern of poorer performance on neuropsychological tests over time, compared to subjects with intact insight. Therefore, before examining WCST performance we categorized subjects with PANSS insight and judgment scores of 3 or lower as intact insight ($n = 63$) while subjects with scores of 4 or higher were classified as having impaired insight ($n = 29$). It was decided a priori that subjects with a score of 3 (mild) would be included in the intact, rather than impaired, insight group because subjects with a mild rating have a relatively clear understanding that they need treatment.

To explore whether this categorization resulted in any unexpected group differences that might confound the planned analyses, $t$ tests were conducted comparing the demographics of both groups. These tests revealed that subjects in the impaired group had significantly lower IQ scores on the Slosson Intelligence Test (Slosson, 1963), but there were no significant differences between groups for measures of psychiatric history, psychosocial function, or level of positive and negative symptoms. A summary of the characteristics of both groups is presented in table 15.1.

The scores of impaired and intact subjects were compared from three administrations: intake, five months, and one year following intake. Specific scores on the 3 WCST variables selected for this study were compared between groups using a repeated measures analyses of covariance, with IQ entered as the covariate. Significant group differences were found on 2 WCST variables studied: categories correct ($F[1,2] = 8.10$, $p <.01$) and perseverative errors ($F[1,2] = 9.39$, $p <.01$), with subjects with impaired insight demonstrating poorer performance on both measures. No significant group effect was observed for the other WCST variable studied: nonperseverate errors, though a trend was observed ($F[1,2] = 2.86$, $p <.10$) indicating that the impaired insight group made more nonperseverative errors than the intact insight group. No time effects or interactions were found, suggesting that the scores of both groups did not improve over time.

These findings replicate those of Young et al. (1993) and support the hypothesis that some cases of impaired insight result from neuropsychological impairments that may specifically be related to fixed frontal deficits. The results indicate that the neuropsy-chological deficits detected at intake were unchanged one year later. Additionally, the WCST performance of impaired and intact groups differed even when the effects of IQ were partialled. We conclude from these findings that deficits associated with impaired insight involve more than a poorer global level of intellectual function. The deficits associated with the impaired subjects in our sample appear to involve a compromise of concept formation, information processing, and deficits in self-monitoring. These deficits may, therefore, be similar to the deficits observed in neurologically impaired patients suffering from anosognosia.

## Improvements in Insight and Psychosocial Rehabilitation

As noted in the background section of this chapter, little is known about the effects of various treatments upon impairments in insight. McEvoy et al. (1993) have suggested that psychosocial rehabilitation may lead to improvements in the level of insight. They hypothesized that enhanced levels of self-esteem, which may result from rehabilitation, could help some patients acknowledge that they need treatment. In other words, patients who deny illness to cope with the desperate reality of their condition and its limitations may be enabled by rehabilitation to acknowledge their actual state and accept help. Support for this hypothesis can be found in a study that reported symptomatic improvement in positive, negative, and general symptoms for patients with schizophrenia as correlated with participation in a vocational rehabilitation (Bell, Milstein, & Lysaker, 1993).

To explore the hypothesis that vocational rehabilitation might lead to improvements in insight, we examined changes in insight in 44 subjects with schizophrenia or schizo-affective disorder and at least moderately impaired insight, who were enrolled in a 26-week vocational rehabilitation program (Lysaker & Bell, 1995). As before, subjects were categorized as having impaired insight if they received a rating of moderate (4) or greater on the PANSS insight and judgment item during the evaluation conducted prior to assignment to a work placement. Subjects were predominantly male, with a mean age of 45, a high school education, and average intelligence. They had an average of 7 lifetime psychiatric hospitalizations and worked a mean of 222 hours in the job placement provided by the rehabilitation placement.

This vocational rehabilitation program included rapid work placement at a job site consistent with the subjects' previous work history and interests and supervision from regular hospital staff. Subjects were also assigned to attend weekly support groups that offered problem solving and attempted to revitalize subjects' identification with a worker role. Brief individual counseling was also available if problems on the job arose. As described above, job placements included working at the V. A. Medical Center alongside regular employees at sites such as the escort service, laundry, pharmacy, electrical shop, and medical administration.

Insight was measured one week before beginning work and five months following enrollment. Improvement was defined as an instance in which a subjects' insight score at five months follow-up was at least one point lower than that subject's score was at intake. Amount of improvement in insight was operationally defined as the difference between the PANSS score at five months and PANSS insight score at intake (e.g., an intake rating of 5 and five-month rating of 3 represents an improvement of 2 points).

Results indicated that insight scores for 61% of subjects improved five months following enrollment in a vocational rehabilitation program. A paired $t$ test examining insight scores confirmed that subjects showed significant improvement from intake ($x$ = 4.5, SD = .66) to five months follow-up ($x$ = 3.6, SD = 1.5; $t$ = 12.4, $p$ <.001). For those subjects whose insight improved, 16 improved 1 point, 4 improved 2 points, and 6 improved 3 points.

To explore the question of which subjects improved, stepwise multiple regressions were conducted predicting the amount of improvement in insight. Cognitive impairment was found to be a uniquely significant predictor of improvement, accounting for over a third of the variance ($R^2$ = .34, $p$ <.001). In particular, better performance on the Digit Symbol Substitution Test of the Weschler Adult Intelligence Scale-Revised (Weschler, 1981), the Slosson IQ, and a higher frequency of perseverative errors on the WCST predicted greater improvement (partial $R^2$ = .16, .11, and .07, respectively). By contrast, measures of psychosocial function and symptomatology (including lifetime number of hospitalizations, age, years of education, years at longest full-time job, and intake PANSS positive, negative, and general scores) were unrelated to change in insight scores.

These results support the hypothesis of McEvoy et al. (1993) that vocational rehabilitation can lead to improvement in certain aspects of insight. They further suggest that the subjects who benefited most from the intervention were those with fewer cognitive deficits. These results parallel other findings linking impairments in insight to cognitive deficits and suggest that impairments in insight associated with lower levels of intelligence, deficits in attention and information processing, and possibly fixed frontal impairments may be especially intractable.

One question raised by these results is, Were the subjects with fewer cognitive deficits suffering from a different form of impaired insight than those who had severe cognitive deficits? Perhaps impaired insight, which is secondary to cognitive deficit, does not respond to rehabilitation, while impaired insight, which stems from other causes, does. One hypothesis is that the impaired insight of the subjects who improved was the result of defensiveness and not neuropsychological deficit. These subjects consequently were able to process their experiences at work and benefit from the support groups. This hypothesis can be considered only tentative at present and awaits the findings of future research.

## Conclusions

Our psychosocial treatment research has found that: (1) impairment in certain aspects of insight predicts poorer compliance with psychosocial treatments in a manner similar to the way these impairments predict poorer medication compliance; (2) impairments in insight are related to functional impairment at work; (3) impairments in insight are associated with persistent neuropsychological deficits, which severely limit the ability to effectively process information; and (4) psychosocial rehabilitation represents a potentially effective treatment for patients with poor insight and lesser levels of cognitive impairment.

These studies suggest that for some patients with schizophrenia, unawareness of illness may stem from neuropsychological impairments. These impairments may be frontally based and directly interfere with the effective processing of information. Individuals with these impairments may, therefore, deny that they need medication and experience difficulty working and or getting along with others secondary to enduring deficits, rather than stubbornness, a willful preference for illness, or defensiveness.

Not all impairments in insight, however, appear to be the result of neuropsychological deficits. We have identified a number of subjects for whom improvements in insight after rehabilitation could be predicted by their relatively better performance on neuropsychological testing. The poorer insight of these subjects could presumably be the result of defensiveness, though that is conjecture at this point.

More research is needed to better identify the group of subjects whose impairments respond to rehabilitation and to examine what accommodations could be made in rehabilitation programs for subjects with more severe neuropsychological deficits. Perhaps rehabilitation that offers continuous feedback and that uses techniques designed to facilitate the processing of this information might lead to similar improvements. Additionally, existing interventions that have as their goal cognitive remediation might result in improved work performance, treatment compliance, and insight for these patients.

*References*

Amador, X., Strauss, D., Yale, S., & Gorman, J. M. (1991). Awareness of illness in schizophrenia. *Schizophrenia Bulletin, 17*(1): 113–132.

Bartko, G., Herczeg, I., & Zador, G. (1988). Clinical symptomatology and drug compliance in schizophrenic patients. *Acta Psychiatrica Scandinavia, 77,* 74–76.

Bell, M. D., Lysaker, P. H., Goulet, J. L., Milstein, R. M., & Lindemeyer, J. P. (1994). Five component model of schizophrenia: Assessing the factorial invariance of the PANSS. *Psychiatry Research, 52,* 295–303.

Bell, M. D., Milstein, R. M., Goulet, J. L., Lysaker, P. H., & Cicchetti, D. (1992). The positive and negative syndrome scale and the brief psychiatric rating scale: Reliability, comparability and predictive validity. *Journal of Nervous and Mental Disease, 180,* 723–728.

Bell, M. D., Milstein, R. M., & Lysaker, P. H. (1993). Pay and participation in work activity: Clinical benefits for clients with schizophrenia. *Psychosocial Rehabilitation Journal, 17,* 173–177.

Bolton, B., & Roessler, R. (1986). *Manual for the work personality profile.* Fayetteville, AR: Arkansas Research and Training Center in Vocational Research.

Braff, D. L., Heaton, R., Kuck, J., Cullum, M., Moranville, J., Grant, I. & Zisook, S. (1991). The generalized pattern of neuropsychological deficits in outpatients with chronic schizophrenia with heterogeneous Wisconsin Card Sorting Test results. *Archives of General Psychiatry, 48,* 891–898.

Greenfeld, D., Strauss, J., Bowers, M., & Mandelkern, M. (1989). Insight and interpretation of illness in recovery from psychosis. *Schizophrenia Bulletin, 15,* 245–252.

Heaton, R. (1981). *Wisconsin Card Sorting Test Manual.* Odessa, FL: Psychological Assessment Resources.

Heinrichs, D., Cohen, B., & Carpenter, W. (1985). Early insight and the management of schizophrenic decompensation. *Journal of Nervous and Mental Disease, 173,* 133–138.

Kay, S., Fiszbein, A., & Opler, L. (1987). The positive and negative syndrome scale (PANSS) for schizophrenia. *Schizophrenia Bulletin, 13,* 261–276.

Kay, S. R., & Sevy, S. (1990). Pyramidical model of schizophrenia. *Schizophrenia Bulletin, 16*, 537–545.

Lin, I., Spiga, R., & Fortsch, W. (1979). Insight and adherence to medication in chronic schizophrenics. *Journal of Clinical Psychiatry, 40*, 430–432.

Lysaker, P. H., & Bell, M. D. (1994). Insight and cognitive impairment in schizophrenia: Performance on repeated administration of the Wisconsin Card Sorting Test. *Journal of Nervous and Mental Disease, 182*, 656–670.

Lysaker, P. H., & Bell, M. D. (1995). Work rehabilitation and improvements in insight in schizophrenia. *Journal of Nervous and Mental Disease*.

Lysaker, P. H., Bell, M. D., Milstein, R. M., Goulet, J. G., & Bryson, G. J. (1995). Insight and treatment compliance in schizophrenia. *Psychiatry*.

McEvoy, J. P., Apperson, L. J., Applebaum, P. S., Ortlip, P., Brecosky, J., Hammil, K., Geller, J. L., & Roth, L. (1989). Insight in schizophrenia. Its relationship to acute psychopathology. *Journal of Nervous and Mental Disease, 177*(1), 43–47.

McEvoy, J. P., Applebaum, P. S., Geller, L. J., & Freter, S. (1989). Why must some schizophrenic patients be involuntarily committed? The role of insight. *Comprehensive Psychiatry, 10*(1), 13–17.

McEvoy, J. P., Schooler, N. R., Friedman, E., Steingard, S., & Allen, M. (1993). Use of psychopathology vignettes by patients with schizophrenia or schizoaffective disorder and by mental health professionals to judge insight. *Journal of Nervous and Mental Disease, 150*, 1649–1657.

McGlashan, T., Levy, S., & Carpenter, W. (1975). Integration and sealing over: Clinically distinct recovery styles from schizophrenia. *Archives of General Psychiatry, 32*, 1269–1272.

Robinson, A., Heaton, R., Lehman, R., & Stilson, D. (1980). The utility of the Wisconsin Card Sorting Test in detecting and localizing frontal lobe lesions. *Journal of Consulting Clinical Psychology, 48*, 605–614.

Slosson, R. (1963). *Slosson intelligence test for children and adults*. East Aurora, NY: Slosson Educational Publications.

Spitzer, R., Williams, J., Gibbon, M., & First, M. (1989). *Structured clinical interview for DSM-III-R*. New York: Biometrics Research Department.

Wechsler, D. *Wechsler adult intelligence scale-revised*. San Antonio, TX: Psychological Corporation.

Wilson, W., Ban, T., & Guy, W. (1986). Flexible system criteria in chronic schizophrenia. *Comprehensive Psychiatry, 27*, 259–265.

Young, D. A., Davila, R., & Scher, H. (1993). Unawareness of illness and neuropsychological performance in chronic schizophrenia. *Schizophrenia Research, 10*, 117–124.

# 16

WILLIAM R. MCFARLANE

ELLEN P. LUKENS

# Insight, Families, and Education

## An Exploration of the Role of Attribution in Clinical Outcome

The problem of insight in patients with schizophrenia has perplexed theoreticians and vexed clinicians for well over a century. The conundrum is all too familiar: these individuals are suffering simultaneously from the most severe of mental illnesses while unaware of a profound discrepancy between their experience and that of their peers.

Until the advent of massive evidence that schizophrenia is partly or perhaps entirely an organic syndrome, it has been assumed that this *grand indifference* was psychologically determined. Lack of insight either protected the person from a self-assessment that might be overwhelmingly demoralizing or it defended against ambivalence and unconscious conflicts that were threatening and anxiety provoking.

This chapter presents evidence to support a broader concept. Poor insight is proposed to be the result of a lack of information about the illness and its treatment, in combination with a neurophysiological disorder of the prefrontal cerebral cortex. This combination makes self-awareness physically difficult to achieve.

In this context, we will propose that education, training, and alterations of the social context foster insight, especially when those interventions involve not only patients but their families, friends, and even other patients and their families. To support this idea, we will present the recent experience and empirical results of the New York State Family Psychoeducation in Schizophrenia Study, as at least preliminary evidence that such an approach has scientific merit. A principal focus of this intervention was to promote knowledge about the illness among families of patients. Therefore, we will discuss the therapeutic effects that follow education—in particular, increased cooperation with treatment among patients.

Although insight has many dimensions, including awareness of illness, acknowledgment of symptoms, and acceptance of treatment, attribution and its relationship to knowledge will be emphasized here. The argument will be made that these two dimensions—attributional style and knowledge about the illness—when considered primarily in relation to families, can determine a major portion of short-term clinical outcome in patients with schizophrenia. Lack of knowledge about the illness is largely a result of earlier clinical ideologies. These ideologies proscribed both professional contact and the sharing of patient information with families. Thus, lack of knowledge is seen as predominately iatrogenic, with the implication that insight, at least in families, is modifiable by clinicians.

The empirical literature suggests a causal sequence leading to lack of insight as follows: (1) family attitudes regarding the illness and behavior toward the patient have a large influence on outcome, especially relapse, in both positive and negative directions; and (2) misattribution about symptoms and confusion about the source of symptoms are associated with negative family attitudes and behaviors, and with lack of information about the complex dimensions of illness. Attempts to modify such attribution through both education and coping skill training have been shown to be markedly effective in lowering relapse rates among patients. The conclusion is that attribution and understanding among family members not only influence patient outcome but are modifiable by education, training, and social support. It would not be surprising if family attitudes and behavior also influenced patients' level of insight into their illness. For this reason, in the next section, we will review the literature as it relates to the relationship between family attitudes and patient outcome. We will argue that by providing families with education, training, and social support, the level of insight in the person suffering from the illness can also be modified.

## Review of the Literature

The foundations for the approach described here lie in research begun in the early 1960s. In 1958, Brown and Rutter, collaborating in London, England, began to focus extensively on the course of mental illness, particularly schizophrenia. They hypothesized that intense and negative interactions might predispose patients with schizophrenia to greater risk of relapse than more low-key and benign interactions. They developed a measurable construct, which they termed *expressed emotion*, that they believed might account for the poorer outcome in certain family constellations. In a carefully designed and executed study, they found that high expressed emotion predicted relapse rates over nine months after the initial assessments, and that those who returned to live with parents or in large boarding homes had worse outcomes than those who lived elsewhere. More precisely, a subfactor, *critical comments*, accounted for most of the predictive power and the variance in relapse.

To measure the kind of relationship between family member and patient, Brown used several measures, which included criticism, overinvolvement, and warmth (Brown & Rutter, 1966; Rutter & Brown, 1966). The ratings for criticism were based on an actual count of statements judged to be critical because of tone of voice *and/or* content (i.e., a clear statement of either resentment, hostility, disapproval, or dislike), as well as an overall measure of harshness of content. Overinvolvement was rated on a 6-point scale and reflected a combined measure of overprotection, intrusiveness, control, and general anxiety regarding the patient. Warmth was represented in terms of a 6-point scale that included sympathy and concern, interest, and appreciation of the individual as a person, and shared enjoyment in mutual activities. A summary variable dichotomized families as demonstrating high or low expressed emotion. High expressed emotion was determined by 7 or more critical comments and/or a summary score for overinvolvement of 4 or more. The main goal in this semistructured interview, termed the Camberwell Family Interview (CFI), was to encourage the respondent to express him or herself in ways that represented inner feelings and attitudes regarding the patient in the three months prior to interview.

The results in this and several replication studies have been noteworthy (Brown, Birley, & Wing, 1972; Vaughn & Leff, 1976; Vaughn, Snyder, Jones, Freeman, & Falloon, 1984; Moline, Singh, Morris, & Meltzer, 1985; Karno & Jenkins, 1987; Tarrier et al., 1989; Nuechterlein, Edell, Norris, & Dawson, 1986; Leff et al., 1987). High levels of expressed emotion of key family members were related to the likelihood of relapse during a follow-up period (usually nine months). Moreover, the patients who did most poorly had family members who were most expressive in terms of affect. These studies have used prospective designs in which past behaviors, emotional response among relatives, and relapse were measured independently. For instance, in a replication conducted by Brown, (Brown et al., 1972), 58% of the patients from families described as high in expressed emotion relapsed during the nine months after discharge from a psychiatric hospitalization, as compared to only 16% in the low expressed emotion group ($p < .001$). In another replication, Vaughn and Leff (1976) found that two factors—regular medication and reduced familial contact—served to mediate between the measure of expressed emotion and relapse over a nine-month period. She subsequently replicated the study in metropolitan Los Angeles, where street drugs complicated the course of treatment and overall outcome (Vaughn et al., 1984). In spite of this, findings were consistent: relapse of psychotic symptoms was high among male patients in households characterized by high levels of expressed emotion, particularly criticism. Later research, on the relationship between attribution and expressed emotion, elucidated this further.

## Types of Attribution by Families

In a study of the relationship between attribution and expressed emotion, Brewin, MacCarthy, Duda, and Vaughn (1991) specifically examined how families understand or explain the illness of schizophrenia in their relative. In a simple count of attributions, they found that 58 relatives made a total of 1,033 different attributions for the illness and for positive and negative symptoms. Among the most common were: "stress, genetic influences, losses and separations, taking recreational drugs, unemployment, insensitive behavior by other people, misinterpretation of a situation, failure to take medication, conscious and unconscious attitudes, bad company, rebelliousness, the menstrual cycle, childishness, attention seeking, current stress, aspects of personality, and the relative's own behavior toward the patient" (p. 549). The authors found that families who attributed the illness to factors external to the patient tended to be overinvolved, while those who viewed the patient as the cause of his or her behavior tended to be critical. Relatives who saw behavior as more personal to, internal to, and controllable by the patient manifested higher criticism and hostility. In particular, they saw negative symptoms as controllable and more personal than illness driven. The role of knowledge of illness in determining not only attribution but also criticism and hostility is illustrated by comments from the father of a 19-year-old recently diagnosed patient:

> I found I was much more irritable with him before we found out that he wasn't well. It was getting quite bad. . . . He was sort of squaring up, and I really felt I'd have liked him to leave. But having found out that he's . . . that it's not his fault, you feel more sorry for him, you try and understand it a bit more. (Brewin et al., 1991, p. 552)

In general, phenomena among the patients that are attributed to controllable, idiosyncratic, or personal factors appear to be associated with higher criticism among family members. Given the power of criticism to predict relapse and course, the linkage becomes circular. As symptoms and bizarre behavior increase, relatives' attributions tend to become more personal, which in turn is associated with criticism from relatives and deterioration in the patient's mental status. This cycle is contingent on relatives' ignorance, disagreement, and confusion about the cause of those same phenomena. If relatives assume that the symptoms of illness are controllable by the patient, they are likely to make attributions of intentionality, responsibility, and outright blame (Fincham, Beach, & Nelson, 1987; Bradbury & Fincham, 1990).

### Attribution and Symptoms

A relationship between criticism by the family toward the patient and longstanding interpersonal deficits in the patient has been observed in other studies, particularly when these deficits are not attributed to the illness process. Two separate content analyses of the Camberwell Family Interview (Vaughn, 1977; Runions & Prudo, 1983) have suggested that critical parents tended to focus on negative personality traits rather than on florid psychotic symptoms. Vaughn, in her early replications of the expressed emotion findings, became curious about the differences between the low and high expressed emotion families, because their elucidation could suggest the source of high expressed emotion. After an extensive content analysis of the comments upon which the critical comments ratings were based, she was able to construct some rather unexpected generalizations. The highly critical relatives were angered by the poor functioning and lack of initiative of their ill relative, and less concerned about the psychotic symptoms and more grossly deviant aspects of their behavior. They also tended to personalize these functional deficits, attributing them to poor character, laziness, manipulativeness, or lack of consideration. In later work, she observed that critical responses seemed to be related to negative symptoms, as well as to the relapse of positive symptoms (Vaughn & Leff, 1981). Based on clinical observation, Beels and McFarlane (1983) described the tendency for families to criticize withdrawal, lack of motivation, and poor hygiene among patients (all considered negative symptoms). Mintz and his colleagues (Mintz, Neuchterlein, Goldstein, Mintz, & Snyder, 1989) explored the relationship between criticism and increasing dysfunction on the part of the patient as measured by certain negative symptoms, particularly apathy, inertia, and lack of affection. He argued that exposure to these kinds of symptoms might lead to increasing criticism among parents, and in turn, decreased mastery on the part of the patient might exacerbate that criticism. Glynn and Liberman (1990) reported that 26 male patients from critical households had higher ratings for thought disorder, anxious depression, and anhedonia-asociality when compared to a control group of 14 male patients in low expressed emotion families. There was no support for a relationship between criticism and other negative symptoms.

Other studies suggest other dimensions of attribution and critical attitudes. In work by Miklowitz (Miklowitz, Goldstein, & Falloon, 1983), criticism tended to be associated with higher premorbid functioning and fewer residual symptoms over time. Earlier findings (Brown et al., 1972; Vaughn et al., 1984; Leff et al., 1987) had also supported this association. The implication in these studies was that critical comments reflect a tendency for parents to react with disappointment to a child of whom more was expected and who is less blatantly and visibly disabled.

Greenley (1986) conducted a content analysis of the original Brown, Monck, Carstairs, & Wing (1962) data and found that families described as high in expressed emotion doubted that the patient had a legitimate illness and were generally more anxious and fearful of the patient, compared to relatives described as low in expressed emotion. In her recent work, Vaughn (1989) described members of families characterized as low in expressed emotion as believing that the patient suffers from a genuine illness, allowing them to combine objective empathy with tolerance of disturbed behavior and an increased ability to remain calm during a crisis. The families with low expressed emotion tended to have a different orientation and appeared to behave differently as well. They were calmer, less preoccupied, and more understanding of the patient's problems. They attributed the patient's deficiencies to forces beyond their control, but believed that those forces were legitimate and in the general category of afflictions such as other chronic medical or neurological disorders. They were much less guilty and ashamed, because they did not see the problem as personal failures on either their or their ill relative's part. They tended to keep a greater interpersonal distance and allow for more withdrawal when needed. Koenigsberg and Handley's (1986) description of low expressed emotion included respect for the patient's desire for privacy and distance, and tolerance of odd or unusual behaviors. Yet Vaughn (1986) observed that when family members expressed little emotion of any kind (to the point that they appear to have no expectations for the patient), there seemed to be an increase in negative symptoms and in social impairment in particular. These findings suggest that the families' level of knowledge and acceptance of schizophrenia as an illness has implications for the course and intensity of the symptoms that the patients present.

### Knowledge and Expressed Emotion

In theory, a family's perception of the patient as truly ill should increase as the patient requires psychiatric care and as the family and patient are exposed to even minimal education about the illness. This is supported by Barrowclough and Tarrier's (1984) finding that relatives' knowledge about schizophrenia was inversely correlated with their level of critical comments. Several studies have intervened to increase families' knowledge and then assessed family attitudes and well-being. Berkowitz (1984) found that education led to greater awareness of diagnosis and more optimism among those families described as high in expressed emotion at baseline. Smith and Birchwood (1987, 1990) presented information to families regarding concepts of schizophrenia, symptoms, treatment outcomes, and hospital and community resources, and assessed family members shortly after the presentation and at a six-month follow-up point. Not surprisingly, 75% of the sample of family members did not understand basic facts about the effects, purpose, mechanisms of action, or side effects of medication at baseline. After the presentation, however, knowledge increased dramatically and was retained after six months.

## Clinical Implications

To summarize, the empirical evidence suggests that a major source of negative attitudes and behavior on the part of relatives—seemingly a major risk factor for relapse—lies in their lack of information regarding schizophrenia. Family knowledge, or the lack of it, is at least partly iatrogenic—the result of longstanding clinical policies among mental health professionals that discouraged sharing diagnoses and other clinical information with patients and their families.

To even begin to struggle with schizophrenia, the family must possess (1) the available knowledge about the illness itself and (2) coping skills that are specific to this or other psychiatric disorders. However, that knowledge and those skills are frequently counterintuitive. Many families have developed, through painful trial and error, methods of dealing with positive and negative symptoms, functional disabilities, and the desperation of their ill relatives.

The psychoeducational approaches have been designed to address specific major psychiatric disorders, so they proceed with the assumption that these disorders tend to elicit responses from family members that can be self-defeating, although understandable. One of the core principles in psychoeducational work states that expecting families to intuitively understand such a mystifying condition and to know what to do about it is unrealistic. Further, general family functioning varies independently of the presence of schizophrenia or other biologically based mental disorders, so that the clinician practicing family psychoeducation can expect to encounter a full range of well-functioning *and* highly dysfunctional families.

The more adaptive families tend to have access to information, and the treatment system is a crucial source of that information. So a critical need is that families and patients have access to the treatment system and to each other to develop more effective means of coping with the day-to-day challenges of managing schizophrenia at home. That access can be provided through multiple-family groups or the family self-help movement. We believe that the family's level of insight regarding the origins of illness, in association with a nonstigmatizing context and tolerant environment, is an important part of this process. It fosters a situation in which the patient can also begin to understand and gain insight regarding the origins of the illness, the impact of schizophrenia on day-to-day functioning, and the importance of treatment compliance and management of symptoms.

The psychoeducational program that we will describe was designed to address such issues. This multiple-family group model has developed as a natural extension of multiple family therapy and psychoeducation. It serves as one example of an intervention designed to promote education, insight, improved communication, and lowered stress in the home environment. This clinical approach combines antipsychotic medication with a program that helps families and patients reduce the level of intensity and complexity in their household. The result is that relapse is delayed, reduced in severity, or for the less severely ill patient, perhaps eliminated entirely. This approach includes two major components: (1) education of family members about the details of the disorder, and (2) support and guidance for family and patients over a fairly prolonged period after an episode. The elements in the approach were drawn from previous experiments that appear to have been successful (Langsley, Machotka, & Flomenhaft, 1971; Beels, 1975; Goldstein, Rodnick, Evans, May, & Steinberg, 1978).

## Elements of the Psychoeducational Multiple-Family Group Model

The basic psychoeducational model consists of four treatment stages that roughly correspond to the phases of an episode of schizophrenia, from the acute phase through the slow recuperative and rehabilitation phases. These stages are (1) joining; (2) survival skills training and workshop; (3) reentry; and (4) social and vocational rehabilitation.

### Joining

Contacts with the families and with the newly admitted individuals are initiated within 48 hours after a hospital admission and diagnosis of *schizophrenia, schizoaffective disorder*, or *schizophreniform disorder*. Initial contacts with the patient are deliberately brief and nonstressful. The aim is to establish minimal rapport and to gain permission to include the family in the ongoing treatment process. Families are contacted either during a visit to the hospital or by telephone. They are made aware that the clinician is willing to collaborate with them in helping their relative recover and avoid further relapse. The family is asked to join with the clinician in establishing a working alliance or partnership. The purpose of this alliance is to provide the best posthospital environment for the patient to recover. The clinician is respectful of the family's distress and offers concrete assistance wherever appropriate. Families are invited to join the clinician for sessions in which the clinician helps them work out a recovery strategy that suits the needs and desires of both the patient and the family. This strategy is designed to be mindful of the limits imposed by the illness itself.

*Joining* in this model refers to a way of working with families that is characterized by collaboration rather than by treatment of the family. Thus, in keeping with the underlying philosophy of the model, the clinician assumes the least pathology in attempting to understand and relate to the family. The joining phase is typically three to seven sessions, but more may be required until a sufficient number of families are engaged. The goal of this phase is to (1) establish a working alliance, (2) become acquainted with any family issues and problems that might contribute to stress either for the patient or for the family, (3) learn of the family's strengths and resources in dealing with the illness, and (4) create a contract with mutual and attainable goals. Joining, in its most general sense, continues throughout the treatment. Therefore, it is the responsibility of the clinician to remain an available resource for the family, as well as their advocate, in dealing with any other system necessitated by the illness of their relative. To foster this relationship, the clinician demonstrates concern for the patient, acknowledges the family's loss, and grants them sufficient time to mourn. The clinician is available to the family outside of the formal sessions, avoids treating the family as a patient or blaming them in any way, helps to focus on the present crisis, and serves as a source of information about the illness. By helping the family members to experience the clinician as an ally, the clinician may also enhance the patient's openness. In this context, the patient may be more able to use the information presented and discussed in the multiple family group setting.

### Survival Skills Training and Workshop

Once the family is joined and while the patient is still being stabilized, the family is invited to a workshop conducted by the clinician and other relevant staff. The purpose of the workshop is to provide information to families so that they can begin to understand the complexity of the illness. These sessions are conducted in a formal, classroomlike atmosphere. The workshop is specifically for family members and friends of the patient; patients usually are not invited, unless they are exceptionally well compensated and are not delusional or denying illness. The clinicians working with the families conduct the workshop, assisted by the psychiatrist(s) treating the patients. Experience suggests that the optimal size is from four to seven families, which coincidentally seems to be the ideal range for an ongoing psychoeducational multiple-family group.

The format for these workshops differs dramatically from therapy sessions. They proceed in an informal lecture and discussion fashion, with a classroom seating arrangement. Audiovisual aids are used extensively, particularly to illustrate concepts of brain function, medication effects, and symptoms and signs. In the author's workshops, the biological information is presented via a professional-quality videotape with frequent breaks for questions and discussion. The family clinicians then present a number of guidelines—survival skills, as Anderson, Reiss, and Hogarty (1986) call them—for the management of schizophrenia (see table 16.1).

Families who successfully complete the social skills training workshop are better equipped to help their ill family member understand his or her experiences as being illness related, and to acknowledge this for themselves. They are also in a position to help other families and unrelated patients to utilize and process this information in the context of a supportive group environment.

### Reentry

Following the workshop, the clinician begins meeting twice monthly with the families and patients in the multiple-family group format. The goal of this stage of the treatment is to plan and implement strategies to cope with the vicissitudes of a person recovering from an acute episode of schizophrenia. Major content areas include medication compliance, helping the patient avoid the use of street drugs and/or alcohol, the general lowering of expectations during the period of negative symptoms, and an increase in tolerance for these symptoms. Two special techniques are introduced to participating

TABLE 16.1     Family Guidelines

Here's a list of things everyone can do to help make things run more smoothly:

1. *Go slow.* Recovery takes time. Rest is important. Things will get better in their own time.
2. *Keep it cool.* Enthusiasm is normal. Tone it down. Disagreement is normal. Tone it down too.
3. *Give each other space.* Time out is important for everyone. It's okay to reach out. It's okay to say no.
4. *Set limits.* Everyone needs to know what the rules are. A few good rules keep things clear.
5. *Ignore what you can't change.* Let some things slide. Don't ignore violence.
6. *Keep it simple.* Say what you have to say clearly, calmly, and positively.
7. *Follow doctor's orders.* Take medications as they are prescribed. Take only medications that are pre-scribed.
8. *Carry on business as usual.* Reestablish family routines as quickly as possible. Stay in touch with family and friends.
9. *No street drugs or alcohol.* They make symptoms worse.
10. *Pick up on early signs.* Note changes. Consult with your family clinician.
11. *Solve problems step by step.* Make changes gradually. Work on one thing at a time.
12. *Lower expectations, temporarily.* Use a personal yardstick. Compare this month to last month rather than last year or next year.

*Source:* Adapted from C. Anderson, D. Reiss, & G. Hogarty (1986). *Schizophrenia and the family: A practitioner's guide to psychoeducation and management.* New York: Guilford Press.

members as supports for the efforts to follow the family guidelines: (1) formal problem solving, and (2) communication skills training. The application of either one of these techniques characterizes each session. Further, each session follows a prescribed, task-oriented format or paradigm, designed to enhance family and patient coping effectiveness and to strengthen the alliance among the families, the patients, and the clinicians.

It is in this context that the group process is particularly important and effective. It allows families and patients to increase their understanding of the problems associated with the illness of schizophrenia. As the group members work together on the formal problem-solving and communication skills training, they provide each other with feedback and observations that are critical to facilitating change and compliance with treatment.

## Social and Vocational Rehabilitation

Approximately one year following an acute episode, most patients begin to evidence signs of a return to spontaneity and active engagement with those around them. This is usually the sign that the negative symptoms are lifting and the patient can now be challenged more intensively. In the multiple-family group, the focus of this phase deals more specifically with the rehabilitative needs of the patient, addressing the two areas of functioning in which there are the most common deficits: social skills and the ability to get and maintain employment. The sessions are used to role-play situations likely to cause stress for the patient if entered into unprepared. Family members actively assist in various aspects of this training endeavor. Additionally, the family is encouraged to rebuild its own network of family and friends, which has usually been weakened as a consequence of the presence of schizophrenia. Regular sessions are conducted on a once-monthly basis, although more contact may be necessary at particularly stressful times.

It is during this stage that patient insight begins to emerge, as a result of a collaborative effort in the treatment to be alert for increased symptoms as a patient's responsibilities and external demands increase. Our experience is that it is more tolerable and hopeful for the patient to define illness as a relative disability than as a catastrophic collapse and an absolute barrier to living life normally. Relatives involved in the rehabilitation process during this time can help a patient understand their limitations (i.e., increase their insight) by providing a supportive, nonstigmatizing environment. They are encouraged to emphasize achievements and functional progress, while helping the patient accept some degree of limitation and the continued need for treatment.

## The New York State Family Psychoeducation in Schizophrenia Study

The New York State Family Psychoeducation in Schizophrenia Study was designed to fully test this model in a community-based sample. The study utilized a two-cell design to experimentally compare psychoeducational multiple-family and psychoeducational single-family treatment over a two-year period. The design included: (1) random assignment, (2) full specification of the test therapies, (3) extensive training and ongoing supervision of experienced therapists by the project's supervisory staff, (4) a standard-dose medication strategy, and (5) wide-ranging measurement of patient and family outcomes.

The total sample consisted of 172 *DSM-III-R* patients with schizophrenic, schizoaffective, or schizophreniform disorders, recruited and treated at six New York State public psychiatric facilities. These facilities encompassed a wide range of the public-service patient population in terms of chronicity, race, ethnicity, social class, and geography. Clinicians at each participating site assessed and treated 24 to 36 patients. There were no significant differences at baseline between the treatment conditions.

### Relapse Outcome

One-year relapse outcome was determined using the Brief Psychiatric Rating Scale (BPRS): 19.0% of multiple-family group (MFG) cases relapsed during the first year as compared to 28.6% of single-family treatment cases. The relapse rates at two years were 28% and 42%, respectively. For cases completing the treatment protocol (80% of the sample) or when controlled for medication compliance, this was a statistically significant difference. Rates of clinically significant relapse (cases that met criteria for seven days) were 16.3% versus 25.6%, respectively, over two years. The multiple-family result—an annual clinically significant relapse rate of under 10%—compares quite favorably to expected relapse rates of about 40% using medication alone or with supportive individual therapy (Hogarty et al., 1979). Among Caucasian families with patients who only partly remitted during the index admission, there was a marked difference in relapse, again favoring the MFG format: 17% versus 59%, at two years, using the more rigorous criteria. That is, in the highest risk subsample, the MFG relapse rates were actually lower than in more well-stabilized patients, while the opposite effect was observed in single-family treatment.

## Rehospitalization Outcome

We also compared the mean number of hospitalizations for the entire sample for two years prior to the study with hospitalizations during the study period. These rates dropped to about one third of the sample's prior rate by the end of the two-year observation and treatment interval.

## Employment Outcome

The sample as a whole increased significantly in employment (full- or part-time competitive or sheltered job) from 17.3% at two months prior to the test treatments to 29.3% during the 18- to 24-month period in treatment (Chi square = 7.63, $p$ = .001). Although multi-family group treatment yielded a higher employment gain than single-family treatment (16% vs. 8%), the difference was not statistically significant.

## Medication Compliance

Furthermore, the family intervention appeared to affect pharmacological treatment. Medication compliance, as assessed by the treating psychiatrists, averaged close to 90% for the entire sample across the two years, increasing slightly over that period. The study was conducted in a large state hospital system, under less than ideal circumstances, yet the outcome was fairly dramatic, suggesting wide applicability to a variety of less financially stressed settings.

## Conclusion

We began this chapter with the proposition that aspects of insight are directly related to the availability of information. The family serves as an important frame of reference for the patient and can directly or indirectly influence the patient's knowledge about his or her illness. As such, family education may be critical to the development of increased insight and cooperation in patients with schizophrenia.

Our experience with psychoeducational interventions for families appears to confirm that some of the difficulties in promoting insight have been iatrogenic. Conversely, the clinical team can directly enhance insight by education and training in the application of skills that flow logically from a more comprehensive, biopsychosocial understanding of schizophrenia. The education-training paradigm also suggests that availability of information and accurate attribution are key aspects of insight. In our study, awareness of illness and acknowledgment of symptoms among both patients and families appear to increase during the treatment process, particularly after the educational presentations. The unusually high and gradually increasing medication compliance rates among patients underscores the links among attribution, awareness, and acknowledgment among family members, on the one hand, and the acceptance of treatment among patients, on the other. The evidence seems to suggest that in the modal case, direct instruction and ongoing skill training by empathic clinicians lead to enhancements of all aspects of insight, and from insight to positive clinical outcomes.

This discussion leaves unanswered one important question: Would more formalized education and training of patients in coping skills have the same effects as they do in families? Currently, there is only anecdotal and clinical report regarding this question, but such evidence suggests that if the timing of these interventions is carefully considered, the answer is positive.

In the majority of cases treated during the two-year period of the New York State study, the patients became increasingly cooperative with treatment, as is suggested by the high rates of medication compliance. In addition, patients who remained stable for at least six months after at least one year in treatment were offered an educational session that included an abbreviated version of the same videotaped informational presentation that had been given to their families at the beginning of the treatment. The result of the indirect and direct educational intervention in the multiple-family groups was that patients began to urge other patients to see the symptomatic underpinnings of their subjective distress. They would also encourage other patients to accept treatment, to regulate their lives to reduce stress, and to gradually increase the demands and expectations they were attempting to meet. Patients appeared to absorb the concepts and suggestions that were presented by the multiple-family group leaders, and to proceed toward acceptance, albeit at widely varying paces. Perhaps because of the substantial cognitive impairments that are inherent to schizophrenia, these patients appeared to require much longer time and more repetitive exposure to information and advice to achieve acceptance than did their family members.

One major advantage of the multiple-family groups is that they evolve toward a culture of compliance and cooperation. In this context, individual members and families have to contend with other ordinary citizens who accept the explanations and treatment offered and over time begin to visibly reap the benefits of doing so. The families and the patients support and encourage insight as it evolves among other group members, through either suggestion or indirect modeling.

A similar process occurred in relation to substance abuse and its effects on functioning and life satisfaction. Throughout the course of treatment, the clinicians made frequent reference to the deleterious effects of substance abuse on subjective and objective well-being. In the problem-solving process, substance abuse was systematically defined as the principal problem as long as it remained a factor in a given patient's clinical status. By the end of the two-year study period, all patients had reduced their abuse to subclinical levels, but that reduction rarely occurred quickly.

Interestingly, it quickly became apparent to the study clinicians that if a given family tended to discount biological explanations and resist treatment, the patient in that family would also discount such explanation. It emerged that families as a whole vary widely in their acceptance of medical authority or even relevance, and when there is a strong family resistance to medical explanations and treatment, it is virtually impossible to promote insight in the patient. Some studies have found that in treating chronic medical disorders—essential hypertension being the classic example—noncompliance and denial are the norm rather than the exception (Glanz & Scholl, 1983; Becker, 1988).

Liberman and his colleagues (1986) have developed systematic educational and behavioral skill training methods that specifically attempt to teach patients about the biological, psychological, and social aspects of schizophrenia. This is followed by training in skills that facilitate discussion with a psychiatrist and/or a nurse about medication, its effects and side effects, and what compliance with a maintenance regimen offers. These methods assume that poor insight is modifiable and that direct education and coaching are the simplest and most effective means for enhancing all aspects of insight. Again, there is some emphasis on attribution, but more weight is given to dealing with the consequences of denial and the advantages of cooperation with treatment. In particular, these behavioral approaches are personalized in such a way that they are meaningful to the specific individual.

In summary, the available evidence suggests that family insight can be enhanced by education and assistance in the practical application of those insights, at least when these interventions involve a group of families. It remains to be seen whether education and skill training can produce comparable increases in insight systematically in patients with schizophrenia. The major obstacle may be the cognitive impairments of the disorder itself. Our experience suggests that this deficiency slows the process of absorption of knowledge and development of insight, but it does not appear to categorically rule out acceptance and understanding of the illness paradigm. Our study provides clear empirical evidence that the consequences of insight, especially cooperation with a medication regimen, can be promoted through education and family support. For that reason, research should focus on trials of education and skill training for persons with the illness at various intervals along the recovery continuum to determine what is the earliest point at which education is both effective and not destabilizing. Further increments of improvement in outcome seem likely to follow such an intervention strategy.

## References

Anderson, C., Reiss, D., & Hogarty, G. (1986). *Schizophrenia and the family: A practitioners guide to psychoeducation and management.* New York: Guilford Press.

Barrowclough, C., & Tarrier, N. (1984). Psychosocial interventions with families and their effects on the course of schizophrenia: A review. *Psychological Medicine, 14,* 629–642.

Becker, L. A. (1988). Family systems and compliance with medical regimens. In C. N. Ramsey (Ed.), *Family systems in medicine* (pp. 416–431). Heidelberg: Springer-Verlag.

Beels, C. C. (1975). Family and social management of schizophrenia. *Schizophrenia Bulletin, 13,* 97–118.

Beels, C. C., & McFarlane, W. R. (1983). Thoughts on family therapy and schizophrenia. In W. R. McFarlane (Ed.), *Family therapy in schizophrenia* (pp. 17–40). New York: Guilford Press.

Berkowitz, R. (1984). Therapeutic intervention with schizophrenic patients and their families: a description of a clinical research project. *Journal of Family Therapy, 6,* 211–233.

Birchwood, M. J. (1990). Families coping with schizophrenia: Coping styles, their origins and correlates. *Psychological Medicine, 20,* 857–865.

Birchwood, M. J., & Smith, J. (1987). Schizophrenia and the family. In J. Orford, (Ed.), *Coping with disorder in the family* (pp. 7–38). Croom Helm: Kent.

Birchwood, M. J., Smith, J., Cochrane, R., Wetton, S., & Copestake, S. (1990). The Social Functioning Scale: The development and validation of a new scale of social functioning for use in family intervention programs with schizophrenic patients. *British Journal of Psychiatry,* 853–859.

Bradbury, T. N., & Fincham, F. D. (1990). Attributions in marriage: Review and critique. *Psychological Bulletin, 107,* 3–33.

Brewin, C. R., MacCarthy, B., Duda, K., & Vaughn, C. E. (1991). Attribution and expressed emotion in the relatives of patients with schizophrenia. *Journal of Abnormal Psychology,* *100,* 546–554.

Brown, G. W., & Rutter, M. (1966). The measurement of family activities and relationships. *Human Relations, 19,* 241–263.

Brown, G. W., Birley, J. L. T., & Wing, J. K. (1972). Influence of family life on the course of schizophrenic disorders: A replication. *British Journal of Psychiatry, 121,* 241–258.

Brown, G. W., Monck, E. M., Carstairs, G. M., & Wing, J. K. (1962). Influence of family life on the course of schizophrenic illness. *British Journal of Psychiatry, 16,* 55–68.

Fincham, F. D., Beach, S., & Nelson, G. (1987). Attribution processes in distressed and nondistressed couples: 3. Causal and responsibility attributions of spouse behavior. *Cognitive Therapy Research, 11,* 71–86.

Glanz, K., & Scholl, T. (1983). Intervention strategies to improve adherance among hypertensives: review and recommendations. *Patient Counseling & Health Education, 1,* 14–28.

Glynn, S., & Liberman, R. (1990). Functioning of relatives and patients facing severe mental illness. In H. P. Lefley & D. L. Johnson (Eds.), *Families as allies in the treatment of the mentally ill: New directions for mental health professionals* (pp. 255–266). Washington, DC: American Psychiatric Press.

Glynn, S., Randolph, E., Eth, S., Paz, G., Leona, G., Shaner, A., & Strachan, A. (1990). Patient psychopathology and expressed emotion in schizophrenia. *British Journal of Psychiatry, 157,* 887–890.

Goldstein, M., Rodnick, E., Evans, J., May, P., & Steinberg, M. (1978). Drug and family therapy in the aftercare treatment of acute schizophrenia. *Archives of General Psychiatry, 35,* 1169–1177.

Greenley, J. (1986). Social control and expressed emotion. *Journal of Nervous and Mental Disease, 174*(1), 24–30.

Hogarty, G. E., Schooler, N. R., Ulrich, R. F., Mussare, F., Herron, E., & Ferro, P. (1979). Fluphenazine and social therapy in the aftercare of schizophrenic patients: Relapse analyses of a two-year controlled study of fluphenazine decanoate and fluphenazine hydrochloride. *Archives of General Psychiatry, 36,* 1283–1294.

Karno, M., & Jenkins, J. H. (1987). Expressed emotion and schizophrenic outcome among Mexican American families. *Journal of Nervous and Mental Disease, 195*(3), 143–51.

Koenigsberg, H., & Handley, R. (1986). Expressed emotion: From predicative index to clinical constrict. *American Journal of Psychiatry, 43,* 1361–1373.

Langsley, D. L., Machotka, P., & Flomenhaft, K. (1971). Avoiding mental hospital admission: A follow-up study. *American Journal of Psychiatry, 127,* 1391–1394.

Leff, J., Wig, N. N., Ghosh, A., Bedi, H., Menon, D. K., Kuipers, L., Korten, A., Ernberg, G., Day, R., Sartorius, N., & Jablensky, A. (1987). Expressed emotion and schizophrenia in North India, III: Influence of relatives' expressed emotion on the course of schizophrenia in Chandigarh. *British Journal of Psychiatry, 151,* 166–173.

Liberman, R. (1986). Coping and competence as protective factors in the vulnerability-stress model of schizophrenia. In M. J. Goldstein, I. Hand, & K. Hahlweg (Eds.), *Treatment of schizophrenia: Family assessment and intervention* (pp. 201–216). Berlin: Springer.

McFarlane, W. R. (1983). *Family therapy in schizophrenia.* New York: Guilford Press.

Miklowitz, D., Goldstein, M., & Falloon, I. (1983). Premorbid and symptomatic characteristics of schizophrenics from families with high and low levels of expressed emotion. *Journal of Abnormal Psychology, 92*(3), 359–367.

Mintz, L., Nuechterlein, K., Goldstein, M., Mintz, J., & Snyder, K. (1989). The initial onset of schizophrenia and family expressed emotion: Some methodological considerations. *British Journal of Psychiatry, 154,* 212–217.

Moline, R., Singh, S., Morris, A., & Meltzer, H. (1985). Family expressed emotion and relapse in 24 urban American patients. *American Journal of Psychiatry, 142*(9), 1078–1081.

Mujica, E., Haas, G. L., Hien, D., Goldman, D., Passik, S., & Rudich, G. (1991). Expressed emotion and positive/negative symptoms in schizophrenia. *American Psychiatric Association*, (poster presentation), New Orleans, LA.

Nuechterlein, K., Edell, W., Norris, M., & Dawson, M. (1986). Attentional vulnerability indicators, thought disorder, and negative symptoms. *Schizophrenia Bulletin, 12*, 408–426.

Runions, J., & Prudo, R. (1983). Problem behaviors encountered by families living with a schizophrenic member. *Canadian Journal of Psychiatry, 28*, 382–386.

Rutter, M., & Brown, G. (1966). The reliability and validity of measures of family life and relationships in families containing a psychiatric patient. *Social Psychiatry, 1*(1), 38–53.

Smith, J., & Birchwood, M. (1987). Specific and non-specific effects of educational intervention with families living with schizophrenic relative. *British Journal of Psychiatry, 150*, 645–652.

Smith, J., & Birchwood, M. (1990). Relatives and patients as partners in the management of schizophrenia: the development of a service model. *British Journal of Psychiatry, 156*, 654–660.

Tarrier, N., Barrowclough, C., Porceddu, K., & Watts, S. (1988). The assessment of psychological reactivity to the expressed emotion of the relatives of schizophrenic patients. *British Journal of Psychiatry, 152*, 618–624.

Tarrier, N., Barrowclough, C., Vaughn, C., Bamrah, J., Porceddu, K., Watts, S., & Freeman, H. (1988). The community management of schizophrenia: A controlled-trial of a behavioral intervention with families to reduce relapse. *British Journal of Psychiatry, 153*, 532–542.

Tarrier, N., Barrowclough, C., Vaughn, C., Bamrah, J., Porceddu, K., Watts, S., & Freeman, H. (1989). The community management of schizophrenia. A two-year follow-up of a behavioral intervention with families. *British Journal of Psychiatry, 154*, 625–628.

Vaughn, C. (1977). Patterns of interactions in families of schizophrenics. In H. Katschnig (Ed.), *Schizophrenia: The other side*. Vienna: Urban & Schwarzenberg.

Vaughn, C. (1986). Patterns of emotional response in the families of schizophrenic patients. In M. Goldstein, I. Hand, & K. Hahlweg (Eds.), *Treatment of schizophrenia* (pp. 97–106). New York: Springer-Verlag.

Vaughn, C. (1989). Annotation: Expressed emotion in family relationships. *Journal of Child Psychology and Psychiatry, 30*(1), 13–22.

Vaughn, C., & Leff, J. (1976). The influence of family and social factors on the course of psychiatric illness: A comparison of schizophrenic and depressed neurotic patients. *British Journal of Psychiatry, 129*, 125–137.

Vaughn, C., & Leff, J. (1981). Patterns of emotional response in relatives of schizophrenic patients. *Schizophrenia Bulletin, 7*(1), 43–44.

Vaughn, C., Snyder, K., Freeman, W., Jones, S., Falloon, I., & Liberman, R. (1982). Family factors in schizophrenic relapse: A replication. *Schizophrenia Bulletin, 8*(2), 425–426.

Vaughn, C. E., Snyder, K. S., Jones, S., Freeman, W. B., & Falloon, I. R. (1984). Family factors in schizophrenia relapse: A replication in California of British research on expressed emotion. *Archives of General Psychiatry, 42*, 1169–1177.

## 17

ANTHONY S. DAVID

# The Clinical Importance
# of Insight

This volume attests to the revival in interest in the concept of insight in psychosis since Aubrey Lewis's first foray into this area in 1934. A number of reviews have preceded it and have paved its way (see, for example, David, 1990; Amador, Strauss, Yale, & Gorman 1991; Ghaemi & Pope, 1994). Assessing insight has always been seen as an important part of phenomenology and psychopathology, and is defined in most textbooks of psychiatry and abnormal psychology, although usage and definitions of the term vary (Marková & Berrios, 1992; Berrios & Marková, chap. 2). The clinical importance of insight is now being studied. Certain themes have been addressed, such as the relationship between insight and treatment compliance (McEvoy, Apperson, et al., 1989a; Buchanan, 1992; McEvoy, chap. 14; McFarlane, chap. 16); acting upon hallucinations (Rogers, Gillis, Turner, & Frise-Smith, 1990) and delusions (Buchanan et al., 1993; Buchanan & Wessely chap. 12; Torrey, chap. 13), and the nature of delusions (Garety, chap. 4); the specificity of poor insight for the diagnosis of schizophrenia (Amador et al., 1994; Wing, Cooper, & Sartorius, 1974; Amador & Kronengold, chap. 4); the relationship of insight with depression (Kiersky, chap. 6) and positive and negative symptoms of schizophrenia (Cuesta & Peralta, 1994; Kemp & Lambert, 1995; Selten, chap. 5); the value of insight as a predictor of outcome (McGlashan, 1981; McEvoy, Appelbaum, Apperson, Geller, & Freter, 1989). Finally, recent work has begun to look at the relationship of insight to cognitive impairment (Young, Davila, & Scher, 1993; McEvoy, Freter, Merritt & Apperson, 1993; Cuesta & Peralta, 1994; Lysaker & Bell (1994; chap. 15) and cerebral ventricular enlargement (Takai, Uematsu, Hirofumi, Sone, & Kaiya, 1992); Some of this data is based on relatively small samples with measures taken at a single point in time.

## The Fractionation of Insight

I have proposed that insight be viewed as three overlapping dimensions, embodied in a brief Schedule for the Assessment of Insight (SAI; David, 1990):

1. The awareness that one is suffering from a mental illness or condition
2. The ability to relabel mental events such as hallucinations and delusions as abnormal
3. Acceptance of the need for treatment

A possible fourth element has been called *hypothetical contradiction* by Brett-Jones, Garety, and Hemsley (1987) and seems to entail a test of perspective taking. Further fractionation is possible: Kemp and David (in press) have suggested that awareness of illness should also encompass awareness of change. It is readily understandable that a person may note a change in him or herself without taking the additional step of illness attribution. Similarly, certain mental events may be relabeled but not others—analogous to the extreme specificity seen in some neurological cases (see Kinsbourne, chap. 9). For example, the patient may recognize memory impairment but not (cortical) blindness, the paradoxical combination first noted by Gabriel Anton at the end of the 19th century (David, Owen, & Forstl, 1993) and extended more recently by Young, De Haan, & Newcombe (1990). The latter studied a woman who, after a stroke, was aware of her rather mild memory loss but not a much more profound facial recognition deficit (see also Barr, chap. 7; Keefe, chap. 8). Finally, acceptance of treatment may include acceptance of *the need for treatment* without actual compliance. There are also instances where behavioral acceptance dissociates from verbalized acceptance, and indeed this verbal-behavior discordance may apply to all of the proposed dimensions of insight.

Although, this fractionation has some face validity and arguments may be advanced in its support, does it (a) have empirical support? and (b) is it of heuristic value?

### Empirical Support

There have been at least three applications of principal components analysis (PCA) to the three dimensions of the insight, and the results are somewhat similar. David, Buchanan, Reed, and Almeida (1992); Peralta and Cuesta (1994); and Aga, Agarwal, & Gupta (1994) found that the different elements of insight all loaded on a single factor. However, all of these studies emphasize the relatively weak correlation with overall psychopathology as rated by scales such as the Brief Psychiatric Rating Scale (BPRS; Overall & Gorham, 1962). David et al. (1992) found a correlation of $r = -.31$ ($n = 91$; $p < .005$) between the Present State Examination (PSE; Wing, et al., 1974) total symptom score and the SAI total score, while Aga et al. (1994), in a study of 59 psychotic inpatients in India, found that the BPRS correlated with the total insight score comparably at $r = .28$, which was not significant after Bonferroni correction. Peralta and Cuesta (1994) used PCA to examine insight and psychopathology using the Scale for the Assessment of Negative Symptoms (SANS; Andreasen, 1984a) and Scale for the Assessment of Positive Symptoms (SAPS; Andreasen, 1984b) and found that while insight produced a factor explaining 19.6% of the variance, negative symptoms, thought disorder, and delusions and hallucinations each loaded on separate factors.

McEvoy, Apperson, et al. (1989) were the first to propose an insight scale (as a single dimension) called the Insight and Treatment Attitudes Questionnaire (ITAQ). In a study of 52 acute or acute-on-chronic schizophrenic patients, they found a variable correspondence between BPRS scores and ITAQ at various time points, including acute admission and follow-up, reaching a maximum of $r = -.35$ ($p = .006$) at 14 days postadmission. Michalakeas et al. (1994) also used the ITAQ to examine insight and psychopathology using the BPRS in 77 patients with schizophrenia and mood disorders. They found that ITAQ and BPRS correlated poorly in the schizophrenic group at various points during the patients' admission, but reached $r = -.4$ ($p < .007$) at discharge. However, the correlations were consistently stronger in the manic group and weaker in the depressives.

Birchwood et al. (1994) adapted the SAI to be used as a self-report measure. Again PCA derived a single factor from the three subscales and found that the scale had the sensitivity to detect change in psychopathology in 31 acute patients undergoing treatment. However, the intercorrelation between components was moderate ($r = .42$ on average). This is in line with data from David et al., (1992), Aga et al., (1994), and Kulhara, Basu, and Chakrabarti (1992). David et al., found that the items intercorrelated at $r$ between 0.51 and 0.26. Kulhara, Basu, et al. (1992) followed 22 inpatients in Chandigarh, India, and calculated correlation coefficients with the BPRS on admission and after one and two weeks as well as intercorrelations among the three dimensions from the SAI. Like David et al., they found that compliance and relabeling showed the weakest, while compliance and illness awareness, the strongest intercorrelation. The relationship with symptom severity, as measured by the BPRS, was significant only after the second week at $r$ between .47 and .26 — again, remarkably similar to David's figures in spite of the different populations under study. Kulhara, Chakrabarti, and Basu (1992) then compared a small group of schizophrenic and affective disorder patients and found that the latter group had better insight.

Amador et al. (1994), in the largest study of its kind to date involving 412 patients with psychotic or severe mood disorders from a variety of centers, used the Scale to Assess Unawareness of Mental Disorder (SUMD) to examine the diagnostic specificity of insight. Unawareness of mental disorder in general, its consequences, and the efficacy of medication, plus six specific symptoms, were inquired about and rated on a 0–3 scale. Overall, the *DSM-III-R* schizophrenic group ($N = 221$) showed the poorest insight even though some 41% of them were aware that they suffered from a mental disorder. Of interest is the proportion of schizophrenic patients who were completely unaware of individual symptoms. This ranged from 28% for asociality to 58% for delusions. Severity of positive symptoms measured by the SAPS (e.g., delusions) correlated with SUMD items with coefficients ranging from .14 to .23 (worse symptoms, less awareness).

*Heuristic Value*

In considering the heuristic value of isolating insight from its nexus within psychopathology and then fractionating insight itself, we are attempting to find a purchase on seemingly intractable philosophical and psychological enigmas. These include the nature of delusions and hallucinations; self-awareness; and self-consciousness in general. If the dissociability of insight components can be established, this opens up various possibilities for understanding and even management. If treatment compliance can be separated—to a degree—from delusions and hallucinations, then it may be possible to improve compliance without having to wait for a panacea to arrive. It is possible that compliance may be a facet of personality and stable across a number of situations, but that it evolves across the individual's life span. Similarly, it could be hypothesized that recognizing that one has an illness is tightly culture bound, and will be aligned with other illness beliefs and models. Hence, this aspect of insight should vary according to culture and perhaps ethnicity (as suggested by Johnson and Orell, in press; see also Perkins & Moodley, 1993a). On the other hand, the neurological analogy with anosognosia may be more applicable to the relabeling of abnormal phenomena and so would be predicted to be relatively hard-wired and universal.

Coming closer to home, diagnostic differences in insight as propounded by Amador et al. (1994) and Amador and Kronengold (chap. 1) may tell us something about the nature of the disorders in question, and schizophrenia in particular. Lack of insight may indeed be a prime symptom of schizophrenia. However, it may be of heuristic interest to pursue the fractionation theme more fully. The relationship between insight and different psychotic symptoms may be studied, with the hope of furthering the understanding of both. For example, an obvious target is hallucinations, although David et al. (1992) found no relation between these in any modality and insight. Fulford (1989; Fulford, chap. 3) has argued that hallucinations are false beliefs about possible perceptions and thus a subset of delusions; Garety and colleagues have concentrated on delusions themselves and have shown that the dimensions of delusional beliefs, such as strength of conviction, preoccupation, and so on, are also dissociable (see Garety & Hemsley, 1987; Kendler, Glazer, & Morgenstern, 1983; Garety, chap. 4).

In the Amador et al. study (1994), hallucinations were regarded as real in 39.5% of schizophrenics (the proportions in the other diagnostic groups were not significantly different). Such awareness did not appear to relate to current or past functioning (as measured by the Global Assessment Scale, GAS; Endicott, Spitzer, & Fleiss, 1976), unlike other positive and negative symptoms. This concurs with data from a recently completed phenomenological survey of 100 psychotic hallucinators (Nayani & David, 1996) with a variety of diagnoses, although most were schizophrenic. They found that the belief that the hallucination "came from outside" did not seem to covary with insight into illness more broadly defined. Insight did not show any association with the ability to control the voices or whether the source of the voice involved a complex delusional framework (plotter, alien beings, etc.), rather than a source involving real people (the subject's mother, doctor, etc.). Insight was, however, positively correlated with the number of coping mechanisms employed by the subject ($r = 0.26$, $p = .001$). Furthermore, the scale devised by Aggernaes (1972) to quantify the reality and sensory characteristics of the hallucination—in a sense, lack of insight or failure to question the belief in the hallucinatory experience—was inversely related to the SAI total insight score, but the association was very weak and thus failed to reach statistical significance. Hence, insight does not appear to be enmeshed in the process whereby perceptions, even those derived from internal cognitive processes such as those underlying, auditory-verbal hallucinations (David, 1994), are apprehended, but occurs in some sense after the fact. Nevertheless, there did seem to be a link between bizarre delusions and lack of awareness of the unreal nature of hallucinations in Amador et al.'s survey.

Insight as currently defined is conceptually related more to positive symptoms—hallucinations, delusions, and productive thought disorder—than to negative or deficit symptoms. Indeed, this accords with lay views of what constitutes mental illness as McEvoy, Schooler, Friedman, Steingard, & Allen (1993) demonstrated by recording judgments of case vignettes. This imbalance is beginning to be redressed (Selten, van den Bosch, & Sijben, chap. 5). Amador et al. (1994) hint that patients with deficit symptoms have poorer insight in general, although the actual awareness of such symptoms was not greatly different and if anything slightly better than their positive counterparts (see chap. 1). Data from a study of late paraphrenia, a condition characterized by florid positive symptomatology, illustrates the positive-negative distinction. Almeida, Howard, Levy, & David (1996) plotted SAPS scores and scores on the High Royds Evaluation of Negativity Scale (HENS; Mortimer, McKenna, Lund, & Mannuzza, 1989) against the SAI total score and found the now expected modest correlation with positive symptoms ($n = 40$; $r = -.48$, $p < .001$). However, HENS scores showed no discernable relationship ($r = -.1$).

The vignette study mentioned above also raised another dissociation, that between self and other perception. Those symptoms that patients rated as indicating mental illness—correctly in the view of the psychiatrists involved—were generally regarded as less applicable to themselves than others (McEvoy, Schooler, et al., 1993). This need not apply just to psychotic symptoms. Social inappropriateness was correctly identified in videotaped role-plays by schizophrenic patients, but they rated their own, at times inappropriate behavior as higher in social appropriateness than judges (Carni & Nevid, 1992). In considering such work, we must not forget that, like many aspects of insight, the perfect self-knowledge that we seem to demand of our patients is an unattainable ideal. To assume that those of us who are not psychotic have the gift to "see ourselves as others see us,"* especially in complex social situations, would be to display a profound lack of insight.

## Against Insight

It is curious to observe the strength of feeling among professionals when the topic of insight is considered. The first of two editorials for *The Lancet* (1990) medical journal belittled academic exploration of the concept, arguing that this was "hifalutin" or pretentious—"academically nourishing but clinically sterile." The attitude put forward was akin to "I know it when I see it," so why bother agonizing over definitions? The second (Joyce, 1993), discarded the cloak of anonymity yet seemed to be in favor of preserving the mystery of insight as though it were somehow poetic and beyond scientific explanation. More cogent criticism came from mental health professionals worried about the judgment of insight, framed by Perkins and Moodley (1993b) as a kind of political coercion of the disenfranchised (the mentally ill) by a politically powerful Eurocentric body, better known as psychiatrists.

---

* Robert Burns, Scots poet (1759–1796)

Ignoring the antipsychiatry rhetoric, these critics do highlight the sociocultural influences on illness beliefs that, as mentioned above, must surely be relevant to insight or elements of it (see Kirmayer & Corin, chap. 10; Kim, chap. 11). Similarly, considering compliance, there may be many reasons, some of them perfectly reasonable — not the least of which are unpleasant side effects why some patients refuse medication. It would be disingenuous to ascribe all of these to a psychopathological symptom we choose to call poor insight. Indeed, the term *treatment compliance*, entomologically reducible to "bending with," is too passive, less attractive than, and perhaps ethically inferior to treatment adherence or "sticking to" (Holm, 1993). However, while Van Putten (1974) drew attention to the adverse influence extrapyramidal side effects (EPS) have on such adherence, he later showed (Van Putten et al., 1976) that, when these were abolished or minimized, some patients continue to refuse medication on account of their denial of illness (or, in some cases, enjoyment of it). It has also been shown that neither EPS (Pan & Tantum, 1989) nor a history of adverse effects (Marder et al., 1983) reliably discriminates between medication compliance and noncompliance in depot clinics and open inpatient units, respectively. Moreover, Marder's group went on to show that the belief that medication was beneficial exerted a strong influence on consent to treatment (see McEvoy, chap. 14) rather than the nature of the experience of medication.

## Insight and Prognosis

In order to convince the skeptic of the clinical importance of insight over and above the other features of psychosis, which may wax and wane with treatment and recovery, it must be shown to be predictive and somewhat enduring. Little is known about what happens to insight, however broadly defined, over time and successive illness episodes, and even less about the dimensions of insight. There is some evidence on compliance (Hoge et al., 1990; Buchanan, 1992) that suggests that patterns of noncompliance repeat themselves in successive relapses of psychosis. McEvoy, Freter, & Merritt, et al. (1993) followed a small group of outpatients and found that initial ITAQ scores in 22 subjects correlated with those one year later at $r = .7$, the mean difference being 0.6 points ($SD = 4.5$). In an earlier study of inpatients, McEvoy, Apperson, and colleagues (1989) found that while psychopathology improves with treatment, insight is slower to change. Some authors have found an inverse association between insight and the number of previous hospitalizations when studied at a single time point. The scenario is of a person who may recover from an illness, yet deny that he or she was ill and refuse or discontinue maintenance therapy and contact with his or her carer, only to relapse and repeat the cycle. However, clinical experience suggests that such a negative cycle need not be inevitable. Some individuals appear to learn from experience and develop insight. When calculating a simple correlation between insight and number of hospitalizations, such individual variation may be obscured (David et al., 1992).

What of overall prognosis? Ever since Emil Kraepelin's attempt to delineate dementia praecox (schizophrenia) from manic depressive insanity at the end of the last century, psychiatrists have looked toward clinical outcome as the most powerful arbiter of validity of any psychopathological construct. Seminal work by Strauss and Carpenter in the mid-1970s (1974) and more recently by Warner (1985) raised a weakness in this method if only illness-related factors were considered, since the premorbid adjustment and the prevailing socioeconomic climate both exert substantial influences on the outcome of psychosis. The extent to which insight into psychosis is determined premorbidly or is intrinsic to the morbid process, or the result of the interface between illness and culture, are all questions for research. As stated, a working hypothesis could be proffered to the effect that illness beliefs are especially malleable by culture; that compliance might be somewhat more of a premorbid characteristic distributed differently among individuals in a population (yet still influenced by learning and experience); and that the ability to relabel psychotic phenomena as symptoms of a disorder is more a cognitive ability vulnerable to disruption by the disorder itself. Since the same array of influences may act differentially upon the presence of delusions, negative symptoms, age of onset, and so on, insight is no more or less worthy of consideration as a prognostic indicator as any other traditional predictor.

## Insight and Compliance

The relationship between treatment compliance and other facets of insight has already been covered in detail (McEvoy, chap. 14). Since treatment with neuroleptic agents undoubtedly confers a better outcome on psychosis, at least in the short and probably medium term, and since insight *has something to do with* compliance (although the two terms are far from synonymous), it follows that insight and prognosis *ought* to be related. Certainly, beliefs about illness and the origin of symptoms, and about the effects of medication on the illness and symptoms, predict medication compliance to a moderate degree (Bartko, Herczeg, & Zador, 1988; Van Putten, 1974; Pan & Tantum, 1989; Lin, Spiga, & Fortsch, 1979; Marder et al., 1983; Adams & Howe, 1993), leaving a stubborn proportion of the variance unexplained. Similarly, educating individuals about illness generally (including the benefits of medication) does increase compliance (Eckman et al., 1992). In our own studies conducted at the Institute of Psychiatry by Roisin Kemp, improvements were seen in attitudes to medication by acute psychotic inpatients, their actual compliance, and insight scores (but not overall psychopathology) after a brief program of compliance therapy based on the principles of motivational interviewing (Miller & Rollnick, 1991). The results were significant in the short term, and seem to hold up at six months posttreatment (Kemp, Hayward, Applewhaite, Everitt, & David, 1996).

It is hard to imagine a modern, naturalistic study of the relationship of insight to prognosis that was not confounded, to some extent, by adherence to medication or other treatments. Historical cohort studies, such as those undertaken by Kraepelin, Bleuler, and Langfeldt in the early 20th century, did not isolate insight as a possible explanatory variable. Poor compliance was clearly not the same source of despair for clinicians then as it is today. This may be because the treatments available were not effective (although many were believed to be so at the time), or perhaps because patients were *submitted* to treatment by their relatives or on the instruction of the psychiatrist, with little regard for their own views. Another reason why insight was not examined as a predictor of outcome may have been because absence of insight was seen as the sine qua non for psychosis (see Berrios & Marková, chap. 2). In his textbook *Dementia Praecox and Paraphrenia* (1919), Kraepelin discussed aspects of what we might term insight under the heading of "judgment": "the faculty of judgement . . . suffers without exception severe injury . . . [in] the judgement of circumstances not hitherto experienced and *in particular of their own state* . . . they not infrequently commit the grossest blunders" (italics added; p. 25).

Later, when discussing course, Kraepelin writes that the initial episode may quickly resolve: "He [the patient] knows time and place and the people round him, remembers all that has happened, even his own nonsensical actions, *admits he is ill . . .*" but, he goes on: "a lack of clear understanding of morbid phenomena as a whole will always be found on more accurate examination" (p. 182).

Later still, Kraepelin discusses the "observation of self" and notes that in patients with dementia praecox, unlike those with manic depressive illness,

> it is only with difficulty that a glance is gained into the occurrences of their inner life, even when the patients are able to give utterance without difficulty to their thoughts, they are taciturn, repellent, evade questions, give indefinite information that tells nothing" (p. 264).

## Insight and Course

Even the classic follow-up studies in the immediate pre- and perineuroleptic era (e.g., Vaillant, 1964; Stephens, Astrup, & Mangrum, 1966) failed to examine the prognostic implications of insight—or if they did, it clearly did not emerge as a significant finding (see Carpenter, Bartko, Strauss, & Hawk, 1978).

Cross-sectional studies are able to show a relationship to current functioning and previous course. Table 17.1 summarizes studies that have done this, using various measures of insight. The first (Roback & Abramowitz, 1979) is atypical, since their concept of insight was more akin to that used in psychoanalysis, which includes viewing symptoms as a reflection of intrapsychic conflicts rather than attributing them to illness. Perhaps this explains why individuals in that study, though rated as better adjusted, felt themselves to be less so and were generally more troubled.

Taylor and Perkins (1991) interviewed 30 residents of a rehabilitation unit for chronic psychiatric disabilities. They were interested in whether denial or exaggeration of mental health problems affected overall functioning and found, to their surprise, that they did not. However, those who denied mental health problems had a longer history of contact with services, but higher self-esteem and less subjective distress. Takai and colleagues (1992) from Gifu, Japan, investigated 57 chronic schizophrenic patients (mean duration of illness, 16 years; age 39). As well as being the first group to show an association between poor insight and cerebral ventricular enlargement using MRI, Takai et al. also demonstrated an association with number of prior hospitalizations ($r = .23$), which remained significant after a multiple regression analysis that controlled for other clinical variables. Work from Australia by O'Connor and Herrman (1993) was aimed primarily at identifying factors related to successful rehabilitation. The SAI was used in 41 schizophrenic patients, and the 21 with low insight scores ($< 9$) spent more than six months in the program, and 8 of them spent more than two years. Other factors, such as cognitive impairment and negative symptoms, were particularly influential. Amador et al., (1993) showed that the number of previous admissions was associated with current awareness of mental disorder and acknowledgment of the possibility of future illness.

TABLE 17.1    Studies Examining the Relationship Between Insight and Clinical Progress

| Authors (Year) | Subjects | Clinical Progress Cross-Sectional Associations |
|---|---|---|
| Roback & Abramowitz (1979) | 24—all but 4 were Sz | Psychological mindedness associated with better adjustment |
| McEvoy, Freter et al. (1989) | 24 *DSM-III* Sz | ITAQ lower scores and involuntary admission |
| Taylor & Perkins (1991) | 30 (90% Sz) | Denial related to longer contact with service but less distress |
| David et al. (1992) | 91 *DSM-III-R* | SAI no correlation with No of hospitalization ($r = .04$); poorer insight with involuntary admission |
| Takai et al. (1992) | 57 *DSM-III-R* chronic Sz | SAI inverse correlation with No of hospitalization ($r = -.23$) |
| Amador et al. (1993) | *DSM-III-R* Sz | SUMD correlated with No of previous hospitalization ($r = .3$) |
| O'Connor & Herrman (1993) | 41 *DSM-III-R* residual Sz | SAI related to length of time in rehabilitation program |
| Peralta & Cuesta (1994) | 115 *DSM-III-R* inpatients | Unawareness of illness or symptoms and more hospitalizations (not treatment refusal) |
| Amador et al. (1994) | 412 *DSM-III-R* psychotic patients | SUMD correlated with current GAS (range $-.13-.32$); and GAS over past year (range $-.15-.26$) |

McEvoy, Appelbaum, et al.'s 1989 study will be discussed further below; regarding current functioning, they showed that 12 patients who required involuntary commitment had significantly lower ITAQ scores than the remainder. Interestingly, a survey of psychiatric admissions to an English county in the 1930s and 1940s analyzed by Shepherd (1957) showed that approximately 50% of patients who were "certified"—that is, involuntary admissions—failed to recover and leave hospital over a five-year period compared to just under 20% of those admitted voluntarily. There may be an element of self-fulfilling prophecy here, in that the act of certification may have determined the length of admission. However, the finding is also understandable in terms of a subgroup of patients lacking in insight having a poorer prognosis.

Peralta and Cuesta (1994) from Spain surveyed 115 inpatients and showed that, while awareness of illness and symptoms did not correlate significantly with global functioning or refusal of treatment, these insight parameters did correlate with the number of previous hospitalizations ($r = -.23$ and $-.3$, respectively). Amador et al. (1994) found modest negative correlations between most items of the SUMD and the GAS, for current functioning, and GAS estimated for the preceding year, in their survey of around 400 patients.

These studies shed light on the relevance of insight to the course of illness, but have tended to concentrate on chronic cases, whose course and outcome are by definition poor, and did so at a single point in time. Table 17.2 summarizes studies that have attempted a more prospective design. Soskis and Bowers (1969) must be credited with one of the first of these. Their patients were assessed three to seven years after discharge, and it was found that those who viewed their illness as a personal experience to be

TABLE 17.2    Prospective Studies Examining the Relationship Between Insight and Clinical Outcome

| Authors (Year) | Subjects | Follow-up (yrs) | Relationship Between Insight and Clinical Outcome |
| --- | --- | --- | --- |
| Soskis & Bowers (1969) | 32 'Sz' center had psycho-therapeutic orientation | 3–7 | Posthospital adjustment if illness seen as learning experience (not No. of admissions) |
| McGlashan et al. (1981) | 30 *DSM-II* Sz | 1 | Soskis & Bowers scale predicted quality of work and less time in hospital |
| Heinrichs et al. (1985) | 38 RDC criteria Sz or Sz-affective | Variable—index adm to next adm | 24 with "early insight on their first relapse"; 2 required readmission; 7 of the remaining 14 readmitted |
| McEvoy, Appelbaum et al. (1989) | 52 *DSM-III* Sz | 2.5–3.5 | Readmission sign associated with ITAQ; trend to predict compliance at 30 days post discharge |
| Buchanan (1992) | 61 RDC Sz | 1 & 2 | 'Do you think you have been unwell/become ill again?' Not assoc with compliance. Previous compliance predicted future compliance at 1 year |
| McEvoy, Freter et al. (1993) | 24 *DSM-III* Sz or Sz-aff outpatients | 1 | ITAQ did not predict exacerbation; 3 readmitted patients had lower initial insight |
| Van Os et al. (1996) | 166 RDC psychotics | 4 (mean) | Duration of hospitalization during follow-up and independent living |
| David et al. (1995) | 150 RDC psychotics (subset of van Os) | 4 (mean) | PSE insight predictive of subsequent insight and attitudes to treatment |

learned from and integrated had better posthospital adjustment. It is possible that these patients would not meet modern criteria for schizophrenia. McGlashan (1981) used methods devised by Soskis and Bowers (1969) to study the effects of attitudes toward recent illness on recovery, and found that a realistic attitude regarding past illness correlated with more desirable employment and social outcomes after one year.

Heinrichs, Cohen, and Carpenter (1985) had the case records of 38 current outpatients rated, blind to course. Some 24 were regarded as having had early insight on their first relapse, and of these, only 2 required readmission subsequently, compared to 7 of the remaining 14. The study was only quasi-prospective, and there was no adjustment for person-years of follow-up. The findings were not explained by medication compliance or severity of illness. The same methodological weaknesses apply to Van Putten et al.'s 1976 study. They were especially interested in medication refusal. Seven cases who were later characterized as persistent refusers (out of 29) had insight as determined by a simple definition (similar to the PSE) rated on admission, while 18 out of 30 compliers were insightful. A truly prospective study was undertaken by Buchanan (1992) on 61 patients from the Maudsley Hospital. Insight was judged on the basis of a number of questions, particularly, Do you think you have been unwell during this admission? and, Do you think you will become ill again?. He found that the answers did not predict later compliance after one or two years, whereas more directly assessed beliefs in treatment efficacy and an optimistic outlook (e.g., faith in chances of recovery) were predictive, at least after one year.

McEvoy, Freter, Everett, et al. (1989) followed 52 schizophrenic patients having rated them on the ITAQ. The authors demonstrated the predictive validity of the measure for rehospitalization (61% were admitted again at least once) as well as compliance. However, they emphasize the importance of other mediating factors, particularly the quality of the aftercare environment. A more recent study by McEvoy, Freter, Merritt, et al. (1993) recruited 24 stable outpatients from the Western Psychiatric Institute and Clinic, Pittsburgh. Eleven had exacerbations over a one-year follow-up period, but initial insight scores, BPRS ratings, and psychometric testing results did not differ between this group and the remainder. There is a hint that the 3 patients who required readmission were less insightful on the ITAQ measure. The small numbers involved preclude firm conclusions on this issue.

## Recent Work

In order to examine predictors of outcome in the functional psychoses, van Os et al. (1996) assembled a large, representative cohort of recent-onset, mixed psychotic patients. In this study, 337 consecutive admissions to two South London hospitals were assessed. Those that had at least one psychotic symptom, according to the Research Diagnostic Criteria (RDC; Spitzer, Endicott, & Robins, 1978), occurring in clear consciousness and an onset of illness within five years of index assessment were extensively investigated ($N = 191$) and followed up after four years (mean length of follow-up, 47 months, $SD = 14$). Data were available on 166 cases (83%).

The authors carried out a factor analysis on the major categories of symptoms derived from the PSE. This revealed seven psychopathological dimensions that corresponded broadly to subsyndromes of acute and chronic schizophrenic illness, mania, depressive psychosis, and delusional states, and explained 63% of the variance. A further factor was lack of insight, based on the PSE interviews, and explained 8% of the total variance. Here, the insight item (no. 104) into psychotic symptoms is measured on a single dimension. Probe questions include, Do you think there is anything the matter with you? and responses are scored 0–3:

    0 = "Full insight . . . able to appreciated the issues involved"
    1 = "As much insight into the nature of the condition as social background and intelligence allow"
    2 = "Agrees to nervous condition but . . . does not really accept the explanation in terms of nervous illness (e.g., gives delusional explanation):
    3 = "Denies nervous condition entirely"

A variety of clinical and social outcome measures were obtained on the cohort. They included the Global Assessment of Functioning-symptomatology (GAF-s; Jablensky et al., 1992), derived from the Global Assessment Scale; World Health Organization Disability Assessment Schedule (DAS; Jablensky, Schwartz, & Tomov, 1980); Iager Negative Symptom Rating Scale (Iager, Kirch, & Wyatt, 1985). To assess the course of illness and associated disabilities longitudinally, a modified version of the Life Chart instrument from the Multi-Center Study on the Course and Outcome of Schizophrenia

(WHO, 1992) was used. This charts the proportion of the follow-up period spent unemployed, in hospital, in prison, or without accommodation.

Using logistic regression techniques, van Os and colleagues (1996) found that initial lack of insight was predictive of the time spent in hospital and living independently over the follow-up period of four years on average, and this effect was independent of *DSM-III-R* diagnosis, sociodemographic factors and other prognostic indicators.

Further analysis of this data set has been undertaken to explore the correlates and associations of insight (David et al., 1995) on the 150 cases who had full data sets including insight measures. This has been made possible by the generous cooperation of the organizers of the Camberwell Collaborative Functional Psychosis Study (see acknowledgments). The comprehensiveness of the current evaluation permitted study of the relationships between insight and diagnostic, sociodemographic, and neuropsychological variables.

The observation frames with respect to insight were: (1) at recruitment of the cohort, *first within-episode comparison*; and (2) follow-up of cohort (those cases who were psychotic, $n = 94$) after four years and included a more detailed assessment of insight, *second within-episode comparison*. Of interest in the current context is the prediction of outcome measures four years later, from insight measured at initial assessment, *longitudinal comparison*. The results are described in more detail in David et al., (1995).

Of the 150 follow-up subjects, 53 (35%) were female; mean age at baseline assessment was 26.4 years (range 16–50; $SD = 6.5$). Regarding diagnoses at baseline assessment, 81 subjects (54%) had a *DSM-III-R* diagnosis of schizophrenia or schizophreniform disorder; 38 (25%) of affective psychosis; 12 (8%) of schizoaffective psychosis; and 19 (13%) of delusional disorder or unspecified functional psychosis. The mean duration of illness prior to baseline assessment was 2.2 years ($SD = 2.0$). Ninety-four (63%) of the 150 subjects with a valid PSE insight rating at index assessment had a second within-episode insight score. The remainder were in remission, so attracting a "not applicable" rating for the item.

### Within-Episode Comparisons

There were no differences in insight score between males and females, *DSM-III-R* schizophrenics versus other psychotics, or whites versus nonwhites (mostly British and Caribbean-born Afro-Caribbeans) at either time point (ethnicity has been found to influence treatment compliance in the U.K.; Sellwood & Tarrier, 1994). Nor were there any differences in age or illness duration between individuals with different scores on the PSE insight item, at either index or follow-up assessment. However, individuals from socioeconomic classes 1 and 2 showed significantly better insight ($p = .01$). Obstetric complications, premorbid adjustment, age of onset, and cerebral atrophy as measured from CT scans did not correlate with insight. However, verbal IQ and, curiously, left-handedness, were related at both assessments (more so initially).

Verbal IQ—assessed using the National Adult Reading Test (NART; Nelson, 1982) and vocabulary subtest of the Wechsler Adult Intelligence Scale (1955)—was assumed to give an estimate of premorbid IQ. In this study it was those with "perfect" insight

TABLE 17.3 Correlation Matrix (Pearson's *r*) Between Measures of PSE Insight Scores at Index and Follow-up, and Scores on the Schedule for the Assessment of Insight (SAI) and Attitudes to Treatment Measured at Follow-up

| | Follow-up Insight Score (PSE 104) | Compliance | Illness Recognition | Relabeling Psychosis | Total SAI Score | Hospital Helpful | Medication Helpful | Day Care Helpful |
|---|---|---|---|---|---|---|---|---|
| Initial Insight Score (PSE 104) | .23* | −.21* | −.22* | −.14 | −.26** | −.21* | −.21* | .09 |
| Follow-up Insight Score (PSE104) | — | −.68*** | −.71*** | −.76*** | −.85*** | −.45*** | −.42*** | −.71*** |
| Hospital # | — | .53*** | .46*** | .28** | .54*** | — | .59*** | .36* |
| Medication | — | .56*** | .57*** | .33** | .61*** | — | — | .39* |
| Day Care # | — | .44** | .58*** | .36* | .59*** | — | — | — |

\# Measures only recorded in patients who had experience in these treatment settings; maximum number of subjects = 94.

*p < .05
**p < .01
***p < .001

TABLE 17.4   The Stability of Insight in 26 Psychotic Subjects Who Were Inpatients on Two Occasions Separated by a Mean of 4 Years

|  | PSE Insight after 4 years (Time 2) | | | | |
|---|---|---|---|---|---|
| PSE Insight @ Index Assessment (Time 1) | Full | Limited | Partial | Nil | Total |
| Full | 1 | – | – | – | 1 |
| Limited | 1 | – | – | 1 | 2 |
| Partial | – | 4 | 4 | 4 | 12 |
| Nil | – | 3 | 4 | 4 | 11 |
| Total | 2 | 7 | 8 | 9 | 26 |

$\chi^2 = 20.1$, $(df = 9)$; $p = .02$

who differed from the remainder in scoring in the above-average range in IQ, while the others with less insight to no insight did not show differences. This may be interpreted as showing that poor insight is not so much a cognitive deficit in psychosis, where it tends to be the norm, but instead, that preserved insight may be thought of as a somewhat rarer cognitive skill. Finally, multiple regression analysis indicated that the social class effect is largely accounted for by IQ (see David et al., 1995, for details).

### Longitudinal Comparison

Insight at index assessment was moderately, but significantly, correlated with insight at follow-up (see table 17.3: Pearson's $r = 0.23$, $p = .039$). There were also significant correlations between PSE insight at follow-up and each dimension of insight from the SAI (David, 1990) and the total score, weighted to take into account patients who may not have been on medication or who were not hallucinated/deluded at their second within episode assessment ($r = 0.26$, $p = 0.004$). Also at follow-up, insight measures from this schedule correlated strongly with whether hospital treatment, day care, and medication were regarded as helpful. Not surprisingly, insight measured by the SAI and PSE correlated very highly ($r = -.85$).

The mean PSE total scores were slightly higher at index (21.9; $SD = 12.5$) than at follow-up assessment (18.2; $SD = 11.4$). At neither time point did these measures correlate with insight scores significantly.

Twenty-six subjects who were psychotic at the time of the second assessment were hospital inpatients. Their mean PSE insight score was 2.27 ($SD = 0.78$) on the first occasion and 1.92 ($SD = 0.98$) on the second, a trend toward improvement; the two scores were moderately correlated ($r = 0.344$, $p = .085$: see table 17.4).

### Conclusions

The work described above adds further weight to the contention that insight encompasses a distinct aspect of psychosis and is clinically important. This is supported by the cross-sectional analyses, which show that rating on a simple index of insight is independent of many basic clinical and demographic variables, such as precise diagnosis, gender, ethnicity, and global severity of psychopathology, at least in this population (see also McGlashan 1981; McEvoy, Apperson, et al., 1989; David, et al., 1992). Hence, insight may be justifiably regarded as a separate aspect of the mental state across persons of different ages and cultures. Intelligence (and socioeconomic status during upbringing) were related, with above-average intelligence and higher social class being associated with full insight despite the presence of psychosis. Multiple regression revealed that the effect of IQ remained after controlling for social class and ethnicity, suggesting that educational opportunity may be less important than basic intelligence in this regard.

We have reviewed the clinical relevance of the insight concept. Insight relates to familiar outcome variables, treatment compliance, and voluntary versus involuntary commitment to hospital. This information needs to be bolstered by more prospective studies and is a relatively new addition to the psychiatric credo. Early work on outcome failed to recognize insight as a possible predictor, although reanalysis of the classical work since Kraepelin by historical scholars may yet reveal important nuggets of information, concealed beneath the arcane technical jargon of the time or disguised within other constructs. In the study described above, a crude index of insight demonstrated predictive validity, in that it was significantly related to certain socially and clinically relevant outcome measures, such as living independently and gainful employment. Again, the novelty of this finding may reside in the sophistication of the techniques employed by van Os and colleagues (1996), in that the independent effects of insight could be examined on a number of outcome measures. It would be wrong to overemphasize the prognostic implications of insight, since it is only one factor among many.

Concurrent validity is provided by the high correlation between the simple PSE insight measure and a fuller schedule for insight assessment. This replicates the study by David et al. (1992) on a different sample. Scores on the schedule were, in turn, consistent with other items dealing with perceived helpfulness of treatment. There are now many insight-assessment instruments to assist (and confuse) researchers (see Amador and Kronengold, chap. 1). The time is ripe for a systematic comparison of all of these. I would favor those instruments that enable the components of insight to be scored separately.

There are few reports that enable firm conclusions to be drawn on the stability of insight across illness episodes. In our study, the correlation between the PSE insight item at index and follow-up, though significantly positive, was weak. In fact, only one subject had perfect insight and only 7 had no insight on both occasions out of a possible 84 subjects who were psychotic and hence rated each time. However, the circumstances of the two ratings were rather different, with the first within-episode assessment based entirely on patients recently admitted to hospital. The simple measure of insight used longitudinally, insofar as it influences compliance, is bound to have an effect on the outcome of psychosis. Nevertheless, poor insight on first or early presentation appears to affect outcome regardless of whether subsequent relapses show the same degree of illness awareness and recognition. This could be taken to imply that remediation that targets poor insight early on in the course of a patient's illness may have a beneficial effect on prognosis. This may act by improving early warning systems in patients and their confidants (Heinrichs et al., 1985). The utility of early intervention in preventing or minimizing relapse is now well established (Birchwood, 1992).

## Final Remarks

Aubrey Lewis ended his 1934 essay on insight with the words: "I should be the last to suggest for these views finality or completeness." I am sure all contributors to this volume would echo that sentiment. However, some things have changed in the 60 or so intervening years. Insight is now firmly anchored on the psychiatric map. The notion of insight in psychotherapy (Reid & Finesinger, 1952)—that is, an understanding of unconscious processes and motivations relevant to current behaviour and relationships—and that of self-deception (McLaughlin & Rorty, 1988) are different matters. These, too, seem ripe for empirical investigation, but will require even greater philosophical hurdles to be overcome than is the case for insight into psychosis. Other conditions on the borders of psychosis, such as anorexia nervosa, seem amenable to study using a framework similar to that described in this chapter (Greenfield, Anyon, Hobart, Quinlan, & Plantes, 1991). Neuropsychiatric disorders such as Alzheimer's disease provide an important testing ground for theories relating to the biological and psychosocial underpinnings for aspects of insight. Awareness of cognitive decline, functional capacity, depression, and even psychotic symptoms may show dissociations within a single individual (Vasterling, Seltzer, Foss, & Vanderbrook, 1995; Mullen, Howard, David, & Levy, 1996).

The concept of insight provides a different vantage point from which the enduring questions of psychosis can be tackled. Such questions include the nature of sanity and madness, the social and cultural considerations of illness, the ethics of treatment; the interface between the individual and the illness, the brain, and the mind. All questions desperately seek insight.

*Acknowledgments*    The recent data reported here are taken from (David et al., 1995) and were collected as part of the Camberwell Functional Psychosis Study, which was supported by grants from the Mental Health Foundation to Professors R. Murray, S. Lewis, and Drs. P. Bebbington and B. Toone. I acknowledge the work of Jim van Os, Peter Jones, Tom Fahy, Alice Forster, and Ian Harvey, who collected and helped analyze the data. I would also like to thank Roisin Kemp, Peter Hayward, Alec Buchanan, Osvaldo Almeida, Tony Nayani, Sonja Johnson, Rob Howard, Marta Amador, Mary Phillips, the many contributors to this book, and finally Xavier Amador for their inspiration and ideas, which I have cynically appropriated and called my own.

*References*

Adams, S. G., & Howe, J. T. (1993). Predicting medication compliance in a psychotic population. *Journal of Nervous and Mental Disease, 181,* 558–560.

Aga, V. M., Agarwal, A. K., & Gupta, S. C. (1994). The relationship of insight to psychopathology in schizophrenia: A cross sectional study. Submitted for publication.

Aggernaes, A. (1972). The experienced reality of hallucinations and other psychological phenomena. *Acta Psychiatrica Scandinavica, 48,* 220–238.

Almeida, O., Howard, R., Levy, R., & David, A. (1996). Insight and paranoid disorders of late life (late paraphrenia). *International Journal of Geriatric Psychiatry, 11,* .

Amador, X. F., Flaum, M., Andreasen, N. C., Strauss, D. H., Yale, S. A., Clark, S. C., & Gorman, J. M. (1994). Awareness of illness in schizophrenia and schizoaffective mood disorders. *Archives of General Psychiatry, 51,* 826–836.

Amador, X. F., Strauss, D. H., Yale, S. A., Flaum, M. M., Endicott, J., & Gorman, J. M. (1993). Assessment of insight in psychosis. *American Journal of Psychiatry, 150,* 873–879.

Amador, X. F., Strauss, D. H., Yale, S. A., & Gorman, J. M. (1991). Awareness of illness in schizophrenia. *Schizophrenia Bulletin, 17,* 113–132.

Andreasen, N. C. (1984a). *Scale for the Assessment of Negative Symptoms (SANS).* Iowa City: University of Iowa.

Andreasen, N. C. (1984b). *Scale for the Assessment of Positive Symptoms (SAPS).* Iowa City: University of Iowa.

Anonymous. (1990). Real insight. Editorial. *Lancet, 336,* 408–409.

Bartko, G., Herczeg, I., & Zador, G. (1988). Clinical symptomatology and drug compliance in schizophrenic patients. *Acta Psychiatrica Scandinavica, 77,* 74–76.

Birchwood, M. (1992). Early intervention in schizophrenia: theoretical background and clinical strategies. *British Journal of Clinical Psychology, 31,* 257–278.

Birchwood, M., Smith, J., Drury, V., Healy, J., MacMillan, F., & Slade, M. A. (1994). A self-report insight scale for psychosis: reliability, validity and sensitivity to change. *Acta Psychiatrica Scandinavica, 89,* 62–67.

Brett-Jones, J. R., Garety, P., & Hemsley, D. (1927). Measuring delusional experiences: A method and its application. *British Journal of Clinical Psychology, 26,* 256–257.

Buchanan, A. (1992). A two-year prospective study of treatment compliance in patients with schizophrenia. *Psychological Medicine, 22,* 787–797.

Buchanan, A., Reed, A., Wessely, S., Garety, P., Taylor, P., Grubin, D., & Dunn, G. (1993). Acting on delusions II. The phenomenological correlates of acting on delusions. *British Journal of Psychiatry, 163,* 77–81.

Carni, M. A., & Nevid, J. S. (1992). Social appropriateness and impaired perspective in schizophrenia. *Journal of Clinical Psychology, 48,* 170–177.

Carpenter, W., Bartko, J., Strauss, J., & Hawk, A. (1978). Signs and symptoms as predictors of outcome: A report for the international pilot study of schizophrenia. *American Journal of Psychiatry, 135,* 940–945.

Cuesta, M. J., & Peralta, V. (1994). Lack of insight in schizophrenia. *Schizophrenia Bulletin, 20,* 359–366.

David, A. S. (1990). Insight and psychosis. *British Journal of Psychiatry, 156,* 798–808.

David, A. S. (1994). The neuropsychological origins of auditory hallucinations. In *The neuropsychology of schizophrenia.* Ed. A. S. David & J. C. Cutting, pp. 269–313. Hove, East Sussex: Erlbaum.

David, A., Buchanon, A., Reed, A., & Almeida, O. (1992). The assessment of insight. *British Journal of Psychiatry, 161,* 599–602.

David, A. S., Owen, A. M., & Forstl, H. (1993). An annnotated summary and translation of "On self-awareness of focal brain diseases by the patient in cortical blindness and cortical deafness" by Gabriel Anton. *Cognitive Neuropsychology, 10,* 263–272.

David, A., Van Os, J., Jones, P., Harvey, I., Forster, A., & Fahy, T. (1995). Insight and psychotic illness: Cross-sectional and longitudinal associations. *British Journal of Psychiatry, 167,* 621–628.

Eckman, T. A., Wirshing, W. C., Marder, S. R., Liberman, R. P., Johnston-Cronk, K., Zimmermann, K., & Mintz, J. (1992). Technique for training schizophrenia patients in illness self-management: A controlled trial. *American Journal of Psychiatry, 149,* 1549–1555.

Endicott, J., Spitzer, R. L., & Fleiss, J. (1976). The Global Assessment Scale. *Archives of General Psychiatry, 33,* 776–771.

Fulford, K. W. M. (1989). *Moral theory and medical practice.* Cambridge: Cambridge University Press.

Garety, P., & Hemsley, D. R. (1987). Characteristics of delusional experience. *European Archives of Psychiatry and Neurological Sciences, 236,* 294–298.

Ghaemi, S. N., & Pope, H. G. (1994). Lack of insight in psychotic and affective disorders: A review of empirical studies. *Harvard Review of Psychiatry, 2,* 22–33.

Greenfield, D. G., Anyon, W. R., Hobart, M., Quinlan, D., & Plantes, M. (1991). Insight into illness and outcome in anorexia nervosa. *Internal Journal of Eating Disorders, 10,* 101–109.

Heinrichs, D. W., Cohen, B. P., & Carpenter, W. T. (1985). Early insight and the management of schizophrenia decompensation. *Journal of Nervous and Mental Disease, 173,* 133–138.

Hoge, S. K., Applebaum, P. S., Lawlor, T., Beck, J. C., Litman, R., Greer, A., Gutheil, T. G., & Kaplan, E. (1990). A prospective, multicenter study of patients' refusal of antipsychotic medication. *Archives of General Psychiatry, 47,* 949–956.

Holm, S. (1993). What is wrong with compliance? *Journal of Medical Ethics, 19,* 108–109.

Iager, A. C., Kirch, D. G., & Wyatt, R. J. (1985). A negative symptom rating scale. *Psychiatry Research, 16,* 27–36.

Jablensky, A., Schwartz, R., & Tomov, T. (1980). WHO collaborative study of impairments and disabilities associated with schizophrenic disorders. A preliminary communication. Objective and methods. *Acta Psychiatrica Scandinavica, 285* (suppl.), 152–163.

Jablensky, A., Sartorius, N., Ernberg, G., Anker, M., Cooper, J. E., Day, R., & Bertelsen, A. (1992). Schizophrenia: manifestations, incidence and cause in different cultures. *Psychological Medicine* (Monograph Suppl.), *20,* 1–97.

Johnson, S., & Orrell, M. (in press). Insight and psychosis: a social perspective. *Psychological Medicine.*

Joyce, C. R. B. (1993). Insight. *Lancet, 341,* 213–214.

Kemp, R., & David, A. (1997). Insight and compliance. In: B. Blackwell (Ed.), *Treatment Compliance and the Therapeutic Alliance,* pp. 61–84. Gordon and Breach Publishing Group: Newark NJ.

Kemp, R., Hayward, P., Applewhaite, G., Everitt, B., & David, A. (1996). Compliance therapy in psychotic patients: A randomised controlled trial. *British Medical Journal, 312,* 345–349.

Kemp, R. A., & Lambert, T. J. (1995), Insight in schizophrenia and its relationship to psychopathology. *Schizophrenia Research, 18,* 21–28.

Kendler, K. S., Glazer, W. M., & Morgenstern, H. (1983). Dimensions of delusional experience. *American Journal of Psychiatry, 140,* 466–469.

Kraepelin, E. (1919). *Dementia praecox and paraphrenia* (R. M. Barclay, Trans.). Edinburgh: E & S Livingston.

Kulhara, P., Basu, D., & Chakrabarti, S. (1992). Insight and psychosis: II. A pilot study comparing schizophrenia in affective disorder. *Indian Journal of Social Psychiatry, 8,* 45–48.

Kulhara, P., Chakrabarti, S., & Basu, D. (1992). Insight and psychosis: I. An empirical inquiry. *Indian Journal of Social Psychiatry, 8,* 40–44.

Lewis, A. (1934). The psychopathology of insight. *British Journal of Medical Psychology, 14,* 332–348.

Lin, I. F., Spiga, R., & Fortsch, W. (1979). Insight and adherence to medication in chronic schizophrenics. *Journal of Clinical Psychiatry, 40,* 430–432.

Lysaker, P., Bell, M., Milstein, R., Bryson, G., & Beam Goulet, J. (1994). Insight and psychosocial treatment compliance in schizophrenia. *Psychiatry, 57,* 307–315.

Marder, S. R., Mebane, A., Chien, C-P., Winslade, W. J., Swann, E., & Van Putten, T. (1983). A comparison of patients who refuse and consent to neuroleptic treatment. *American Journal of Psychiatry, 140,* 470–472.

Marková, I. S., & Berrios, G. E. (1992). The meaning of insight in clinical psychiatry. *British Journal of Psychiatry, 160,* 850–860.

McEvoy, J. P., Apperson, L. J., Appelbaum, P. S., Ortlip, P., Brecosky, J., Hammill, K., Geller,

J. L., & Roth, L. 1989. Insight into schizophrenia. Its relationship to acute psychopathology. *Journal of Nervous and Mental Disease, 177*, 43–47.

McEvoy, J. P., Appelbaum, P. S., Apperson, L. J., Geller, J. L., & Freter, S. (1989). Why must some schizophrenic patients be involuntarily committed? The role of insight. *Comprehensive Psychiatry, 30*, 13–17.

McEvoy, J., Freter, S., Everett, G., Geller, J., Appelbaum, P. S., Apperson, J., & Roth, L. (1989). Insight and the clinical outcome of schizophrenic patients. *Journal of Nervous and Mental Disease, 177*, 48–51.

McEvoy, J. P., Freter, S., Merritt, M., & Apperson, L. J. (1993). Insight about psychosis among outpatients with schizophrenia. *Hospital and Community Psychiatry, 44*, 883–884.

McEvoy, J. P., Schooler, N. J., Friedman, E., Steingard, S., & Allen, M. (1993). Use of psychopathology vignettes by patients with schizophrenia or schizoaffective disorder and by mental health professionals to judge patients' insight. *American Journal of Psychiatry, 150*, 1649–1653.

McGlashan, T. (1981). Does attitude toward psychosis relate to outcome? *American Journal of Psychiatry, 138*, 797–801.

McLaughlin, B. P., & Rorty, A. O. (1988). *Perspectives on self-deception.* Berkeley: University of California Press.

Michalakeas, A., Skoutas, C., Charalambous, A., Peristeris, A., Marinos, V., Keramari, E., & Theologou, A. (1994). Insight in schizophrenia and mood disorders and its relation to psychopathology. *Acta Psychiatrica Scandinavica, 90*, 46–49.

Miller, W. R., & Rollnick, S. (1991). *Motivational interviewing: Preparing people to change.* New York: Guilford Press.

Mortimer, A. M., McKenna, P. J., Lund, C. E., & Mannuzza, S. (1989). Rating of negative symptoms using the High Royds Evaluation of Negativity (HEN) scale. *British Journal of Psychiatry, 155* (suppl. 7), 89–91.

Mullen, R., Howard, R., David, A., & Levy, R. (1996). Insight in Alzheimer's disease. *International Journal of Geriatric Psychiatry, 11*, 645–651.

Nayani, T., & David, A. (1996). The auditory hallucination: A phenomenological survey. *Psychological Medicine, 26*, 29–38.

Nelson, H. E. (1982). *National Adult Reading Test (NART):* Test manual. Windsor: NFER-Nelson.

O'Connor, R., & Herrman, H. (1993). Assessment of contributions to disability in people with schizophrenia during rehabilitation. *Australian and New Zealand Journal of Psychiatry, 27*, 595–600.

Overall, J. E., & Gorham, D. R. (1962). The brief psychiatric rating scale. *Psychological Reports, 10*, 799–812.

Pan, P-C., & Tantum, D. (1989). Clinical characteristics, health beliefs and compliance with maintenance treatment: A comparison between regular and irregular attenders at a depot clinic. *Acta Psychiatrica Scandinavica, 79*, 564–570.

Peralta, V., & Cuesta, M. J. (1994). Lack of insight: Its status within schizophrenic psychopathology. *Biological Psychiatry, 36*, 559–561.

Perkins, R. E., & Moodley, P. (1993a). Perception of problems in psychiatric inpatients: Denial, race and service usage. *Social Psychiatry and Psychiatry Epidemiology, 28*, 189–193.

Perkins, R., & Moodley, P. (1993b). The arrogance of insight. *Psychiatric Bulletin, 17*, 233–234.

Reid, J. R., & Finesinger, J. E. (1952). The role of insight in psychotherapy. *American Journal of Psychiatry, 108*, 726–734.

Roback, H. B., & Abramowitz, S. I. (1979). Insight and hospital adjustment. *Canadian Journal of Psychiatry, 24*, 233–236.

Rogers, R., Gillis, J. R., Turner, R. E., & Frise-Smith, T. (1990). The clinical presentation of command hallucinations in a forensic population. *American Journal of Psychiatry, 147,* 1304–1307.

Sellwood, W., & Tarrier, N. (1994). Demographic factors associated with extreme non-compliance in schizophrenia. *Social Psychiatry and Psychiatric Epidemiology, 29,* 172–177.

Shepherd, M. (1957). A study of the major psychoses in an English county. *Maudsley Monographs, No. 3.* London: Chapman & Hall.

Soskis, D., & Bowers, M. (1969). The schizophrenic experience: A follow-up study of attitude and post-hospital adjustment. *Journal of Nervous and Mental Disease, 149,* 443–449.

Spitzer, R., Endicott, J., & Robins, E. (1978). Research diagnostic criteria: rationale and reliability. *Archives of General Psychiatry, 35,* 773–782.

Stephens, J. H., Astrup, C., & Mangrum, J. C. (1966). Prognostic factors in recovered and deteriorated schizophrenics. *American Journal of Psychiatry, 122,* 1116–1121.

Strauss, J., & Carpenter, W. (1974). The prediciton of outcome in schizophrenia. *Archives of General Psychiatry, 31,* 37–42.

Takai, A., Uematsu, M., Hirofumi, U., Sone, K., & Kaiya, H. (1992). Insight and its related factors in chronic schizophrenic patients: A preliminary study. *European Journal of Psychiatry, 6,* 159–170.

Taylor, K. E., & Perkins, R. E. (1991). Identity and coping with mental illness in long-stay psychiatric rehabilitation. *British Journal of Clinical Psychology, 30,* 73–85.

Vaillant, G. E. (1964). Prospective prediction of schizophrenic remission. *Archives of General Psychiatry, 11,* 509–518.

van Os, J., Fahy, T., Jones, P., Harvey, I., Sham, P., Lewis, S., Toone, B., Williams, M., & Murray, R. (1996). Psychopathological syndromes in the functional psychoses: associations with course and outcome. *Psychological Medicine, 26,* 161–176.

Van Putten, T. (1974). Why do schizophrenic patients refuse to take their medication? *Archives of General Psychiatry, 31,* 67–72.

Van Putten, T., Crumpton, E., & Yale, C. (1976). Drug refusal in schizophrenia and the wish to be crazy. *Archives of General Psychiatry, 33,* 1443–1446.

Vasterling, J. J., Seltzer, B., Foss, J. W., & Vanderbrook, V. (1995). Unawareness of deficit in Alzheimer's disease. *Neuropsychiatry, Neuropsychology and Behavioral Neurology, 8,* 26–32.

Warner, R. (1985) *Recovery from schizophrenia: Psychiatry and the political economy.* London: Routledge & Kegan Paul.

Wechsler, D. (1955). *Wechsler Adult Intelligence Scale: Manual.* New York: Psychological Corporation.

Wing, J. K., Cooper, J. E., & Sartorius, N. (1974). *The measurement and classification of psychiatric symptoms.* Cambridge: Cambridge University Press.

Young, A. W., De Haan, E. H. F., & Newcombe, F. (1990). Unawareness of impaired face recognition. *Brain and Cognition, 14,* 1–18.

Young, D. A., Davila, R., & Scher, H. (1993). Unawareness of illness and neuropsychological performance in chronic schizophrenia. *Schizophrenia Research, 10,* 117–124.

JOHN S. STRAUSS

# Epilogue

When the group of us who carried out the International Pilot Study of Schizophrenia wanted to rate insight, it was all so simple. We had one item to check, "Insight." But even then we'd have experiences such as when I asked a patient "Do you hear voices when no one's there?" and he responded, "Yes, but don't tell the ward staff. They don't want me to talk about voices, so I tell them no." And he was right; they didn't want him to talk about his voices. He was trying to teach me about the interpersonal aspects and social context of insight, but at that point I was mostly just interested in making a rating. Insight: No   Yes   Maybe. And now in this volume spread out in front of us is the vast panoply of the concept, from psychological to descriptive to social to biological; from causal sequence, social ⇒ psychological ⇒ biological to causal sequence, biological ⇒ psychological ⇒ social; from the multidimensional aspects of insight to the cross-cultural and historical differences of the concept over time.

It is overwhelming. And yet we must try not to escape to one or another simplistic notion. It is interesting, understandable, and a bit sad how torn probably all of us are, as reflected in this volume, between taking a broad overview, perhaps underestimating the complex details, or carrying out a precise examination of only a small part of the concept—as if we could understand the biology or meaning of a concept like insight, then everything else would be relatively trivial. But the importance, the value, the beauty of the phenomenon of insight is that it will not just lie down and behave for us in this way. If we focus on the biological, the social relativism is lurking not far off, waiting to be noticed and making a solely biological explanation inadequate. And if we focus only on the social, those neurological patients with insight problems are not far away, either. And we can't even assume that because insight is so complex it's not worth

352

pursuing; insight has been viewed as a key factor in mental illness. Not only has it been seen as important diagnostically, but even among nonprofessionals there is the common view: if you think you're crazy, you're not. And as Berrios and others in this volume point out, insight—at least in some of its definitions—is often perceived as something almost defining the human psyche in both health and disorder. For these and other reasons noted in this book, the concept of insight itself is probably at or near the center of our field, requiring us to somehow deal with a wide range of historical concepts, of domains, of people, and of cultures if we are to approximate an understanding of its mysteries.

Again and again, perhaps to escape such demands, we retreat to the world of single causes, of unique causal directions (e.g., biological $\rightarrow$ psychological) and of simplistic definitions of insight—definitions that in practice often sound like, "You don't have insight if you don't believe what I believe, although I don't have the insight to note my belief *is* a belief rather than some absolute truth." Of course, this problem of perspective has plagued humanity, not only in the mental health field but also in the clash of religious, political, and other systems.

The problem created by insight as a dependent variable, defined at least partially as disagreeing with socially established reality, cannot be underestimated. A severe problem is also generated by the mere fact that possessing insight into one's own severe mental disorder involves major social and psychological implications. "Having insight" in most societies means accepting the lowest of all status, and especially with schizophrenia, a status that many people believe (incorrectly) is essentially hopeless, a status that frequently also involves being discounted as a meaningful human being, becoming in our parlance a schizophrenic. Many, perhaps all of us, have had the experience of being destructively labeled—personally or professionally—and of the pain such labeling involves. But the labels "mental illness" and "schizophrenia" render trivial the labels that most of us have experienced. It is understandable that people might go out of their way to avoid such labeling, such acceptance.

In reviewing the contributions to this volume, I thought first I might comment from some lofty or Stygian distance on each of them, their strengths and their weaknesses (as if I knew). Then, missing in the volume an extensive reflection on the subjective complexities of insight, the experience of insight, the description in depth of the writer's own, or even a patient's perspective, I thought I might describe my own experiences, as in people telling me, "John, why can't you ever see that you (e.g., when I write a paper and suggest things) leave out so much of what you know? It's like you don't get it, no matter how often I remind you." We all have our experiences of what we hope are normal lacks. But it seemed best to start off by noting how overwhelmed I was by the diversity, complexity, and importance of the various contributions, and I urge us all to note this complexity and diversity and to feel the need to develop even more advanced models and approaches for bringing these orientations and findings together. Somehow, these various approaches themselves need to be considered as data, and an overarching approach could be to consider these "data" together. In such an analysis (or synthesis), it must be remembered that the dependent variable—insight—itself varies according to the cultural context, assessment, situation, and psychological level at which it is assessed (e.g., overt self-report, observed behavior). Thus, the model needed for comprehending insight may be more a cannonical correlation, where element combinations vary on both sides of the equation, than a multiple regression, where the dependent variable has only a limited dimension of variability.

My own suggestion for beginning to deal with such complexities regarding insight is to promote one of the directions that several authors in this volume have begun to undertake: insight as a process. Although it is useful to use insight as a static label, a rating, or even a multidimensional rating (e.g., Greenfeld, Strauss, & Bowers, 1989; Amador, Strauss, Yale, & Gorman, 1991), still, as Kraepelin, Freud, Piaget, and so many others have suggested, it is difficult to understand a concept in human behavior without noting its evolution over time. It is essential to consider the concept as a process that has an evolution, since in that evolution may lie hidden many of the determinants, effects, and even clues to the very nature of the phenomenon.

In thinking about insight as a process, for example, I recalled one subject in our study of improvement in schizophrenia—a woman with whom I conducted follow-up research interviews when she was a patient in a state hospital. In a portion of one of these interviews, she described a delusion of hers:

P.S. (patient): I have felt the past couple months that I'm pregnant. And I hear a voice from the child in me. It talks to me. And I don't know, doctor, I'm Jewish, too, and I don't know. I think why the delusion? I think I'm pregnant with the Christ child. And I haven't had sex in two years.

J.S. (Dr. Strauss, interviewer): What do you make of that?

P.S.: I don't know.

J.S.: You've had that thought before, as I recall, huh?

P.S.: Yes, I have. A couple of times in the past years. But I swear to God I haven't had sex since two Julys ago with my husband. And here I am feeling pregnant.

J.S.: So this seems kind of strange, or like you're uncertain about that, yeah. I've seen that.

P.S.: Are you a medical doctor?

J.S.: Yeah.

P.S.: You want to just feel it and see if you can . . . ?

J.S.: No.

P.S.: You're too—yeah, I understand.

J.S.: Well, 'cause I really want to do this in terms of the research interview. So you're sort of three quarters convinced that it's true, but one quarter not so sure, huh? And you don't think that's connected with being under stress at all, huh?

P.S.: No.

J.S.: This seems to trouble you in some way, this thinking about it.

P.S.: Only that no one's going to believe me.

J.S.: Oh, that's the main thing. I was not sure . . .

P.S.: It makes me kind of lonely.

J.S.: I thought you also questioned it.

P.S.: It's impossible to be pregnant without sex. [Laughs]

J.S.: Yeah, one would think so.

P.S.: I've been sleeping in my Levis every night, so I know nothing happened in the middle of the night, too.

J.S.: It's hard, isn't it, when you sort of believe something and yet you know that maybe it doesn't make sense and you think well maybe it does make sense.

P.S.: I even feel pregnant. I've been pregnant and I know what it feels like, and I think I am.

In Paiget's studies of the processes of human mental functioning, he often paid particular attention to transitional stages—the young boy, for example, who when he is pouring water from a narrow beaker into a wide one says (with astonishment), "The water level has gone down. There's less water! But there shouldn't be less water; all I did was pour it." This boy is struggling with his evolution from the previous stage, where height of water was the only criterion for quantity, to the more advanced stage, where height and diameter of the water column are both considered in evaluating quantity. Mrs. S. seemed to be undergoing a similar process, struggling with her feeling (delusion) that she was pregnant, but also somewhat anchored in the other realities of her life that would indicate that she wasn't. Such transitions are just one key to the study of process, to determining opposing or interacting forces, the impact of context and situation, or the many other varying factors that may be important in insight.

Could such transitions be built more frequently into the studies described in this volume in the effort to understand and delineate process? I think so. In some instances such an effort would require intensive studies of individual participants in research. It is an approach that our field, our understanding of insight, probably cannot do without, our preoccupation with using almost exclusively large-sample studies to develop our science notwithstanding.

Adding intensive single-person studies to our armamentarium could open up more broadly our window on understanding process, especially if combined with becoming less embarrassed scientifically about considering our own experiences as individuals and including other richer encounters with subjectivity. We in the mental health field have worked hard on our biology, hard on our descriptive characterizations, hard on our epidemiology. But like a horse with quarter anosognosia, we barely notice the fourth leg. The fourth leg is subjectivity, the detailed experience and its evolution in the person—the person with mental disorder or any other person.

How is it that we maintain our relative anosognosia for subjectivity? We do ask people what they feel and think. But that is often as far as we see or go. Would Dostoyevsky have stopped his narration of Raskolnikov in *Crime and Punishment* with a questionnaire? Would Shakespeare have said to Hamlet, "To be or not to be? Check (for British subjects, "tick") the box that most nearly expresses how you feel." Could Hamlet really be done in 30 seconds, as the Reduced Shakespeare Players, who ironically summarize the Bible in a few minutes and the Shakespeare tragedies in less time, would have us believe? Is the rest really just a waste of time? We in the mental health field sometimes act as though that were so. Often we do subjectivity by multiple choice. Some of the subjective variance of the dependent variable insight might be a function of who asks and how, as in the example of the research interview in contrast to the ward staff cited at the beginning of this chapter. To some extent, insight is influenced by what level of subjectivity we investigators will accept. For example, does the person not mixing with other people indicate perhaps that he or she notices at some level of consciousness that he or she is different and has problems, no matter what the individual may say outwardly?

How to use such clinical process data in developing our understanding of insight or any other complex phenomenon is in my view one of the most challenging and exciting aspects of research in a human science such as ours. Many of the answers to this question are still to be discovered, and will require creative and dedicated thinking and exploration. The usual recipes are reasonable enough (for example, to use intensive, single-subject studies to identify variables and sequences to be tested with large N studies, or to use large-sample studies for predicting individual person sequences and thus test their clinical value). But these are really only the most basic of ways in which intensive clinical studies and large-sample stochastic studies can be used to inform each other and help us approximate knowledge.

Elsewhere, we have suggested at least one approach for moving from intense individual studies to more large-sample approaches (Strauss & Hafez, 1981). For Ms. S., for example, it may be useful to begin by noting the existence of the transitional process, then to attempt to define it more operationally, and then to begin to test to see how long it lasts, see what variables affect it, and theorize about the process that it may reflect—for example, the struggle between her concrete world experience (not having had sex for two years) and her belief system (that she is pregnant). The origins of her belief system and the key variables in her concrete world experiences might then be explored. Would having her become more involved in the concrete world—for example, through a job—increase its salience? Would a particular job, such as one involving physical tasks or tasks that are mentally absorbing, have more impact on pushing her toward focusing on her concrete world experiences? Would such jobs have prolonged effects—that is, would they progressively reduce her delusional belief even during the hours when she is not working? This is one possible approach to bridging the gap between intensive individual studies involving qualitative focus and those involving more quanitative methods. But it is only one approach. In human science research, each problem is at least somewhat unique. Experience with the clinical situation and with research methods allows ongoing development of methods and understanding of the problem in creative ways that focus on the reality of the clinical phenomenon as it occurs in the real world and use of as much research rigor involving sampling, measurement, and analysis as is compatible with the progressively evolving understanding of the real phenomenon.

Dr. Kim (chapter 11, this volume) states in his modest way that "a certain number of Japanese psychiatrists seem to balance a meditative way of understanding patients with a modern scientific knowledge of mental disorders" (p. 227). I think the next stage in developing an even more modern scientific approach to our field, and to understanding insight, would be if we could, like Piaget's developing child, begin to think in more complex ways, to embrace a broader range of research paradigms, a broader view of the nature of data to include that "meditative way." Such breadth, including both large-sample studies and intensive studies of individuals including ourselves, would allow us to take the next steps toward understanding insight, recognizing after all that we are dealing not with just any science but with a human science. We have not been able yet really to comprehend and integrate what it might mean to have a phenomenon that is neurophysiologically, psychologically, and culturally determined through some evolutionary interactional process. Employing just one item to rate insight was very useful in the past. But in the future we must think more broadly and richly in our field if we are to make the progress for which this volume provides many of the elements.

*References*

Amador, X. F., Strauss, D. H., Yale, S. A., Gorman, J. M. (1991). Awareness of illness in schizophrenia. *Schizophrenia Bulletin, 17,* 113–132.

Greenfeld, D., Strauss, J. S., & Bowers, M. (1989). Insight and interpretation of illness in recovery from psychosis. *Schizophrenia Bulletin, 15*(2), 245–252.

Strauss, J. S., & Hafez, H. (1981). Clinical questions and "real" research. *American Journal of Psychiatry, 138*(12), 1592–1597.

# Index

action
  affectivity and, 250–51, 259
  delusional, 241, 244–63, 281
  normal beliefs and, 242–44
action failure, 58–62, 156, 186–87
affect
  delusion-based action and, 250–51, 259
  flattened, 21, 28, 83, 252
  inappropriate/incongruent, 9, 21
agnosia. See autonoetic agnosia
alien control, delusions of, 70
alien hand syndrome, 11, 112, 122
allopsychosis, 123, 125–26
alogia, 83
altered sensation, 68–69
ama'e, 224
ambiguity, 183–84
amygdala, 130
analogical reasoning, 203
anastrophe, 42
anhedonia, 22, 23, 83
anosodiaphoria, 7, 28, 109
anosognosia, 124, 335
  autonoetic agnosia and, 145–65, 308
  behavioral vs. verbal aspects, 110–11
  denial personalities and, 97

  domain specificity, 27
  earliest accounts of, 7, 8
  as heterogeneous, 28
  Japanese view of, 224–25
  neuropsychological theories on, 120–21
  overview, 25–29, 109–10
  unawareness as key element, 87, 107, 258
anterior cingulate gyrus, 150, 152, 161–62, 165
anticipatory representation, 186
Anton's syndrome, 87, 112, 333
apathy, 83, 116
apophany, 42
attention deficits, 81, 83, 153–54, 158, 159
attribution of illness, 16, 24
  awareness and, 197–98, 333
  by family, 318–22
  labeling and stigmatization, 206–7
  measurement, 17–19
  medical vs. value-based models, 55, 199
auditory hallucinations
  actions based on, 249
  as characteristic of typical schizophrenia, 21, 126, 143
  delusional elaboration of, 50–51, 335

358